Infection Prevention and Control in the Hospital

Guest Editor

KEITH S. KAYE, MD, MPH

INFECTIOUS DISEASE CLINICS OF NORTH AMERICA

www.id.theclinics.com

Consulting Editor
ROBERT C. MOELLERING Jr, MD

March 2011 • Volume 25 • Number 1

SAUNDERS an imprint of ELSEVIER, Inc.

W.B. SAUNDERS COMPANY
A Division of Elsevier Inc.
1600 John F. Kennedy Blvd., Suite 1800, Philadelphia, PA 19103-2899.
http://www.theclinics.com

INFECTIOUS DISEASE CLINICS OF NORTH AMERICA Volume 25, Number 1
March 2011 ISSN 0891–5520, ISBN-13: 978-1-4557-0462-0

Editor: Barbara Cohen-Kligerman
Developmental Editor: Donald Mumford

Infectious Disease Clinics of North America (ISSN 0891–5520) is published in March, June, September, and December by Elsevier Inc., 360 Park Avenue South, New York, NY 10010-1710. Periodicals postage paid at New York, NY and additional mailing offices. Subscription prices are $251.00 per year for US individuals, $435.00 per year for US institutions, $124.00 per year for US students, $297.00 per year for Canadian individuals, $538.00 per year for Canadian institutions, $355.00 per year for international individuals, $538.00 per year for international institutions, and $171.00 per year for Canadian and international students. To receive student rate, orders must be accompanied by name of affiliated institution, date of term, and the *signature* of program/residency coordinator on institution letterhead. Orders will be billed at individual rate until proof of status is received. Foreign air speed delivery is included in all *Clinics* subscription prices. All prices are subject to change without notice. **POSTMASTER:** Send address changes to *Infectious Disease Clinics of North America,* Elsevier Health Sciences Division, Subcription Customer Service, 3251 Riverport Lane, Maryland Heights, MO 63043. **Customer Service: 1-800-654-2452 (US). From outside of the US and Canada, call 1-314-447-8871. Fax: 1-314-447-8029. E-mail: JournalsCustomerService-usa@elsevier.com (print support) or JournalsOnlineSupport-usa@elsevier.com (online support).**

Infectious Disease Clinics of North America is also published in Spanish by Editorial Inter-MÅdica, Junin 917, 1ᵉʳ A 1113, Buenos Aires, Argentina.

Reprints. For copies of 100 or more, of articles in this publication, please contact the Commercial Reprints Department, Elsevier Inc., 360 Park Avenue South, New York, New York 10010-1710. Tel. (212) 633-3812, Fax: (212) 462-1935, E-mail: reprints@elsevier.com.

Infectious Disease Clinics of North America is covered in *MEDLINE/PubMed (Index Medicus), Current Contents/Clinical Medicine, Science Citation Alert, SCISEARCH,* and *Research Alert.*

Printed and bound by CPI Group (UK) Ltd, Croydon, CR0 4YY

Transferred to Digital Print 2011

Contributors

CONSULTING EDITOR

ROBERT C. MOELLERING Jr, MD

Shields Warren-Mallinckrodt Professor of Medical Research, Harvard Medical School; Department of Medicine, Beth Israel Deaconess Medical Center, Boston, Massachusetts

GUEST EDITOR

KEITH S. KAYE, MD, MPH

Professor of Medicine; Corporate Director, Department of Medicine, Unit of Infection Prevention, Epidemiology, and Antimicrobial Stewardship, Detroit Medical Center and Wayne State University, University Health Center, Detroit, Michigan

AUTHORS

GEORGE J. ALANGADEN, MD

Professor, Department of Medicine, Division of Infectious Diseases, Wayne State University; Director, Infection Control and Epidemiology, Harper University Hospital and Karmanos Cancer Center, Detroit, Michigan

DEVERICK J. ANDERSON, MD, MPH

Assistant Professor of Medicine, Division of Infectious Diseases, Duke University Medical Center, Durham, North Carolina

MAUREEN BOLON, MD, MS

Assistant Professor of Medicine, Division of Infectious Diseases, Department of Medicine, Northwestern University Feinberg School of Medicine, Chicago, Illinois

CAROL E. CHENOWETH, MD

Professor, Division of Infectious Diseases, Department of Internal Medicine; Department of Infection Control and Epidemiology, University of Michigan Health System, Ann Arbor, Michigan

TEENA CHOPRA, MD

Division of Infectious Diseases and Infection Control, Wayne State University, Detroit, Michigan

EVELYN COOK, CIC

Nurse Clinician, Department of Medicine, Duke Infection Control Outreach Network, Durham, North Carolina

SARA E. COSGROVE, MD, MS

Associate Professor of Medicine, Division of Infectious Diseases; Director, Antimicrobial Stewardship Program; Associate Hospital Epidemiologist, The Johns Hopkins Medical Institution, Baltimore, Maryland

ELAINE FLANAGAN, RN, BSN, MSA, CIC
Department of Infection Prevention and Hospital Epidemiology, Detroit Medical Center, Detroit, Michigan

WILLIAM P. GOINS, MD, MPH
Assistant Professor of Medicine, Division of Infectious Diseases, Department of Medicine, Baylor College of Medicine, Houston, Texas

STEPHAN HARBARTH, MD, MS
Infection Control Program, University of Geneva Hospitals and Medical School, Geneva, Switzerland

COURTNEY HEBERT, MD
Section of Infectious Diseases and Global Health, University of Chicago, Chicago, Illinois

BENEDIKT HUTTNER, MD
Infection Control Program, University of Geneva Hospitals and Medical School, Geneva, Switzerland

KEITH S. KAYE, MD, MPH
Professor of Medicine; Corporate Director, Department of Medicine, Unit of Infection Prevention, Epidemiology, and Antimicrobial Stewardship, Detroit Medical Center and Wayne State University, University Health Center, Detroit, Michigan

EBBING LAUTENBACH, MD, MPH, MSCE
Associate Professor of Medicine and Epidemiology, Department of Medicine (Infectious Diseases), Center for Clinical Epidemiology and Biostatistics, University of Pennsylvania School of Medicine, Philadelphia, Pennsylvania

ANDIE S. LEE, MD
Infection Control Program, University of Geneva Hospitals and Medical School, Geneva, Switzerland

DROR MARCHAIM, MD
Clinical Fellow, Department of Medicine, Unit of Infection Prevention, Epidemiology, and Antimicrobial Stewardship, Detroit Medical Center, Wayne State University, Detroit, Michigan

LONA MODY, MD, MSc
Division of Geriatric Medicine, University of Michigan Medical School; Geriatrics Research, Education and Clinical Center, Veterans Affairs Ann Arbor Healthcare System, Ann Arbor, Michigan

WILLIAM A. RUTALA, PhD, MPH
Department of Hospital Epidemiology, University of North Carolina Health Care; Division of Infectious Diseases, University of North Carolina School of Medicine, Chapel Hill, North Carolina

SANJAY SAINT, MD, MPH
Professor, Division of General Medicine, Department of Internal Medicine, University of Michigan Health System; Veterans Affairs Ann Arbor Healthcare System, Ann Arbor, Michigan

H. KEIPP TALBOT, MD, MPH
Assistant Professor of Medicine, Division of Infectious Diseases, Department of Medicine, Vanderbilt University School of Medicine, Nashville, Tennessee

THOMAS R. TALBOT, MD, MPH
Associate Professor of Medicine, Division of Infectious Diseases, Department of
Medicine, Vanderbilt University School of Medicine, Nashville, Tennessee

PRANITA D. TAMMA, MD
Pediatric Infectious Diseases Fellow, Department of Pediatric Infectious Diseases,
The Johns Hopkins Medical Institution, Baltimore, Maryland

DAVID J. WEBER, MD, MPH
Department of Hospital Epidemiology, University of North Carolina Health Care;
Division of Infectious Diseases, University of North Carolina School of Medicine,
Chapel Hill, North Carolina

STEPHEN G. WEBER, MD, MS
Section of Infectious Diseases and Global Health, University of Chicago, Chicago, Illinois

KEITH F. WOELTJE, MD, PhD
Professor of Medicine in Infectious Diseases, Washington University School of Medicine;
Director, Clinical Advisory Group, BJC HealthCare, Center for Clinical Excellence,
St Louis, Missouri

JERRY M. ZUCKERMAN, MD
Assistant Professor of Medicine, Department of Medicine, Jefferson Medical College;
Medical Director, Infection Prevention and Control Department, Albert Einstein Medical
Center, Philadelphia, Pennsylvania

Contents

Infection control is the discipline responsible for preventing nosocomial infections. There has been an increasing focus on prevention rather than control of hospital-acquired infections. Individuals working in infection control have seen their titles change from infection control practitioner to infection control professional and most recently to infection preventionist (IP), emphasizing their critical role in protecting patients. The responsibilities of IPs span multiple disciplines including medicine, surgery, nursing, occupational health, microbiology, pharmacy, sterilization and disinfection, emergency medicine, and information technology. This article discusses the structure and responsibilities of an infection control program and the regulatory pressures and opportunities the program faces.

The toll of health care–associated infections on patients and the seeming ease of the procedure thought best able to prevent them have focused a spotlight onto hand hygiene performance. Poor performance of hand hygiene by health care workers inspires outrage in the general public. Much is understood regarding barriers to and motivators of hand hygiene performance. Guidelines encouraging use of alcohol-based hand hygiene agents have facilitated hand hygiene improvement efforts. These efforts and evidence that improved hand hygiene performance is associated with a reduction in health care–associated infections should encourage those in the hand hygiene campaigns.

Failure to perform proper disinfection and sterilization of medical devices may lead to introduction of pathogens, resulting in infection. New techniques have been developed for achieving high-level disinfection and adequate environmental cleanliness. This article examines new technologies for sterilization and high-level disinfection of critical and semicritical items, respectively, and because semicritical items carry the greatest risk of infection, the authors discuss reprocessing semicritical items such as endoscopes and automated endoscope reprocessors, endocavitary probes, prostate biopsy probes, tonometers, laryngoscopes, and infrared coagulation devices. In addition, current issues and practices associated with environmental cleaning are reviewed.

David J. Weber and William A. Rutala

Approximately 80,000 central venous line–associated bloodstream infections (CLA-BSI) occur in the United States each year. CLA-BSI is most commonly caused by coagulase-negative staphylococci, *Staphylococcus aureus, Candida* spp, and aerobic gram-negative bacilli. These organisms commonly gain entrance in into the bloodstream via the catheter-skin interface (insertion site) or via the catheter hub. Use of strict aseptic technique for insertion is the key method for the prevention of CLA-BSI. Various methods can be used to reduce unacceptably high rates of CLA-BSI, including use of an antiseptic- or antibiotic-impregnated catheter, daily chlorhexidine baths/washes, and placement of a chlorhexidine-impregnated sponge over the insertion site.

Carol E. Chenoweth and Sanjay Saint

Catheter-associated urinary tract infections (CAUTIs) account for approximately 40% of all health care-associated infections. Despite studies showing benefit of interventions for prevention of CAUTI, adoption of these practices has not occurred in many healthcare facilities in the United States. As urinary catheters account for the majority of healthcare-associated UTIs, the most important interventions are directed at avoiding placement of urinary catheters and promoting early removal when appropriate. Alternatives to indwelling catheters such as intermittent catheterization and condom catheters should be considered. If indwelling catheterization is appropriate, proper aseptic practices for catheter insertion and maintenance and use of a closed catheter collection system are essential for preventing CAUTI. The use of antimicrobial catheters also may be considered when the rates of CAUTI remain persistently high despite adherence to other evidence-based practices, or in patients deemed to be at high risk for CAUTI or its complications. Attention toward prevention of CAUTI will likely increase as Center for Medicare and Medicaid Services and other third-party payers no longer reimburse for hospital-acquired UTI.

Jerry M. Zuckerman

Health care–acquired pneumonia (HAP) is associated with significant morbidity and mortality. These infections most frequently arise from a patient's indigenous flora, although occasionally they result from exposure to environmental pathogens such as *Legionella* and *Aspergillus*. This article reviews infection prevention strategies to reduce the incidence of HAP. Successful implementation of these prevention strategies usually requires a multidisciplinary approach and standardization of protocols. This article also discusses strategies to prevent transmission of *Mycobacterium tuberculosis* within health care settings.

result in increased patient morbidity, mortality, and health care costs. Approximately 20% of patients with healthcare–associated pneumonia have viral respiratory infections, with 70% of these infections caused by adenovirus, influenza virus, parainfluenza virus, and respiratory syncytial virus (RSV). These infections typically reflect the level of viral activity within the community. This article focuses on the epidemiology, transmission, and control of health care–associated RSV and influenza virus.

Erratum

Dr Cheston B. Cunha, author of "The First Atypical Pneumonia: The History of the Discovery of *Mycoplasma pneumoniae*" (*Infectious Disease Clinics of North America* volume 24, number 1, pages 1–5, March 2010) notes that it has been brought to his attention by Leonard Hayflick, PhD, that there were some errors in the history that appeared in this article.

It was Dr Hayflick who was the first to suggest that a mycoplasma might be the etiological agent of primary atypical pneumonia and also the first to culture the agent (*M pneumoniae*). In the review, Dr Hayflick was not given proper credit for his seminal work. The following points should have been included:

M pneumoniae was first cultured by Dr Hayflick. As stated in the original publication of the discovery, "The isolation of the Eaton agent and their subsequent passage series were initiated by one of us (L.H.) from a frozen pool…this material was tested five times on agar plates and on each occasion 5–10 colonies were observed…"[1]

The new mycoplasma medium was developed by Dr Hayflick while working at the Wistar Institute in Philadelphia and not in Chanock's laboratory at the NIH as stated. Dr Hayflick discovered the necessary growth factors for the cultivation of this mycoplasma species.[2]

It was incorrectly stated that "Eaton and Chanock found that unless media contained serum or egg yolk, no organismal growth could be seen." Rather, Dr Hayflick discovered that agar and broth media supplemented with horse serum and yeast extract were necessary for *M pneumoniae* culture.

The essential growth supplements for culturing *M pneumoniae* were developed by Dr Hayflick and were not, as stated, from Difco. The essential mycoplasma growth supplements were horse serum and fresh Baker's yeast extract. Called "Hayflick medium," these supplements are still used for *M pneumoniae* culture.

Dr Hayflick, not Eaton and Chanock, as stated, was responsible for the isolation of *M pneumoniae*. Neither Eaton nor Chanock worked with mycoplasmas until taught how to do so by Dr Hayflick and they did not, as stated in the review "…confirm the Mycoplasma genus once the organism could be cultured using the specially prepared agar."

Importantly, it was a PhD researcher, ie, Dr Hayflick, not, as stated, a physician who was responsible for the discovery of *M pneumoniae*.

The foregoing points should correct aspects of the microbiological portion of the article regarding the importance of Dr Hayflick's seminal contribution to suggest that the etiological agent of primary atypical pneumonia might be a mycoplasma and then to succeed in cultivating what later was named by him and others as *M pneumoniae*.

References

1. Chanock RM, Hayflick L, Barile MF. Growth on artificial medium of an agent associated with atypical pneumonia and its identification as a PPLO. Proc Natl Acad Sci 1962;48:41–9.
2. Hayflick L. Tissue cultures and mycoplasmas. Texas Rep Biol Med 1965;23:(Suppl 1): 285–303.

Selected references

Those seeking further information on the microbiological aspects of *M pneumoniae* may find the following sources of interest.

Baernstein HD Jr, Quilligan JJ Jr. Cultivation of Mycoplasma pneumoniae (Eaton agent). J Bacteriol 1963;86:339.
Chanock RM. *Mycoplasma pneumoniae*: proposed nomenclature for atypical pneumonia organism (Eaton agent). Science 1963;140:662.
Eaton MD, Low IE. Propagation of *Mycoplasma pneumoniae* and other fastidious strains of PPLO. Ann NY Acad Sci 1967 July 28;143:375–83.
Edward DG, Freundt EA, Chanock RM, et al. Recommendations on nomenclature of the order Mycoplasmatales. Science 1967;70:1694–6.
Hayflick L, Chanock RM. Mycoplasma species of man. Bacteriol Rev 1965;29:185–221.
Hayflick L, Stanbridge E. Isolation and identification of mycoplasma from human clinical materials. Ann NY Acad Sci 1967;143:608–21.

ACCESS THE CLINICS ONLINE!

Activate your subscription at:
www.theclinics.com

Preface

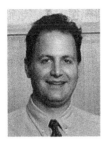

Keith S. Kaye, MD, MPH
Guest Editor

Infection prevention and control has grown and changed significantly since it first became nationally recognized in the early 1970s. Initially, infection control was focused on occupational health and infection surveillance in the hospital. More recently, there has been a growing emphasis on prevention and process in the hospital and also in a multitude of other health care settings. Over the past few years there has been an increased recognition of the quality and cost implications associated with health care–associated infections. Now more than ever infection prevention has been thrust into the spotlight with regards to patient safety, financial accountability, and regulatory readiness. While individual textbooks, articles, and other resources are available to address questions and issues pertaining to infection prevention and control, this issue of *Infectious Disease Clinics of North America* serves as an inclusive, relatively concise and focused primer on infection control.

A multitude of topics are reviewed, including building an infection control program, the economics of an infection control and prevention program, hand hygiene, sterilization and disinfection, device-related infections, multi-drug-resistant bacteria, tuberculosis, influenza and other viral illnesses, fungal infections, antimicrobial stewardship, informatics in infection control, and infection control and prevention in outpatient and long-term care settings.

This issue is intended to serve as a useful reference and primer for infection prevention and control. I want to thank the authors who have contributed valuable time and effort to this issue. We hope that you will enjoy it and find it to be a wonderful resource for helping to build and sustain an Infection Prevention and Control program.

Keith S. Kaye, MD, MPH
Department of Medicine, Unit of Infection Prevention
Epidemiology and Antimicrobial Stewardship
Detroit Medical Center and Wayne State University
University Health Center, 4201 Saint Antoine
Suite 2B, Box 331, Detroit, MI 48201, USA

E-mail address:
KKaye@dmc.org

Infect Dis Clin N Am 25 (2011) xiii
doi:10.1016/j.idc.2010.12.001
0891-5520/11/$ – see front matter © 2011 Elsevier Inc. All rights reserved.

id.theclinics.com

Building a Successful Infection Prevention Program: Key Components, Processes, and Economics

Evelyn Cook, CIC[a],*, Dror Marchaim, MD[b], Keith S. Kaye, MD, MPH[b]

KEYWORDS

• Infection control • HAIs • Program • Infection prevention

Infection control is defined as the discipline responsible for preventing nosocomial infections. Over the past several decades, infection control has grown from a largely anonymous field to a rapidly growing multidisciplinary field of incredible importance with regard to the safety of patients and health care workers and regulation and accreditation of health care facilities and finances. There has been an increasing focus on prevention rather than control of hospital-acquired infections. Individuals working in infection control have seen their titles change from infection control practitioner to infection control professional and most recently to infection preventionist (IP), emphasizing their critical role in protecting patients. The responsibilities of IPs span multiple disciplines including medicine, surgery, nursing, occupational health, microbiology, pharmacy, sterilization and disinfection, emergency medicine, and information technology. This article discusses the structure and responsibilities of an infection control program and the regulatory pressures and opportunities the program faces.

THE EMERGENCE AND DEVELOPMENT OF REGULATION AND REQUIREMENTS OF INFECTION PREVENTION AND CONTROL

The Centers for Disease Control and Prevention (CDC) reports that an estimated 1.7 million infections occur annually in US hospitals with 99,000 associated deaths. The Study for Efficacy of Nosocomial Infection Control (SENIC) estimated the cost of

[a] Department of Medicine, Duke Infection Control Outreach Network, Durham, NC, USA
[b] Department of Medicine, Unit of Infection Prevention, Epidemiology and Antimicrobial Stewardship, Detroit Medical Center, Wayne State University, 4201 Saint Antoine, Suite 2B, Box 331, Detroit, MI 48201, USA
* Corresponding author.
E-mail address: cook0084@mc.duke.edu

Infect Dis Clin N Am 25 (2011) 1–19
doi:10.1016/j.idc.2010.11.007
0891-5520/11/$ – see front matter © 2011 Elsevier Inc. All rights reserved.

health care–associated infections (HAIs) to be $4.5 billion in 1992. Adjusting for inflation, this cost reached approximately $6.65 billion in 2007.[1]

Infection prevention and control efforts have historically focused on monitoring and preventing HAIs locally, but recently, HAI prevention has become a national priority, resulting in a significant evolution of infection prevention and control.[2] It is important and informative to review the emergence and development of infection prevention and control in US hospitals. Infection prevention and control has grown in response to consumer and health care worker demands for improved patient safety and a safer working environment.

Infection control was in its infancy in the 1970s. Regulatory oversight of hospital-acquired infections dramatically increased in the late 1980s and early 1990s because of health care worker safety concerns, pertaining to the risk of occupational exposure to human immunodeficiency virus and hepatitis B virus. Health care workers banded together, urging federal legislation be enacted, requiring employers to provide greater protection for health care workers against these 2 blood-borne pathogens. In 1991, the Occupational Safety and Health Administration (OSHA) released Standard-29 CFR Bloodborne Pathogens-1910.1030. Any employee with occupational exposure to blood or other potentially infectious materials is included in the scope of this standard.[3]

Implementation of the OSHA regulation required investment of the health care resources in time, materials, and money. Infection control departments were not only delegated the initial responsibility for implementation of this standard but also continued to be accountable for oversight and compliance monitoring related to infection prevention of health care workers. For example, closely following the Bloodborne Pathogens legislation, OSHA proposed another legislative mandate aimed at increasing respiratory protection (use of respirators requiring fit testing) for workers at significant risk of incurring *Mycobacterium tuberculosis* (eg, tuberculosis) infection. Again, this proposed legislation was delegated to infection control departments for oversight and implementation. Although the proposed rule specific to tuberculosis was rescinded in 2003, respiratory protection is broadly regulated by OSHA under the general industry standard for respiratory protection. Components of this program include medical clearance to wear a respirator and provision and use of appropriate respirators.[4,5] Infection prevention and control professionals have been charged with ensuring compliance with both these federally mandated health care worker safety initiatives, without the provision of additional resources.

Although OSHA's focus on employee safety issues brought infection prevention to the forefront of health care, other agencies have focused on HAIs as a major patient safety initiative. Although infection prevention and control in the United States has focused on the prevention and surveillance of HAIs for decades, efforts and regulation by certain agencies have brought infection control into the spotlight over the past several years. For example, in 2005, the Institute for Healthcare Improvement (IHI) targeted 3 major categories of infections (surgical site infections, central line–associated bloodstream infections, and ventilator-associated pneumonia) in its initial campaign.[6] In December 2006, the IHI launched a second campaign with the goal of protecting patients from 5 million incidents of medical harm from December 2006 to December 2008. In addition to the major categories of infections listed earlier for the first campaign, the second campaign focused on hand hygiene and a reduction in methicillin-resistant *Staphylococcus aureus* (MRSA) infections.[7] IHI was perhaps the first organization to successfully solicit hospital administration, presidents, and chief executive officers to participate in its campaign, challenging them to commit resources to reduce HAIs. Infection prevention and performance improvement departments were delegated the responsibility for implementation of the IHI recommendations.

The Department of Health and Human Services Centers for Medicare and Medicaid Services (CMS) in consultation with the CDC was required to select 2 hospital-acquired conditions to target for reduction by October 1, 2007. These conditions had to meet the following criteria: (1) should be of high cost, high volume, or both; (2) should require a higher-paying diagnosis related group, when present as a secondary diagnosis; and (3) could reasonably have been prevented if optimal health care practices had been followed. Following this directive, CMS chose catheter-associated urinary tract infections, vascular catheter–associated infection, and surgical site infection after coronary artery bypass graft surgery as hospital-acquired infections that would not be reimbursed unless they had been present on admission. Although this initial list became effective from October 1, 2008, in 2009, additional surgical site infections were added to the list of conditions (including surgical site infections following orthopedic procedures [spinal fusion and surgeries of the shoulder and elbow] and bariatric surgery for obesity).

Because of these changes in reimbursement, there has been significant pressure on experts in the field of infection prevention to achieve zero rates of HAIs. Although not all HAIs are preventable, the Association for Professionals in Infection Control and Epidemiology (APIC) and other experts agree that the primary goal of infection prevention should be the elimination of all preventable infections. The focus should be on "getting to zero" HAIs by optimizing processes pertaining to the prevention of HAIs.

In response to this serious problem plaguing health care organizations, the Joint Commission (JC), which is responsible for hospital accreditation, has brought infection control to the forefront. On January 22, 2003, the JC issued an infection control–related sentinel event alert recommending that hospitals comply with the CDC's new hand hygiene guidelines and they manage all identified cases of death and major permanent loss of function attributed to a nosocomial infection as sentinel events.[8] Subsequently, in 2004, the JC made these recommendations a part of the National Patient Safety Goals (Goals No. 7a and 7b).[9] In 2005, the JC infection control standards were revised, raising the expectations of the organization's leadership related to infection control and prevention.[10]

In 2009, JC again broadened the scope of infection prevention accreditation and expanded the National Patient Safety Goal No. 7 to focus on reducing the risks associated with multidrug-resistant organisms, catheter-associated bloodstream infections, and surgical site infections.[11]

Regulatory efforts are now also shifting to outpatient arenas. CMS recently added new regulations, pertaining to infection control, to its rules and regulations for ambulatory surgical centers. The additional regulation requires that an infection control program be maintained to minimize infections and communicable diseases. Required elements for infection control in ambulatory surgery centers include maintaining a sanitary environment, staff education and training on infection control, and providing an action plan for identifying, preventing, and managing infections and communicable diseases.[12]

HAIs are also receiving more attention from the congress. Legislative efforts are under way at the federal and state levels to mandate public reporting of HAIs. More than 50% of states have passed some form of legislation related to mandatory reporting of HAIs. Federal bills, as do some state bills, require use of the CDC's National Healthcare Safety Network for reporting data.

Health care facilities are struggling to accommodate the ever-increasing regulatory requirements and regulations regarding the reporting of HAIs and performance measures. Unfortunately, some health care facilities lack the basic infrastructure to support implementation of these guidelines.[2]

In summary, this is an exciting but challenging time for IPs. Regulatory focus on infection prevention and public reporting of HAIs is a double-edged sword: although there is increased responsibility and pressure placed on infection prevention and control, IPs are also presented with the unique opportunity to impact and reshape the way health care is delivered and to create a safer environment for patients.

INFECTION PREVENTION AND CONTROL PROGRAM
Mission, Vision, and Values

Infection prevention and control programs vary according to the size and scope of the particular organization. However, there are 3 essential and fundamental concepts to all programs: mission statement, vision, and core values.

The mission statement should be a reflection of the primary goals of the organization or needs that should be addressed by infection prevention. The JC standards require health care organizations to identify risks for acquiring and transmitting infections.[13] This standard explicitly describes the mission of infection prevention programs and their link to the organization's primary mission, for example, provision of safe quality patient care. A typical mission statement for any infection prevention program may be Our facility maintains an organized, effective hospital-wide program designed to systematically identify and reduce the risk of acquiring and transmitting infections among patients, visitors and health care workers. This program involves the collaboration of many programs and services within the hospital and is designed to meet the intent of the Joint Commission standards.

While the mission statement describes the "why," the vision statement describes future goals for the organizations. Organizational leaders have historically used strategic planning sessions to gather input from primary stakeholders to help determine an organization's vision and goals. Infection prevention departments can use a similar approach and invite key stakeholders, such as critical care and surgical staff, to participate. The vision or goals should be included in the infection prevention plan. As an example, a program's vision or goal may be that no patient in the critical care unit will acquire ventilator-associated pneumonia.

The next component integral to a successful infection prevention program is core values. A core value statement describes "how" the program functions on a daily basis and may serve as the blueprint for the program. Core values, or objectives, identify how the department will reach established goals and achieve the vision of the program. For example, a core value might be that the IHI ventilator-associated pneumonia bundle will be implemented, and compliance with all bundle elements will be monitored and reported to the appropriate stakeholders.

Infection Prevention and Control Committee

The SENIC project found that the 4 components of highly effective infection prevention surveillance programs were (1) surveillance with feedback to health care workers; (2) an intense infection control program including best practices with sterilization, disinfection, asepsis, and handling of medical devices; (3) an infection prevention nurse to supervise the program; and (4) a physician epidemiologist or microbiologist with special skills in infection prevention.

The IP, physician epidemiologist, and often a data analyst and an administrative assistant form the central infection prevention team and are the core component of the larger multidisciplinary Infection Prevention and Control Committee (IPCC). These core members are responsible for conducting surveillance, helping the organization maintain regulatory compliance, and performing key programs geared toward HAI prevention. Typically, this core group meets routinely (eg, weekly), reviews data, identifies issues, and develops and oversees quality improvement programs. This group also develops agendas for larger IPCC meetings and brings forth proposals to the IPCC for approval and feedback.

The organization's governing body typically delegates authority and responsibility for the infection prevention program to the IPCC. The IPCC is the central decision- and policy-making body whose primary purpose is to advocate for infection prevention and control[14] and should have the authority to take immediate action if patient, visitor, or health care worker safety is endangered with regard to infection prevention. In most health care organizations, IPCC is designated as a medical staff committee and has reporting obligations to hospital and medical staff leadership. The chairperson should be a physician who has knowledge and/or a special interest in infection prevention.

The IPCC is multidisciplinary, with representation from a variety of specialties and services. At a minimum, services should include infection prevention, administration, nursing, medical staff, microbiology, employee/occupational health, surgical services, environmental services, and pharmacy. Other disciplines within the organization are considered ad hoc members and should be invited to attend the committee meeting based on agenda items and need. IPCC should meet on a regular basis (such as monthly or quarterly) at a predetermined time and location.

Before the IPCC meeting, the core or central infection prevention team should meet to review surveillance findings, address any unusual events, and achieve consensus among team members on proposed actions or recommendations. A meeting agenda should be circulated to IPCC members before the meeting, with action and/or approval items so designated. It is imperative that complete and accurate minutes of the committee's discussion, actions, and recommendations be recorded for each meeting and reported to all appropriate stakeholders, based on the organizational infrastructure. These minutes are often extremely useful for documentation of responsibility and ownership of particular projects and problems. All IPCC minutes should be marked as peer review and/or confidential. **Box 1** provides a summary of the responsibilities of the IPCC members.

KEY MEMBERS OF THE INFECTION PREVENTION TEAM AND/OR PROGRAM
Hospital Physician Epidemiologist or Medical Director of Infection Prevention

Hospital epidemiologists are typically physicians, often specializing in infectious diseases with expertise in infection prevention and act as watchmen for the modern health system.[15] They provide an oversight for infection control in larger health care facilities. Some hospitals, such as smaller community hospitals, might not have a fully trained physician epidemiologist or infectious diseases physician on staff, so other members of the medical staff (eg, the hospital pathologist) might serve as the medical director of infection prevention and chairperson of the IPCC. Medical staff leadership is essential to achieve the infection prevention goals and objectives. **Box 2** summarizes the major responsibilities of the hospital epidemiologist.

Data Programmer and Analyst

Data programmers and analysts are essential for the development and maintenance of databases used in infection prevention. These individuals collaborate with the infection prevention department regarding database structure and organization of data

---

Box 1
Primary responsibilities for IPCC

1. Identify strategies designed to reduce or eliminate the risk of hospital-acquired infection and/or HAIs
2. Review findings related to hospital-acquired infections and HAIs
3. Review findings related to outbreak investigations
4. Review relevant infection prevention and control guidelines
5. Review findings related to monitoring of antibiotic-resistant organisms (infection and/or colonization)
6. Make recommendations and take action based on findings from aforementioned activities
7. Address issues related to emerging and reemerging communicable diseases
8. Make recommendations for new procedures, policies, and/or activities, as appropriate
9. Participate in the review and revision of the infection prevention and control program and risk assessment as warranted to improve outcomes
10. Approve all hospital-wide infection prevention and control policies

---

related to the infection prevention activities and assist in preparing visual presentation of those data (ie, graphs, tables).

Administrative Assistant

Effective administrative assistants possess the essential qualities needed to enhance the effectiveness and productivity of infection prevention programs. They should be highly skilled in organizing and scheduling appointments and/or meetings for the hospital epidemiologist and/or the IPs. These individuals often serve as the "gatekeeper" and organizer for the infection prevention department and assist in eliminating unnecessary interruptions and unscheduled appointments.

Box 2
Primary responsibilities of the hospital physician epidemiologist or medical director of infection prevention

- Provide medical and technical advice and support within the department as well as the health care facility
- In collaboration with the IP, establish long- and short-term goals for the department
- Provide expertise about HAIs, emerging communicable diseases, postexposure management, isolation precautions, and construction and environmental issues/concerns
- Oversee development of programs designed to prevent and/or reduce the transmission of epidemiologically important microorganisms within the facility (ie, antibiotic-resistant organisms) and/or other projects with which the department may be involved
- Participate in and oversee the analysis of surveillance findings and development of interventional strategies
- Assist with the preparation of data and policy revisions for presentation to the IPCC
- Serve as the liaison between the infection prevention department and other members of the medical staff
- Communicate infection control and prevention data to the IPCC, the members of the medical staff, the quality of care team, and other internal committees/teams, as appropriate

IP

Authority for daily oversight and management of the infection prevention program is typically delegated to the IP. Based on the size and complexity of the facility, an IP may perform other key functions in addition to infection prevention. Some of the more common functions assigned to the IP include employee health and nursing education. IPs predominately have backgrounds in nursing, medical technology, microbiology, and/or public health.[14] Additional certification in infection prevention may either be required or preferred. Clinical experience, managerial experience, and good communication skills are also prerequisites for an IP position. Daily responsibilities are multifaceted and require strong organizational skills. **Box 3** lists some of the major responsibilities of IPs in the hospital. IPs must also have the ability to lead and manage a multitude of diverse health care workers. Recognizing the difference between leadership and management and how they apply to specific situations is essential to implementing change.

Leadership is the art of influencing behavior and most facilities have "informal" leaders within each department. These local leaders often have the ability to influence the behavior of others they work with. IPs should recruit these individuals to be infection prevention champions.

Management refers to achieving desired results through efficient use of human and material resources.[16] **Box 4** depicts various management styles and characteristics of IPs. An IP should exhibit good management skills when working with individuals within his or her own department or who work on units for which the IP is responsible.

Meeting Management

Meetings require an enormous amount of human resources and when executed suboptimally, they often do not achieve the desired goals. The IPCC is only one of many multidisciplinary groups whose activities involve infection prevention. IPs can facilitate efficient and effective meetings by using key strategies. **Box 5** lists various strategies for conducting effective and efficient meetings.

Box 3
Primary responsibilities of IPs

- Application of epidemiologic principles in surveillance activities, including data collection and analysis as directed by the infection prevention and control plan and risk assessment

- Assist with product evaluation

- Develop and present educational programs designed for employee and patient education

- Consult with internal and external customers on issues related to infection prevention

- Review hospital- and department-specific IP policies and procedures

- Conduct outbreak investigations

- Conduct infection control risk assessment for all construction activities

- Report IP surveillance findings to the IPCC, hospital leadership, specific hospital departments and committees, public health department (local and state and referring/receiving health care facilities, as appropriate)

- Assist other departments by serving as a resource for continuous compliance with federal/state (eg, OSHA, Department of Health Service Regulation) and accreditation (eg, JC) standards because these standards pertain to infection prevention and control activities

> **Box 4**
> **Management styles and characteristics of IPs**
>
> Autocratic
>
> The IP independently solves problems, without input or advice from others. This style may be necessary when patient and/or employee safety is at risk and decisions must be made quickly.
>
> Consultative
>
> IPs will share problems with peers and solicit their ideas before making a decision. IPs use this approach most often.
>
> Democratic
>
> The democratic style is when the IP shares problems with the group and together they make decisions as a team. Multidisciplinary teams often use this style.

Infection Prevention Staffing

Staffing for infection prevention continues to be a challenge for most infection prevention programs. There continues to be a lack of strong recommendations from recognized experts in the field, such as the CDC.

In the early 1970s, the CDC's SENIC project recommended that hospitals have at least 1 full-time equivalent (FTE) infection control professional for every 250 occupied beds.[17] Later, in the 1990s, participation in the National Nosocomial Infections Surveillance (NNIS) System required 1 FTE infection control professional for the first 100 beds and then another for each additional 250 beds.[18] In 2002, the Association for Professionals in Infection Prevention and Epidemiology initiated a Delphi project on staffing. This project noted that staffing recommendations should consider not only the number of occupied beds but also the scope of the program, the complexity of the health care organization, patient characteristics, and the unique needs of the facility and recommended a ratio of 0.8 to 1.0 IPs per 100 occupied beds.[14] One US state has incorporated staffing requirements into their acute care licensure rules. This state requirement uses a formula that incorporates inpatient and outpatient volume, reimbursement information, and case mix index.

Despite various recommendations and need for increased IP staffing, many organizations have understaffed infection prevention programs. Although not substitutes for trained preventionists, adjuncts to the IP, such as electronic surveillance systems, unit-based nurse liaisons, and nurse advisors, can help to facilitate the work of IPs.

Budget

Budget preparation is an essential component of any efficient program. IPs may have total responsibility for budget preparation, or in some institutions, they may be responsible for providing input. Chief executive officers often use budget variances as the financial metric for the infection prevention program. Basic components of any budget include labor, capital, and miscellaneous expenses. Elements of each component are described in **Box 6**. The cost of HAIs has become an integral component of financial planning for organizations. Decreased reimbursement and nonpayment for certain conditions have forced hospital administrations to confront the financial impact of HAIs. Economic and financial impact of HAIs is discussed in detail later.

Surveillance

Surveillance is defined as the "ongoing systematic collection, analysis and interpretation of health data essential to the planning, implementation and evaluation of public

Box 5
Strategies for conducting effective and efficient meetings

1. Be prepared

   All items included on the agenda should be reviewed in advance. Surveillance data should be evaluated for accuracy and completeness and presented in a visual easy-to-understand format. Items requiring approval should be distributed in advance.

2. Have an agenda

   The agenda should be distributed before the meeting. Most institutions distribute the agenda no less than 1 week before the meeting to give members an opportunity to review and be prepared to discuss issues.

3. Start and end on time

   This simple concept demonstrates respect for members' time and work schedule. When meetings do not begin and end on time, members become disengaged and often will stop attending.

4. Meet only when necessary

   The frequency of meetings should be based on the facility's activities and needs. Meeting schedules vary from monthly to quarterly. Appropriate frequency of meetings also helps with starting and ending them on time. Some states have included a specific requirement for the frequency of IPCC meetings. Be aware of state requirements, and be sure that the schedule is in compliance.

5. Include all issues and solicit inputs relevant to all committee members

   Members want to be part of the team and when they do not feel included, they will be less likely to offer new ideas and input.

6. Stay on target

   Stick to the agenda items as outlined. Some facilities actually time the agenda with an estimated allotment for each discussion or activity. Issues that cannot be resolved or that generate more discussion than anticipated can be tabled or deferred until the next meeting.

7. Capture action items

   JC will expect to see closure to action items. The minutes should reflect approval, rejection, or deferral of action items and the supporting rationale.

8. Get feedback

   An effective way of improving the flow and productivity of a meeting is to request feedback from the members. It is generally more successful if this strategy is included as an agenda item and feedback is solicited immediately after the meeting. Feedback can be obtained through written or verbal communication after the meeting as well.

9. A secret "ninth" key

   Having the meeting at mealtime will typically improve attendance, and providing food is an inexpensive way to demonstrate appreciation for the committee member's time.

health practice, closely integrated with the timely dissemination of these data to those who need to know and the ongoing dissemination of information to those who need to know."[19] A study designed to provide a snapshot of the staffing and structure of hospital-based programs in the United States reported that IPs spent the largest percentage of time (mean, 44.5%) on surveillance activities.[18] **Box 7** lists the

---

Box 6
Budget: major components

Labor expenses

    Include staffing expenses for IPs, clerical support, data entry/analyst support, hospital epidemiologist, or IPCC physician chair support. Consideration should also be given to the labor expenses required if an outbreak investigation would be necessary.

Capital expenses

    Most organizations have a minimum cost that items must incur before qualifying as a capital expense. These are big-ticket items, and requests requiring capital expenses should be well thought out and have supportive rationale.

Miscellaneous expenses

    All other expenses fall into this category and typically include education, travel, journals, professional memberships, and other elements.

---

percentage of time spent on each task, as reported by the preventionists. The type of surveillance activities conducted are influenced by

- Organizational demographics (critical access center vs community hospital vs academic medical center)
- Community demographics (urban or rural)
- Types of procedures and services provided
- Infection prevention risk assessment
- Annual evaluation of the infection prevention plan and goals.

CDC and JC recommend that surveillance be focused on high-risk high-volume activities. CMS expects that a log of all incidents related to infections and communicable diseases be maintained, pertaining to patients and health care workers.[20] Surveillance for HAIs should be performed by screening a variety of data sources such as laboratory, radiological, and pathologic reports; admissions/discharge records; pharmacy databases; and patient charts including history and physical examinations, progress notes, and vital sign records. Often, effective surveillance

---

Box 7
Activities reported by IPs regarding how they spent their time

Activity	Percentage of Time				
	Median	Mean	SD	Minimum	Maximum
Collecting, analyzing, and interpreting data on the occurrence of infections	49.0	44.5	14.3	7	80
Policy development and meetings	14.0	15.0	8.8	0	55
Daily isolation issues	10.0	12.9	9.0	0	50
Teaching infection prevention and control policies and procedures	10.0	13.0	6.2	1	35
Others (eg, product evaluation, employee health, and emergency preparedness)	5.0	8.8	8.2	0	60
Activities related to outbreaks	5.0	6.1	4.8	0	40

From Stone PW, Dick A, Pogorzelska M, et al. Staffing and structure of infection prevention and control programs. Am J Infect Control 2009;37(5):354; with permission.

requires the application of clinical criteria to laboratory-based surveillance data. Concurrent surveillance, conducted while the patient is still in the hospital, is preferred to retrospective surveillance. Retrospective surveillance should only be used when patients are discharged before all the pertinent data can be obtained during hospital admission.[21] IPs should consult with the physician epidemiologist if clinical questions or judgment is needed to appropriately interpret patient data.

There are various types of surveillance philosophies and methodologies. Total- or whole-house surveillance is the collection of infection prevention data throughout the facility. All HAIs are identified, analyzed, and reported. If this methodology is chosen, care should be taken not to report an overall or hospital rate of infection. Rates should be reported separately for specific HAIs and may be stratified by service and/or department. Typically, whole-house surveillance is conducted for invasive infections such as catheter-associated bloodstream infection and infections caused by multidrug-resistant organisms such as MRSA.

Focused or targeted surveillance is conducted only in a particular type of unit or part of an organization in which high-risk and/or high-volume activities occur regarding HAIs. Rather than identifying every device-associated infection in the hospital, an infection prevention program might focus on efforts to detect device-related infections in the critical care areas or burn units and/or hematology wards. Rates are then calculated and reported by the device, unit, and/or service. In the 1990s, CDC shifted the NNIS System from whole-house surveillance to targeted surveillance for certain types of HAIs, such as catheter-associated urinary tract infections.[22]

Combination surveillance strategy is used by many infection prevention programs. This strategy uses a combination of targeted and modified total-house surveillance. Many programs monitor targeted events in defined populations while also monitoring selected events house wide.[22]

Regardless of the type of surveillance methodology used, data must be collected, analyzed, and presented using a consistent and standardized approach. Data that are not reliable or valid are ineffectual and do not engender confidence in the infection prevention program.

Surveillance priorities should include the following: device-associated infections, particularly in the intensive care unit (such as catheter-associated bloodstream infections, catheter-associated urinary tract infections, and ventilator-associated pneumonia); infections associated with procedures (surgical site infections); and infections related to epidemiologically important microorganisms (multidrug-resistant organisms). Surveillance data pertaining to HAIs are usually presented as rates. When calculating meaningful infection rates, it is important to select the most appropriate available denominator. Whenever possible, the denominator should reflect the exposure risk, that is, number of surgical procedures, number of device-days, or number of patient-days in a given unit or in the hospital.

Examples of numerators, denominators, and rate calculation include

- Device-associated infections: rate of infections per 1000 device-days
  (No. of device-associated infections/No. of device-days) × 1000
- Surgical site infections: rate of surgical site infections per 100 procedures
  (No. of surgical site infections/No. of surgical procedures) × 100
- Multidrug-resistant organism infections: rate of infection per 1000 patient-days
  (No. of infection/patients-days) × 1000.

Other surveillance methodologies include the use of active surveillance for certain populations and/or pathogens. Active surveillance proactively identifies the reservoir of an organism in asymptomatically colonized patients. Diagnostic testing is generally performed by culturing samples from the body site most specific for the organism, for example, culturing the samples from nares for MRSA and the perirectal area for vancomycin-resistant enterococci. Cultures are generally performed on high-risk patients during admission to the facility, and if culture results are negative, the process is repeated on some routine basis (typically weekly) during the hospitalization until a positive result is obtained or the patient is discharged. Active surveillance may provide the opportunity for interventions such as maintaiing the patient on contact isolation. Active surveillance data should be trended and reported to the IPCC and the various hospital departments or units. Active surveillance is discussed in detail in the article by Harbarth elsewhere in this issue.

In May 2009, APIC issued a position paper in support of using automated surveillance technologies as an essential part of the infection prevention and control activities.[23] Automated surveillance is defined as the process of obtaining useful information for infection prevention surveillance from hospital databases through the systematic application of medical informatics and computer science technologies.[23] This methodology can increase the ability of infection prevention programs to conduct broader surveillance programs, to rapidly identify trends in infections, and most importantly, to free time and effort of IPs so that they can spend less time entering and mining data and more time rounding, educating, analyzing, and implementing programs. These automated systems are discussed in further detail in the article by Woelje and Lautenbach elsewhere in this issue.

Outbreak Investigation

Outbreaks of both infectious and noninfectious adverse events can occur in any health care setting and pose a threat to patient safety. An outbreak is defined as an increased occurrence of a disease and/or infection above the usual or expected frequency. In some cases, even a single case may constitute an outbreak (eg, smallpox). Outbreaks are usually identified when the rate or number of infections is more than the endemic infection rate, which is defined as the usual or expected occurrence of a disease and/or infection. An endemic infection rate represents a baseline or background rate, which may fluctuate slightly from month to month.[24]

The ultimate goal of any outbreak investigation is to identify factors contributing to the outbreak and to stop or reduce the risk for further occurrences.[24] One of the key components for investigating an outbreak is developing a case definition detailing specific criteria for the definition of a case. Initially, it may be a broad definition that is refined as the investigation proceeds and a specific agent or diagnosis is confirmed. **Box 8** lists the components of an outbreak investigation.

Quality Improvement: Role of the IP

The process of measuring quality of care and reporting the findings is not a new concept.[25] Florence Nightingale collected mortality data and related it to the lack of sanitary conditions.[25] In the early twentieth century, Dr Ernest Codman proposed to his surgeon colleagues that they should measure their surgical site infection rates and disclose them to the public.[25] IPs have the responsibility to perform broad continuous quality improvement services using systematic programs and tools and determine outcomes.[26]

Using a multidisciplinary team approach, systems should be designed to monitor processes as well as outcomes. Direct patient care staff should be included as partners and team members in the infection prevention program and provided with training regarding quality concepts and team-building skills. Infection prevention programs should design systems and processes to ensure timely feedback of infection prevention data to all disciplines as appropriate. Feedback should include outcome measures, infection rates, and process measures such as compliance with hand hygiene or compliance with the central line insertion bundle. Surveillance activities provide value only when findings are used as a mechanism to improve the quality of care that is provided to patients.

ECONOMICS AND BUSINESS PLAN

Society as a whole would definitely benefit from a reduced incidence of nosocomial infections and reduced transmission of highly resistant pathogens within health care institutions. Unfortunately, there are currently no direct reimbursement programs related to hospital-based infection prevention and control. Hospitals are required by regulatory bodies to have an infection control program but must fund their own infection prevention and control programs often based on their administrators' subjective discretions. Therefore, in order for infection control programs to achieve desirable goals, it is critical that hospital epidemiologists and IPs convince their administrators of the beneficial effects of investing in infection control activities and demonstrate that these activities will ultimately lead to improved patient care and reduced hospital costs.[27] In one report, infection control programs were demonstrated to be much more cost-effective than many other commonly applied health care practices such as Papanicolaou test screening to diagnose cervical cancer, mammographic screening to diagnose breast cancer, and cholesterol screening programs in high-risk populations. In this report, infection control was estimated to be extremely cost-effective, requiring only $2000 to $8000 per year of life saved.[28] Unfortunately, hospital administrators are routinely faced with demands to reduce costs and are subjected to continuous inspection and monitoring of their financial expenses and balances.[29] Because infection control programs are typically categorized as cost centers and not as revenue generators, they are often identified as potential areas for budget cuts.[30] In fact, many infection control programs have faced downsizing in recent years.[27,31,32] This downsizing has occurred during a period during which the roles and responsibilities of hospital epidemiologists have continuously and rapidly increased. Apart from traditional infection control activities, infection control programs and IPs often have responsibilities related to antimicrobial stewardship programs, patient safety, employee health, and emergency preparedness.[27]

The best way for infection control programs to obtain adequate funding from hospital leadership is to construct a business case and to assess and demonstrate the cost-effectiveness of an infection control program or intervention. The business case for infection control should incorporate all the various components of the institutional infection control program. Recent guidelines published by the Society for Healthcare Epidemiology of America (SHEA) provide guidance regarding constructing a business case for infection control that can assist hospital epidemiologists in justifying and expanding their programs.[27] These guidelines also provide references and tools to assist infection control programs in developing a business plan that supports a specific intervention.[27] There are multiple other published economic analyses and data that can be used to support business cases for a wide range of infection control interventions and practices.[27,29,30,33–50] Data such as published costs of hospital-acquired infections and infections caused by multidrug-resistant pathogens are often key ingredients to justifying interventions to decrease the incidence of hospital infections.[47,50] Although published costs and cost-effectiveness analyses have

---

Box 8
Primary components of an outbreak investigation

- Establish or verify the diagnosis of reported cases

  Identify agent if possible. Describe the initial magnitude of the problem and what brought the problem to the attention of the infection control/employee health department.

  Confirm laboratory or other clinical findings.

  Review microbiological/laboratory records to confirm increased frequency of certain pathogens.

  Consult with staff to identify lapses in infection control techniques.

- Confirm that an outbreak exists

  Develop a case definition to estimate the magnitude of the problem.

  Compare the current incidence with usual or baseline incidence (endemic rate).

  Formulate a line listing tailored to the illness and population affected.

- Search for additional cases

  Notify the laboratory staff, physicians, and/or other personnel to immediately report additional cases.

  Search for other cases by retrospective review, laboratory reports, and other sources.

  Continue to add cases to the line list as they are identified.

- Characterize cases by person, place, and time

  Person: includes patient characteristics such as age, disease, exposures, treatments, and risk factors.

  Place: consider patient location, that is, hall, unit, or room. Check and confirm status of air exchange, pattern of flow, and other environmental issues because they are related to the outbreak.

  Time: identify the exact period of the outbreak by going back to the first case or indication of the outbreak. Identify the probable period of exposure based on the diagnosis. Plot data on an epidemic curve.

- Take immediate control measures, if indicated

  Institute control measures such as increased attention to hand hygiene and/or additional use of personal protective equipment.

  Confiscate specific suspected products if identified (ie, patient care items).

- Formulate tentative hypothesis (best guess)

  Review data to determine common host factors and exposures.

  Determine nature of the organism, and base a hypothesis on the source or reservoir, mode of transmission, or exposure risk factors.

- Institute preliminary control measures

  Institute control measures based on what is known about the outbreak.

  Consider whether outside assistance is needed.

- Monitor and evaluate effectiveness of the control measures

  Monitor compliance with control measures.

  Evaluate effectiveness of the control measures in controlling the outbreak.

  Consider additional measures if outbreak continues.

- Communicate findings

    Date of final report

    Reported to

    Reported by

    Findings

    Future recommendations

limitations regarding applicability and generalizability, hospital epidemiologists and IPs can still use these analyses to make persuasive cases for hospital support.

Preparation of a successful business plan takes planning and when possible, input from financial professionals. It is important to make an honest assessment of the infection control situation. Most hospital epidemiologists and IPs want to increase the resources available for infection control activities, but it is important to avoid overestimating benefits and the rapidity with which benefits might be achieved or avoid underestimating staff costs and efforts required for success.[27] Overestimation of efficacy in an initial analysis may provide resources in the short-term but it will undermine efforts and necessary trust for success in the long-term after actual resource audits are performed.[27] The SHEA guidelines outline a 9-step approach for completing a business case analysis, so that all crucial components can be assessed and included.[27] Some key components include identifying the right audience and key stakeholders to support and approve a business proposal. In addition, meeting key leaders and administrators early in the process, and getting feedback and input to help effectively frame the business case before a formal presentation is often beneficial. Whenever possible, the infection control team should seek input and support from business and financial leaders in the organization. The 9 steps include the following:

1. Frame the problem and develop a hypothesis about potential solutions.
2. Meet with key administrators before initiation of the proposal to obtain agreement that the issue is of institutional interest, gain leadership support, and identify critical individuals and departments who may be affected by the proposal and whose needs should be included in the business case analysis.[27]
3. Determine the annual cost using local institutional budgets or surveys available online.[51]
4. Determine what costs can be avoided through reduced infection rates using local data and the medical literature available on various infection control cost savings.[52–68]
5. Determine the costs associated with the infections of interest at the hospital. Attributable costs are preferable to overall costs, and variable costs are preferable to fixed costs. In infection prevention, the greatest opportunity to improve hospital profits comes from reducing excess length of stay; therefore, some argue this should be the main component for cost reduction calculations.[69]
6. Calculate the financial impact of the program or intervention by adding the estimated cost savings or additional profits and subtracting the costs of the up front development and implementation.
7. Include additional financial or health benefits such as reduced morbidity and mortality, reduced legal costs, and enhanced reputation for the institution. To identify as many indirect benefits as possible, mathematical models might be used.[70]

8. Make the case for the business case: communicate the findings effectively to the institution's critical stakeholders at an executive level meeting.
9. Prospectively collect cost and outcome data once the program is implemented.

In the era of limited resources, infection control programs and initiatives are subjected to continuous threat and budget reductions. Hospital epidemiologists should be familiar with the basics involved with preparing a business case and should try to establish relationships with financial experts and administrators who can provide advice and assist in business case preparation. Although most infection control professionals do not have formal economic or business training, fiscal analysis and responsibility has become a critical part of hospital epidemiology. The role of effective business plans and cost justifications will continue to grow in importance for infection control programs. Despite limitations, the medical literature provides economic data that can assist the hospital epidemiologist and IPs in constructing a business plan for establishing and maintaining an infection control program.

REFERENCES

1. Scott RD. The direct medical cost of healthcare associated infections in US hospitals and the benefits of prevention. In: Prevention CfDCa, editor. 2009. Available at: http://www.cdc.gov/ncidod/dhqp/pdf/Scott_CostPaper.pdf. Accessed November 3, 2010.
2. Yokoe DS, Mermel LA, Anderson DJ, et al. A compendium of strategies to prevent healthcare-associated infections in acute care hospitals. Infect Control Hosp Epidemiol 2008;29(Suppl 1):S12–21.
3. Occupational exposure to bloodborne pathogen–OSHA. Final rule. Fed Regist 1991;56:64004 Standard 1910.1030.
4. Occupational exposure to tuberculosis. Fed Regist 2003;68:75767–75 Standard 1910;12/31/2003:OSHA.
5. 2007 Guideline for isolation precautions: preventing transmission of infectious agents in healthcare settings. In: (HICPAC) CfDCaP-HICPAC, editor. 2007. Available at: http://www.cdc.gov/hicpac/2007IP/2007isolationPrecautions.html. Accessed November 3, 2010.
6. Saving 100,000 lives campaign. Available at: http://www.ihi.org/IHI/Programs/Campaign/. Accessed November 3, 2010.
7. Protecting 5 millions lives from harm. Available at: http://www.ihi.org/IHI/Programs/Campaign/. Accessed November 3, 2010.
8. Infection control related sentinel events. Available at: http://www.jointcommission.org/SentinelEvents/SentinelEventAlert/sea_28.htm. Accessed January 22, 2003.
9. 2004 National Patient Safety Goals. Available at: http://www.jointcommission.org/PatientSafety/NationalPatientSafetyGoals/2004_npsgs.htm. Accessed November 3, 2010.
10. Gourley D. Joint Commission places infection control under the microscope. 2004. Available at: http://www.highbeam.com/doc/1G1-139951600.html. Accessed November 3, 2010.
11. The Joint Commission. Hospital accreditation program: 2009 National Patient Safety Goals. Reduce the risk of healthcare associated infections. Oakbrook Terrace (IL): The Joint Commission; 2009. p. 11–7. Available at: http://www.jointcommission.org/PatientSafety/NationalPatientSafetyGoals/09_npsgs.htm. Accessed November 3, 2010.

12. Conditions for coverage- infection control. Fed Regist 2008;73(223). Availabe at: http://www.access.gpo.gov/su_docs/fedreg/a081118c.html. Accessed November 3, 2010.
13. Assessing risk is a starting point, vol. IC.01.03.01. 2009.
14. Friedman C. Infection prevention and control programs. In: Carrico R, editor. APIC text of infection control and epidemiology, vol. 1. 3rd edition. Washington, DC: APIC; 2009. p. 1–4.
15. Strausbaugh LJ. Anxiety on the watchtower: the hospital epidemiologist and emerging infectious diseases. Curr Infect Dis Rep 2003;5(6):451–3.
16. Nutty C. Project management and communication. Certification study guide. 3rd edition. APIC; 2007. Available at: http://ecdc.europa.eu/ipse/Working%20packages/WP1/Core%20Curriculum%20Report.pdf. Accessed November 3, 2010.
17. Haley RW, Quade D, Freeman HE, et al. The SENIC project. Study on the efficacy of nosocomial infection control (SENIC project). Summary of study design. Am J Epidemiol 1980;111(5):472–85.
18. Stone PW, Dick A, Pogorzelska M, et al. Staffing and structure of infection prevention and control programs. Am J Infect Control 2009;37(5):351–7.
19. Gaynes R, Richards C, Edwards J, et al. Feeding back surveillance data to prevent hospital-acquired infections. Emerg Infect Dis 2001;7(2):295–8.
20. Hospital interpretive guidelines, vol. 42 CFR 482.42 (a)(2). Department of Health & Human Services (DHHS) Centers for Medicare and Medicaid; 2008. Available at: http://www.cms.gov/manuals/downloads/som107ap_a_hospitals.pdf. Accessed November 3, 2010.
21. Patient safety component protocol: National Healthcare Safety Network (NHSN) Manual. 2008. Available at: http://www.dhcs.ca.gov/provgovpart/initiatives/nqi/Documents/NHSNManPSPCurr.pdf. Accessed November 3, 2010.
22. Arias KM. Surveillance. In: Carrico R, editor. APIC text of infection control and epidemiology, vol. 1. 3rd edition. Washington, DC: APIC; 2009. p. 3–5.
23. Greene L, Cain TA, Khoury R. APIC position paper: the importance of surveillance technologies in the prevention of healthcare-associated infections. Am J Infect Control 2009;37(6):510–3.
24. Srinivasan. Outbreak investigation. In: Carrico R, editor. APIC text of infection control and epidemiology, vol. 1. 3rd edition. Washington, DC: APIC; 2009. p. 1–4.
25. Nadzam D, Soule B. Performance measures. In: Carrico R, editor. APIC text of infection control and epidemiology, vol. 1. 3rd edition. Washington, DC: APIC; 2009. p. 1–9.
26. Altpeter T. Quality concepts. In: Carrico R, editor. APIC text of infection control and epidemiology, vol. 1. 3rd edition. Washington, DC: APIC; 2009. p. 1–8.
27. Perencevich EN, Stone PW, Wright SB, et al. Raising standards while watching the bottom line: making a business case for infection control. Infect Control Hosp Epidemiol 2007;28(10):1121–33.
28. Fraser VJ, Olsen MA. The business of health care epidemiology: creating a vision for service excellence. Am J Infect Control 2002;30(2):77–85.
29. Maragakis LL, Perencevich EN, Cosgrove SE. Clinical and economic burden of antimicrobial resistance. Expert Rev Anti Infect Ther 2008;6(5):751–63.
30. Murphy DM. From expert data collectors to interventionists: changing the focus for infection control professionals. Am J Infect Control 2002;30(2):120–32.
31. Burke JP. Infection control - a problem for patient safety. N Engl J Med 2003;348(7):651–6.
32. Calfee DP, Farr BM. Infection control and cost control in the era of managed care. Infect Control Hosp Epidemiol 2002;23(7):407–10.

33. Freedberg KA, Paltiel AD. Cost effectiveness of prophylaxis for opportunistic infections in aids. An overview and methodological discussion. Pharmacoeconomics 1998;14(2):165–74.
34. Davey P, Craig AM, Hau C, et al. Cost-effectiveness of prophylactic nasal mupirocin in patients undergoing peritoneal dialysis based on a randomized, placebo-controlled trial. J Antimicrob Chemother 1999;43(1):105–12.
35. Richter A, Brandeau ML, Owens DK. An analysis of optimal resource allocation for prevention of infection with human immunodeficiency virus (HIV) in injection drug users and non-users. Med Decis Making 1999;19(2):167–79.
36. Reid RJ. A benefit-cost analysis of syringe exchange programs. J Health Soc Policy 2000;11(4):41–57.
37. Walker D, Fox-Rushby JA. Economic evaluation of communicable disease interventions in developing countries: a critical review of the published literature. Health Econ 2000;9(8):681–98.
38. Wilkinson D, Floyd K, Gilks CF. National and provincial estimated costs and cost effectiveness of a programme to reduce mother-to-child HIV transmission in South Africa. S Afr Med J 2000;90(8):794–8.
39. Lelekis M, Gould IM. Sequential antibiotic therapy for cost containment in the hospital setting: why not? J Hosp Infect 2001;48(4):249–57.
40. Akalin HE. Surgical prophylaxis: the evolution of guidelines in an era of cost containment. J Hosp Infect 2002;50(Suppl A):S3–7.
41. Floyd K, Blanc L, Raviglione M, et al. Resources required for global tuberculosis control. Science 2002;295(5562):2040–1.
42. Hutton G, Wyss K, N'Diekhor Y. Prioritization of prevention activities to combat the spread of HIV/AIDS in resource constrained settings: a cost-effectiveness analysis from Chad, Central Africa. Int J Health Plann Manage 2003;18(2):117–36.
43. Kampf G. The six golden rules to improve compliance in hand hygiene. J Hosp Infect 2004;56(Suppl 2):S3–5.
44. Currie CS, Floyd K, Williams BG, et al. Cost, affordability and cost-effectiveness of strategies to control tuberculosis in countries with high HIV prevalence. BMC Public Health 2005;5:130.
45. Muniyandi M, Ramachandran R, Balasubramanian R. An economic commentary on the occurrence and control of HIV/AIDS in developing countries: special reference to India. Expert Opin Pharmacother 2006;7(18):2447–54.
46. Wilson AP, Hodgson B, Liu M, et al. Reduction in wound infection rates by wound surveillance with postdischarge follow-up and feedback. Br J Surg 2006;93(5):630–8.
47. Anderson DJ, Kirkland KB, Kaye KS, et al. Underresourced hospital infection control and prevention programs: penny wise, pound foolish? Infect Control Hosp Epidemiol 2007;28(7):767–73.
48. Graves N, Halton K, Lairson D. Economics and preventing hospital-acquired infection: broadening the perspective. Infect Control Hosp Epidemiol 2007;28(2):178–84.
49. Perencevich EN, Thom KA. Commentary: preventing Clostridium difficile-associated disease: is it time to pay the piper? Infect Control Hosp Epidemiol 2008;29(9):829–31.
50. Kaye KS. The financial impact of antibiotic resistance. In: Soule BM, Weber S, editors. What every health care executive should know: the cost of antibiotic resistance. Oakbrook Terrace (IL): Joint Commission Resources; 2009. p. 29–42.
51. 2006 APIC member salary and career survey. Available at: http://www.apic.org/Content/NavigationMenu/MemberServices/2006SalarySurveyResults/2006_Salary_Survey.htm. Accessed September 1, 2006.

52. Coskun D, Aytac J, Aydinli A, et al. Mortality rate, length of stay and extra cost of sternal surgical site infections following coronary artery bypass grafting in a private medical centre in Turkey. J Hosp Infect 2005;60(2):176–9.
53. Rello J, Ollendorf DA, Oster G, et al. Epidemiology and outcomes of ventilator-associated pneumonia in a large US database. Chest 2002;122(6):2115–21.
54. Carmeli Y, Troillet N, Karchmer AW, et al. Health and economic outcomes of antibiotic resistance in *Pseudomonas aeruginosa*. Arch Intern Med 1999;159(10):1127–32.
55. Carmeli Y, Eliopoulos G, Mozaffari E, et al. Health and economic outcomes of vancomycin-resistant enterococci. Arch Intern Med 2002;162(19):2223–8.
56. Cosgrove SE, Kaye KS, Eliopoulous GM, et al. Health and economic outcomes of the emergence of third-generation cephalosporin resistance in *Enterobacter* species. Arch Intern Med 2002;162(2):185–90.
57. Cosgrove SE, Carmeli Y. The impact of antimicrobial resistance on health and economic outcomes. Clin Infect Dis 2003;36(11):1433–7.
58. Engemann JJ, Carmeli Y, Cosgrove SE, et al. Adverse clinical and economic outcomes attributable to methicillin resistance among patients with *Staphylococcus aureus* surgical site infection. Clin Infect Dis 2003;36(5):592–8.
59. Cosgrove SE, Qi Y, Kaye KS, et al. The impact of methicillin resistance in *Staphylococcus aureus* bacteremia on patient outcomes: mortality, length of stay, and hospital charges. Infect Control Hosp Epidemiol 2005;26(2):166–74.
60. Schwaber MJ, Navon-Venezia S, Kaye KS, et al. Clinical and economic impact of bacteremia with extended- spectrum-beta-lactamase-producing enterobacteriaceae. Antimicrob Agents Chemother 2006;50(4):1257–62.
61. Giske CG, Monnet DL, Cars O, et al. Clinical and economic impact of common multidrug-resistant gram-negative bacilli. Antimicrob Agents Chemother 2008; 52(3):813–21.
62. Warren DK, Shukla SJ, Olsen MA, et al. Outcome and attributable cost of ventilator-associated pneumonia among intensive care unit patients in a suburban medical center. Crit Care Med 2003;31(5):1312–7.
63. Hugonnet S, Eggimann P, Borst F, et al. Impact of ventilator-associated pneumonia on resource utilization and patient outcome. Infect Control Hosp Epidemiol 2004;25(12):1090–6.
64. Blot SI, Depuydt P, Annemans L, et al. N Clinical and economic outcomes in critically ill patients with nosocomial catheter-related bloodstream infections. Clin Infect Dis 2005;41(11):1591–8.
65. Coello R, Charlett A, Wilson J, et al. Adverse impact of surgical site infections in English hospitals. J Hosp Infect 2005;60(2):93–103.
66. Hollenbeak CS, Murphy DM, Koenig S, et al. The clinical and economic impact of deep chest surgical site infections following coronary artery bypass graft surgery. Chest 2000;118(2):397–402.
67. Tambyah PA, Knasinski V, Maki DG. The direct costs of nosocomial catheter-associated urinary tract infection in the era of managed care. Infect Control Hosp Epidemiol 2002;23(1):27–31.
68. Lai KK, Fontecchio SA. Use of silver-hydrogel urinary catheters on the incidence of catheter-associated urinary tract infections in hospitalized patients. Am J Infect Control 2002;30(4):221–5.
69. Ward WJ Jr, Spragens L, Smithson K. Building the business case for clinical quality. Healthc Financ Manage 2006;60(12):92–8.
70. Perencevich EN, Fisman DN, Lipsitch M, et al. Projected benefits of active surveillance for vancomycin-resistant enterococci in intensive care units. Clin Infect Dis 2004;38(8):1108–15.

Hand Hygiene

Maureen Bolon, MD, MS

KEYWORDS

- Hand hygiene • Hand washing
- Health care workers • Antisepsis

The crucial role of hand hygiene in the prevention of health care–associated infection (HAI) was initially established independently by Oliver Wendell Holmes and Ignaz Semmelweis in the 1840s.[1] Semmelweis, whose insights predated the germ theory by several decades, is credited with recognizing that the hands of medical staff were contaminated while performing autopsies and consequently were responsible for the transmission of "cadaverous particles" during obstetric examinations, leading to puerperal sepsis and death.[2] He further demonstrated that hand antisepsis with chlorinated lime resulted in a dramatic decline in maternal mortality. More than a century later, Mortimer and colleagues[3] established the importance of hand hygiene in preventing *Staphylococcus aureus* transmission in a neonatal unit. When cared for by nurses who did not perform hand hygiene, infants in this study were more likely to acquire *S aureus* than those cared for by nurses who performed hand hygiene with hexachlorophene. As was the case in Semmelweis' time, evidence of the benefits of hand hygiene have not translated into immediate adoption of the practice. The later part of the twentieth century and the early part of the twenty-first century have seen major advances in medical science, including in the field of health care epidemiology. Despite these advances and the development of well-accepted guidelines regarding the practice of hand hygiene, rates of hand hygiene performance by health care workers remain disappointingly low.

HUMAN SKIN AND SKIN FLORA

Human skin is colonized with bacteria. Counts vary depending on body location; in the context of a discussion of HAI, the pertinent figures relate to the bacterial counts on the hands of health care workers, which have been reported to range from 3.9×10^4 to 4.6×10^6 colony-forming units (CFUs)/cm^2.[1] Two classifications of skin flora have been delineated: transient flora and resident flora. Transient flora are those most frequently associated with HAIs and are, therefore, the primary target of hand hygiene within the health care setting. Transient flora reside in the uppermost level of the stratum corneum and are acquired by direct contact with patients or with environmental surfaces associated with patients.[1] These loosely adherent organisms can consequently be

Department of Medicine, Division of Infectious Diseases, Northwestern University Feinberg School of Medicine, 645 North Michigan Avenue, Suite 900, Chicago, IL 60611, USA
E-mail address: m-bolon@northwestern.edu

Infect Dis Clin N Am 25 (2011) 21–43
doi:10.1016/j.idc.2010.11.001
0891-5520/11/$ – see front matter © 2011 Elsevier Inc. All rights reserved.

transmitted to other patients or to the environment if they are not removed by mechanical friction or the detergent properties of soap and water or killed by antiseptic agents.[4] Numerous pathogens have been identified among the transient flora of health care workers' hands, including S aureus, Klebsiella pneumoniae, Acinetobacter spp, Enterobacter spp, and Candida spp. Health care workers with skin damage or chronic skin conditions are more likely to be colonized with pathogenic organisms in greater quantities (both the number of different organisms and the bacterial counts), which can make them more likely to transmit infectious pathogens.[5,6] Resident flora are the low-pathogenicity, permanent residents of the deeper layers of the skin.[4,7] These organisms cause infection only when a normal barrier is disrupted, such as with the placement of an intravenous catheter. Resident flora cannot be removed solely by mechanical friction; thus, an antiseptic agent must be used before the performance of invasive procedures. Surgical hand antisepsis is a special case, in that the goal is to reduce resident flora for the duration of the surgical procedure to prevent contamination of the surgical field if a glove becomes punctured or torn.[1]

In order to interrupt transmission of HAIs spread via health care workers' hands, it is useful to consider the sequence of events necessary for this to occur[1]:

1. Organisms present on a patient's skin or in the proximity of a patient are transferred to the hands of a health care worker.
2. Organisms must be capable of surviving for a short period on the hands of a health care worker.
3. Hand hygiene is inadequate, performed with an inappropriate agent, or omitted entirely.
4. Contaminated hands of a health care worker must come in direct contact with another patient or with an inanimate object that comes in direct contact with the patient.

The contribution of contact with the immediate patient environment (as opposed to the patient directly) to the contamination of health care workers' hands must be emphasized. Viable organisms are present in the 10^6 skin squames that humans shed daily; these may proceed to contaminate patient gowns, bed linen, and furniture.[1] Organisms that are resistant to desiccation, such as staphylococci and enterococci, may thereby join transient flora on the hands of health care workers.

The many terms describing the processes of hand hygiene are listed in **Table 1**. The microbial impact of the three categories of hand hygiene agents (plain soap, alcohol-based hand rub, and antimicrobial soap) is discussed in this article. Hand washing with plain soap removes dirt and transient flora via a detergent effect and mechanical friction. The log reduction of hand flora increases with duration of hand washing, but because the duration of hand washing averages from 6 to 24 seconds in observational studies of health care workers, a realistic expectation is a reduction of 0.6 to 1.1 $\log_{10}$ CFUs after a typical 15-second hand washing episode.[1,7] There is some concern that the trauma caused by frequent hand washing may increase counts of skin flora and episodes of transmission by encouraging desquamation of the epithelial layer of skin and shedding of resident flora.[4,5] In contrast to plain soap, alcohol-based hand rubs work by killing the organisms on the skin rather than physically removing them. The antimicrobial activity of alcohols is attributed to the denaturation of proteins. Although activity varies by compound and concentration, alcohols are active against gram-positive cocci, gram-negative bacilli, Mycobacterium tuberculosis, many fungi, and viruses.[1,4] With a proper 30-second application, alcohol-based hand rubs lead to a bacterial reduction of 3.2 to 5.8 $\log_{10}$ CFUs.[7] Alcohols are considered somewhat less active against nonenveloped viruses, such as hepatitis A virus, rotavirus,

Table 1 Hand hygiene terms	
Plain soap	A detergent-based soap without antimicrobial properties. Action is achieved by physically removing dirt and microorganisms.
Alcohol-based hand rub	A waterless, alcohol-containing agent that kills microorganisms but does not physically remove soil or organic material.
Antimicrobial soap	An agent that possesses bactericidal activity against skin flora. Action is achieved via (1) physical removal of dirt and microorganisms and (2) killing of microorganisms.
Hand hygiene	Any method intended to remove or destroy microorganisms on the hands.
Hand washing	A method involving the use of water and plain soap to generate a lather, which is then distributed across all surfaces of the hands and rinsed off by water.
Hand antisepsis	Hand hygiene using either antimicrobial soap or an alcohol-based hand rub to physically remove and/or kill microorganisms.
Surgical scrub or surgical hand rub	Either antimicrobial soap or an alcohol-based hand rub that is used before surgery to kill transient organisms and reduce resident flora for the duration of a surgical procedure.

Data from Boyce JM, Pittet D. Guideline for hand hygiene in health-care settings. Recommendations of the Healthcare Infection Control Practices Advisory Committee and the HICPAC/SHEA/APIC/IDSA hand hygiene task force. MMWR Recomm Rep 2002;51(RR–16):1–45 [quiz CE1–4]; and Larson EL. APIC guideline for handwashing and hand antisepsis in health care settings. Am J Infect Control 1995;23(4):251–69.

enteroviruses, and adenovirus. Alcohols have poor activity against bacterial spores, such as those of *Clostridium difficile*. The antimicrobial action of antimicrobial soaps also varies by agent. The properties of chlorhexidine are elaborated, because it is one of the more commonly used agents. Chlorhexidine is a cationic bisguanide that derives its antimicrobial action by disrupting cell membranes and precipitating cell contents.[4] Chlorhexidine is considered to have good activity against gram-positive cocci and somewhat less activity against gram-negative bacilli, fungi, and viruses. Chlorhexidine has minimal antimycobacterial activity and is not active against spore-forming bacteria. A distinguishing feature of chlorhexidine is its persistence, a property that makes it a good candidate for surgical hand antisepsis. Bacterial reduction of 2.1 to 3 $\log_{10}$ CFUs has been observed with shorter applications (less than 1 minute) of chlorhexidine.[8]

EVOLUTION OF GUIDELINES

Hand hygiene practices in the United States have been shaped by guidelines issued by the Centers for Disease Control and Prevention (CDC). The earliest guidelines encouraged the use of plain soap and promoted the use of waterless agents only when sinks were not available.[9] In 1995, guidelines were issued by the Association for Professionals in Infection Control (APIC).[4] Hand washing with plain soap was advised for general patient care and removing visible soil. Hand antisepsis with antimicrobial soap or alcohol-based hand rub was recommended in the following circumstances: (1) before performance of invasive procedures, such as surgery or the placement of intravenous catheters, indwelling urinary catheters, or other invasive devices; (2) when persistent antimicrobial activity is desired; and (3) when the reduction of resident flora is important. Opportunities for hand washing with plain soap and water or hand antisepsis with an alcohol-based hand rub included before and after patient contact and after contact with a source of microorganisms (body fluids and substances, mucous membranes, nonintact skin, and inanimate objects that are likely to be contaminated). The role of hand antisepsis with either antimicrobial soap or a waterless agent was further expanded in the recommendations issued by the Healthcare Infection Control Practices Advisory Committee (HICPAC).[10,11] In these documents, hand antisepsis was recommended on exiting the room of a patient with a multidrug-resistant pathogen.

In 2002, the CDC released an updated hand hygiene guideline and, for the first time, endorsed the use of alcohol-based hand rubs for the majority of clinical interactions, provided that hands are not visibly soiled.[1] In addition to the previous recommendation that hand hygiene should be performed before and after patient contact, more comprehensive guidance regarding situations that should prompt hand hygiene was detailed (**Box 1**). After the release of the 2002 CDC guidelines, hand hygiene practices in United States health care facilities changed dramatically as institutions adopted alcohol-based hand rubs, which had been used in Europe for several decades.[12]

Many other national and international bodies issue guidelines for hand hygiene in health care settings. It would be a significant omission not to mention the contribution of the World Health Organization (WHO) to this effort. The WHO First Global Patient Safety Challenge was launched in 2005, a major focus of which is the promotion of hand hygiene practices in the health care setting.[13] As a follow-up, the WHO released hand hygiene guidelines in 2009, with indications for hand hygiene similar to those of the CDC. To assist campaign implementation, the WHO toolkit was developed with freely available materials. These materials are formulated to be applicable to both developed and developing nations as well as in poorly-resourced settings and attempt to take into account cultural and religious influences on hand hygiene practices. The WHO toolkit also provides a simplified and elegant construct to assist health care workers in recognizing hand hygiene opportunities, "Your Five Moments for Hand Hygiene": (1) before patient contact, (2) before aseptic task, (3) after body fluid exposure, (4) after patient contact, and (5) after contacts with patient surroundings.[14]

ALCOHOL-BASED HAND RUBS

After the directive of the 2002 CDC Guideline for Hand Hygiene in Health-Care Settings, alcohol-based hand rubs became the preferred agent for hand hygiene in situations when hands are not visibly soiled. As such, these agents deserve a more detailed look. The reduction in bacterial counts achieved after application of an alcohol-based hand rub varies depending on the alcohol used; n-propanol is more bactericidal than isopranolol, which is more bactericidal than ethanol.[8,15] Efficacy is also related to concentration of the alcohol, with higher concentrations having greater bactericidal effect (up to 95%). Greater flammability limits the use of the higher concentrations of alcohol. In the United States, alcohol-based hand rubs are typically comprised of 60% to 95% ethanol or isopranolol.[1] As discussed previously, alcohols have wide antimicrobial spectra and are fast acting, which makes them ideal for routine hand antisepsis. They lack persistent activity but may be incorporated into surgical hand rubs with another antimicrobial agent possessing persistent activity, such as chlorhexidine. Alcohol-based hand rubs are among the best tolerated agents for hand hygiene, in large part due to the addition of emollients.[1,15] They are superior

Box 1
Centers for Disease Control and Prevention indications for hand hygiene

When hands are visibly dirty or contaminated with proteinaceous material or are visibly soiled with blood or other body fluids, wash hands with either a nonantimicrobial soap and water or an antimicrobial soap and water (categorization of recommendation: IA)

If hands are not visibly soiled, use an alcohol-based hand rub for routinely decontaminating hands in all other clinical situations (described later) (IA). Alternatively, wash hands with an antimicrobial soap and water in all clinical situations (described later) (IB).

Decontaminate hands before having direct contact with patients (IB).

Decontaminate hands before donning sterile gloves when inserting an intravascular catheter (IB).

Decontaminate hands before inserting indwelling urinary catheters, peripheral vascular catheters, or other invasive devices that do not require a surgical procedure (IB).

Decontaminate hands after contact with a patient's intact skin (IB).

Decontaminate hands after contact with body fluids or excretions, mucous membranes, nonintact skin, and wound dressings if hands are not visibly soiled (IB).

Decontaminate hands if moving from a contaminated body site to a clean body site during patient care (II).

Decontaminate hands after contact with inanimate objects (including medical equipment) in the immediate vicinity of the patient (II).

Decontaminate hands after removing gloves (IB).

Before eating and after using a restroom, wash hands with a nonantimicrobial soap and water or with antimicrobial soap and water (IB).

Antimicrobial-impregnated wipes may be considered as an alternative to washing hands with nonantimicrobial soap and water. Because they are not as effective as alcohol-based hand rubs or washing hands with an antimicrobial soap and water for reducing bacterial counts on the hands of health care workers, they are not a substitute for hand antisepsis (IB).

Wash hands with nonantimicrobial soap and water or with antimicrobial soap and water if exposure to *Bacillus anthracis* is suspected or proved (II).

No recommendation can be made regarding the routine use of nonalcohol-based hand rubs for hand hygiene in health care settings. Unresolved issue.

CDC/HICPAC system for categorizing recommendations

Category IA. Strongly recommended for implementation and strongly supported by well-designed experimental, clinical, or epidemiologic studies

Category IB. Strongly recommended for implementation and supported by certain experimental, clinical, or epidemiologic studies and using theoretic rationale.

Category IC. Required for implementation, as mandated by federal or state regulation or standard.

Category II. Suggested for implementation and supported by suggestive clinical or epidemiologic studies or a theoretic rationale.

No recommendation. Unresolved issue. Practices for which insufficient evidence or no consensus regarding efficacy exist.

From Boyce JM, Pittet D. Guideline for hand hygiene in health care settings. Recommendations of the Healthcare Infection Control Practices Advisory Committee and the HICPAC/SHEA/APIC/IDSA hand hygiene task force. MMWR Recomm Rep 2002;51(RR–16):1–45 [quiz: CE1–4].

even to plain soap, the detergent effect of which causes loss of protein and lipids in the stratum corneum layers and consequent drying effect through water loss.[8] Furthermore, the incidence of allergic reactions due to alcohols is believed nonexistent, although there remains the possibility of allergy to an emollient component.[7,16] An additional important benefit of alcohol-based hand rubs is the relative time saved in the performance of hand hygiene compared with the use of soap and water. Hand hygiene performance with an alcohol-based hand rub is typically estimated to require one-third the length of time of a hand wash procedure. In an oft-cited study, health care workers were timed performing hand washing, including travel to and from the sink.[17] The average duration of the hand washing procedure was 61.7 seconds, with a range of 37 to 84 seconds. The same investigators modeled the total time required for hand hygiene. If health care workers were 100% compliant with hand hygiene requirements, a 12-person team would spend 16 hours performing hand washing but just 3 hours using an alcohol-based hand rub. Because time constraints are one of the most frequently cited explanations for failure to perform hand hygiene, it is expected that the change from hand washing to alcohol-based hand rub should improve hand hygiene performance. This issue is examined in more detail below.

Several concerns accompanied the initial introduction of alcohol-based hand rubs in the United States. Fire safety concerns were raised given the known flammability of alcohols. In some locales, fire marshals disallowed the placement of dispensers in hallways,[18] which had the effect of limiting health care worker access to hand hygiene agents. Although flash fires related to use of alcohol-based hand rubs have been infrequently reported in the literature,[19] accumulated experience both in Europe and the United States indicates that these are unusual occurrences.[18,20]

Given the known inactivity of alcohols against *C difficile* spores, there was some initial concern that the move away from hand washing to alcohol-based hand rubs would have the unintended consequence of increased *C difficile* infection rates. Early indications are that this has not occurred. In a study conducted soon after the introduction of alcohol-based hand rubs at a large community teaching hospital, Boyce and colleagues[21] reported a 10-fold increase in the use of alcohol-based hand rubs from 2000 to 2003 and a commensurate increase in the proportion of hand hygiene episodes using alcohol-based hand rubs (from 10% to 85%). Despite this, they noted no increase in *C difficile* infection over this period. Other investigators have similarly failed to demonstrate a correlation between alcohol-based hand rub use and *C difficile* infection.[22] Current guidelines do not specify deviation from routine hand hygiene practices when caring for individuals with *C difficile* infection; however, hand washing with soap and water is currently recommended when caring for patients with *C difficile* infection during outbreaks or settings of hyperendemicity.[23] This approach, as part of a bundle of other infection control measures, has been reported as successful in reducing *C difficile* infection rates during outbreaks of hypervirulent strains of the organism.[24]

STUDIES OF HAND HYGIENE EFFICACY
Impact on Microbial Contamination

Traditionally, the antimicrobial efficacy of hand hygiene products is evaluated following one of two possible methods of hand contamination: artificial contamination or actual clinical practice. To obtain approval by the Food and Drug Administration, antiseptic hand hygiene agents must demonstrate a reduction in the colony counts of a reference *Escherichia coli* strain inoculated onto hands as dictated in the Tentative Final Monograph (TFM).[25] Many studies have demonstrated the superior activity of alcohol-based products for reducing bacterial counts of artificially contaminated hands relative to plain soap or antimicrobial soaps.[1] This has also been demonstrated for antimicrobial-resistant organisms, such as methicillin-resistant *S aureus* (MRSA).[26] As expected, alcohol-based hand rubs are inferior to plain soap and water and antimicrobial soaps for elimination of *C difficile* from artificially contaminated hands.[27] One criticism of studies of artificial contamination is that they do not reflect realistic scenarios of either hand contamination or hand hygiene practices, because hand hygiene performance by volunteers in a study is likely more thorough and of longer duration than that of health care workers in clinical practice. Although studies of the impact of hand hygiene on the hand flora of health care workers in clinical practice have also demonstrated the superiority of alcohol-based hand hygiene,[1,28,29] there remains concern that these studies may also not reflect real-life hand hygiene behaviors because the participants knew they were being studied. Nonetheless, some of these studies do allow insights into the contribution of hand hygiene technique to bacterial reduction. Several investigators have identified lapses in the application of alcohol-based hand rub products by health care workers using direct observation and through the use of fluorescent dye and UV light to evaluate whether or not the hand rub was applied to all surfaces of the hands.[1,28–33] Some of these studies have further confirmed that poor technique can significantly affect the bacterial reduction achieved by alcohol-based hand rubs, although one study showed that the efficacy of hand washing was more sensitive to poor technique than alcohol-based hand rubs.[31] These studies highlight that for alcohol-based hand rubs to achieve optimal effect, health care workers must be trained in proper technique. At minimum, proper technique entails the use of adequate volume of solution, application of the solution for a proper length of time, covering all surfaces of the hands, and starting the procedure with dry hands.

It would be an oversight not to mention the controversy surrounding the formulation of hand rubs as either gels or rinses. Rinses are more commonly used in European health care settings, whereas gels have been more predominant in the United States. Although all gel products marketed in the United States meet the standards of efficacy established in the TFM, some of them do not meet the European standards. Although the TFM specifies a required log-reduction in an indicator organism after the use of an antiseptic agent, European Norm (EN) 1500 requires that waterless products must have equivalent performance to a reference agent, 60% isopropanol.[34] Several studies have demonstrated the failure of commercially available alcohol hand gels to meet the EN 1500 requirements, which has led some to conclude that these products are not suitable for hand antisepsis.[29,35,36] Advocates for gels respond that adherence may be improved with this easier-to-use and better-tolerated formulation. A recent study comparing isopropyl rinse and gel in clinical practice (both formulations met the EN 1500 standard) did demonstrate significantly better hand hygiene compliance with the gel product as well as a reduction in skin drying.[37] This controversy remains unresolved, but it is important to acknowledge that both the TFM and EN 1500 standards are somewhat arbitrary, because it is unknown what level of bacterial reduction is necessary to reduce transmission of infection in the health care setting.[1,38]

Hand Hygiene Adherence

There is little question that rates of hand hygiene performance by health care workers are dismal. The oft-cited figure for adherence is 40%, which is derived from the average adherence reported in 34 studies performed from 1981 to 2000.[1] Baseline adherence in those studies ranged from 5% to 81%. Several investigators have identified that health care workers are more likely to perform hand hygiene after activities rather than before activities and are more likely to perform hand hygiene after contact with body fluids.[39,40] Anticipated baseline rates and health care worker tendencies are important to keep in mind when approaching the large literature on hand hygiene interventions, but before addressing this, further elaboration is required regarding the methods for measuring hand hygiene adherence.

Three methods are most commonly used in the evaluation of health care worker adherence with hand hygiene practices: direct observation of hand hygiene opportunities, self-report of adherence, and indirect measures of hand hygiene product usage. Each of these methods has advantages and disadvantages in terms of accuracy, reproducibility, and ease of measurement. Direct observation is considered the gold standard for assessing hand hygiene compliance.[41,42] This metric is generally presented as number of hand hygiene episodes divided by number of hand hygiene opportunities. Direct observation of hand hygiene is the only method that can provide information on when and why hand hygiene lapses occur, which allows focusing on individuals or groups of individuals requiring further motivation. Direct observation also allows identification of problems with technique or performance that require further education and reinforcement. Direct observation is labor intensive, however, and, as such, it is possible to capture only a minority of hand hygiene episodes that occur. This factor leads to selection bias, particularly if observations are limited to weekday or daytime shifts. Finally, the act of observation can influence the behavior of those being observed and in itself affect the outcome being studied, a phenomenon known as the Hawthorne effect. One group estimated that the Hawthorne effect increased hand hygiene compliance by 55%,[43] which is surely a desirable impact but not one that is likely to be sustained. Assessing hand hygiene adherence by self-report, usually by administering questionnaires to health care workers is among the least costly methods. There are conflicting reports on how well self-report agrees with actual hand hygiene performance,[44,45] but in general, self-report is believed to overestimate hand hygiene adherence.[41] Evaluation of product consumption is an appealing method for determining hand hygiene adherence because of its fairly low cost. A metric of hand hygiene performance can be derived by monitoring volume of product use and dividing by volume dispensed and number of patients to quantify the number of hand hygiene episodes per patient day. Alternatively, hand hygiene product dispensers can be fitted with electronic monitoring devices to quantify the number of hand hygiene episodes that are occurring within a defined time period.

Some investigators have failed to demonstrate a correlation between hand hygiene adherence as measured by direct observation and product usage,[46,47] although one group pointed out that in their study direct observations only captured a minority of hand hygiene events (0.4%) and thus may not have accurately represented adherence rates.[47] There remain concerns that evaluations of product usage do not identify which health care workers are not performing hand hygiene and do not allow assessment of hand hygiene technique. Additionally, product use by patients or visitors cannot be distinguished from that of the health care workers. To establish the methods currently used by health care facilities to monitor hand hygiene adherence, a recent international survey indicated that most facilities were relying on direct observations of hand hygiene opportunities, with less attention given to hand hygiene technique.[48] Product use was monitored as an adjunct. These investigators highlighted several areas of concern, including the fact that time devoted to training observers was typically under an hour and most programs did not evaluate interobserver validity.

The study of barriers to optimal hand hygiene performance helps inform interventions intended to improve performance. Barriers and risk factors have been comprehensively reviewed by other investigators[39]; a few issues are highlighted. With multiple demands on their time, the time required for hand hygiene performance is a frequently discussed barrier to acceptable hand hygiene adherence. As discussed previously, one of the benefits of alcohol-based hand rubs is the time savings in their application. . Yet, given the hands-on nature of care in a modern hospital, countless hand hygiene opportunities occur throughout the day. One group estimated that despite the use of an alcohol-based hand rub, 230 minutes per patient per day would need to be devoted to hand hygiene in an ICU.[49] The inconvenience of hand hygiene due to inaccessibility of sinks, towels, or product dispensers is another issue that may increase the time to perform hand hygiene and reduce adherence. Although sink accessibility would be anticipated to have an impact on hand washing compliance, two groups have reported no effect on hand hygiene adherence when sink accessibility improved after construction of new hospital facilities.[50,51] Irritant contact dermatitis is a common occurrence among health care workers, with a reported prevalence of 10% to 45%.[5,16] Accordingly, skin irritation and dryness may discourage the performance of hand hygiene, even with alcohol-based products, despite the fact that true allergies are thought not likely due to alcohols and studies have shown beneficial effects of alcohol-based hand rubs on skin water loss.[7,16,52] For this reason, provision of lotions to reduce the occurrence of dermatitis merits a category IA recommendation in the CDC guidelines.[1] Fortunately, skin care products are not thought to adversely affect the antimicrobial properties of alcohol-based hand rubs.[53]

Glove use by health care workers often occurs in patient care, whether because of standard precautions or because of the performance of invasive procedures. Gloves are not considered an adequate barrier to the contamination that occurs during patient care, hence, the recommendation that hand hygiene should be performed after glove removal.[1] There is controversy about whether or not the act of wearing gloves stimulates or discourages hand hygiene; studies have demonstrated both outcomes.[1,50,51,54] A related issue is whether or not contact precautions, the use of gowns and gloves by health care workers to prevent transmission of infectious agents, have an impact on hand hygiene adherence. One recent study showed no impact of gown use on hand hygiene rates.[55] Thus, it seems premature to characterize either glove or gown use as definite barriers to hand hygiene performance.

The professional role of the health care worker has been repeatedly found to be a factor in hand hygiene performance; unfortunately, physicians who have completed their training have been identified as possessing the lowest hand hygiene adherence rates by several investigators.[56,57] Because attending physicians often serve as role models for trainees, students, and other professionals, their poor hand hygiene performance can adversely affect that of these individuals. In an observational study of resident hand hygiene practices, hand hygiene adherence increased from 14% to 65% if the senior member of the team practiced hand hygiene.[58] Conversely, if the senior member of the team did not practice hand hygiene, no other member of the team did. Other groups have found that role models have a predominantly negative impact on the hand hygiene of their trainees.[50] In direct surveys of trainees, role modeling has been identified as important in influencing the practice of hand hygiene.[58,59] Pittet and colleagues[60] administered a survey to physicians to explore barriers and motivators of hand hygiene adherence. Among other findings, the belief that one is a role model for other colleagues did positively influence hand hygiene performance, whereas high workload was a risk factor for nonadherence. On a more optimistic note, educational infection control sessions have been found to effectively influence physician adoption of alcohol-based hand rubs.[61] The change observed after educational infection control sessions was more dramatic among physicians than any other group, a difference that was postulated as due to the fact that physicians are more comfortable changing practice when faced with evidence-based recommendations.

Improving Hand Hygiene Adherence

At its root, the practice of hand hygiene can be considered a behavior to be encouraged among health care workers. The practice of hand hygiene occurs outside the health care setting as well, and the variance in practices learned in the home and the expectations within the health care setting explains in part the poor adherence rates among health care workers. Under one rubric, there are two types of hand hygiene behaviors: inherent and elective. Inherent hand hygiene occurs when hands are perceived as physically dirty, either because of sensation, odor, or contact with an "emotionally dirty area," such as the groin or axilla.[62] Inherent hand hygiene is the predominant form of hand hygiene practiced in the community and elicits maximal adherence in both community and health care settings. Conversely, elective hand hygiene practice comprises all other opportunities, including those that should follow many patient and environmental contacts within the health care setting. Although these contacts do not trigger a self-protective response to perform hand hygiene, elective hand hygiene is desirable for preventing transmission to patients.

The theory of planned behavior is a social cognitive model that has been applied to evaluate precipitants of health care worker hand hygiene performance.[63] This approach has identified the importance of perceived social pressure and perceived ease of performance on the motivation to perform hand hygiene whereas beliefs about infections and their prevention are less influential.[64] Although behavioral theory has contributed to understanding of motivators of hand hygiene practice, some investigators have noted that health care workers' intentions do not consistently translate into practice.[65] What seems clear is that an effective hand hygiene intervention should not be limited to a focus on individuals, because removal of impediments within the health care environment and improvements in the institutional climate also contribute to a successful campaign.

In terms of interventions intended to improve hand hygiene adherence, the introduction of alcohol-based hand gel as the preferred agent for hand hygiene has become one of the best studied interventions. Introducing an alcohol-based hand hygiene product is anticipated to be effective in that it represents an easily accessible or even portable agent that can be applied in less time than hand washing, thus reducing the primary barriers to hand hygiene. Many investigators have found that the introduction of an alcohol-based hand rub did improve hand hygiene adherence.[66–70] One of these studies also demonstrated a reduction in HAI rates (discussed in more detail later).[67] Conversely, some investigators have noted limited or no success in improving hand hygiene rates after the introduction of alcohol-based hand rubs.[71,72] A common theme in failed interventions is the lack of an accompanying educational program or an ineffective educational program to promote the use of these agents.[70,72]

Reporting and feedback of individual or unit level performance is a common strategy for motivating practice improvements. One large, multicenter project ascertained hand hygiene performance based on product usage and provided regular feedback on hand hygiene adherence.[73] These investigators demonstrated significant improvements in hand hygiene performance both in ICU and non-ICU settings (median percentage change of 63% and 92%, respectively) over a 12-month period. Notably, the use of indirect measures of hand hygiene performance allowed significant cost savings over direct hand hygiene observations.

Yet another means of encouraging practice is to provide those engaged in patient care with immediate prompts to perform hand hygiene. Several interventions using audible, automatic reminders have reportedly been successful in motivating hand hygiene. One group of investigators noted an improvement in hand hygiene when prerecorded messages encouraging hand hygiene were broadcast on the unit with a frequency of 1 to 15 minutes.[74] It may be relevant that the broadcasted messages were voice recordings of local hospital leadership. Two other groups reported improvement in hand hygiene rates with point-of-care audible reminders triggered by missed hand hygiene opportunities.[75,76] Both studies used devices that monitored room exit as well as hand hygiene performance. Researchers raised concerns regarding the ability to capture multiple individuals exiting a patient room simultaneously as well as the inability to distinguish between health care worker and patient or visitor hand hygiene opportunities. It is not yet clear whether or not this technology would have a sustainable impact on hand hygiene adherence.

As the group most likely to benefit from improved health care worker hand hygiene practices, patients may have a role in encouraging hand hygiene. Both the CDC and WHO guidelines recommend that patients be involved in promoting health care worker hand hygiene (category II recommendation in both guidelines).[1,13] Although a phone survey of US households indicated that 80% of those surveyed would ask a health care worker to perform hand hygiene,[77] there are many factors that may thwart this intention. Surveys of patients reveal a potential willingness to mention hand hygiene to health care workers that is not always mirrored by actual execution of a request.[78] More successful strategies have involved positive reinforcement (ie, thanking a health care worker for performing hand hygiene), providing posters or placards for patients to display that encourage hand hygiene, or requests from the health care workers themselves to be asked about hand hygiene.[79,80] Health care workers do seem amenable to patient prompting to perform hand hygiene.[78] Concerns remain as to whether this is a realistic expectation for patients who are too ill or intimidated by caregivers to participate, but in some settings this may constitute one aspect of an overall safety culture.

Health Care–Associated Infections

Given the dramatic reduction in puerperal sepsis observed by Semmelweis after the introduction of hand antisepsis, it might come as a surprise to learn that the question of whether improved hand hygiene is associated with a decline in HAI remains an active area of inquiry. A recent Cochrane review attempted to synthesize the many studies published on the topic but arrived at no conclusion because only two studies were believed adequate for inclusion.[81] **Tables 2** and **3** present a non-exhaustive compilation of contemporary studies demonstrating successful interventions to improve hand hygiene. The studies listed in **Table 2** were unable to demonstrate a resultant reduction in the chosen metric for HAI, whereas those in **Table 3** reported improvement in at least one metric of HAI that was thought associated with improved hand hygiene practice. Although this is not a formal meta-analysis, there does not seem to be any systematic difference in the level of hand hygiene adherence or degree of change of hand hygiene adherence in studies that showed a decrease in infection compared with those that did not. Infection was not a primary outcome for several of the studies that failed to show an association between hand hygiene performance and infection; furthermore, follow-up was brief in the same studies. There were a wide variety of infectious outcomes

Table 2
Studies that do not demonstrate a reduction in HAIs after interventions to improve hand hygiene performance

Reference, Year Published	Setting	Metric of Hand Hygiene Performance (and Reported Improvement)	Infection Outcome	Comment
Lam et al,[90] 2004	1 NICU in a hospital in Hong Kong	HH adherence (from 40% to 53% before patient contact; from 39% to 59% after patient contact)	HAIs	Short duration of follow-up (6 months); infection was not a primary outcome
Rupp et al,[82] 2008	2 ICUs in a US hospital	HH adherence (from 37%–38% to 68%–69%)	Device-associated infections; MDRO infections; C difficile infections	Low baseline infection rates; study underpowered to detect a difference in infection rates; no active surveillance
Picheansathian et al,[91] 2008	1 NICU in a hospital in Thailand	HH adherence (from 6.3% to 81.2%)	Nosocomial infection rate	Limited data presented on the infection outcome; infection was not a primary outcome
Venkatesh et al,[76] 2008	1 Hematology-oncology unit in a US hospital	HH adherence (from 36.3% to 70.1%)	Nosocomial transmission of VRE	Short duration of follow-up (6 months); infection was not a primary outcome

Abbreviations: HAIs, health care–associated infections; HH, hand hygiene; NICU, neonatal intensive care unit; MDRO, multidrug-resistant organism; VRE, vancomycin-resistant enterococci.
Data from Allegranzi B, Pittet D. Role of hand hygiene in healthcare-associated infection prevention. J Hosp Infect 2009;73:305–15.

considered in the various studies, both those that demonstrated improvement in infection and those that did not. In several studies, it was not clear that standard definitions, such as those developed by the National Healthcare Safety Network, were used to describe infectious outcomes. Lastly, as discussed previously, there are inherent limitations in the measurement of hand hygiene adherence, which undermine the reliability of the dependent variable in such studies.

A common refrain in reviews and editorials is the flawed nature of these studies, which must, by necessity, be conducted without a placebo group of health care workers who do not wash their hands. As is the nature of many infection control studies, many are uncontrolled or before-and-after studies. In many cases the hand hygiene improvement interventions are multicomponent, for instance, a new hand hygiene product may be introduced along with a campaign to improve hand hygiene. As such, it is difficult to tease out which aspect is responsible for a change in infection rates. Furthermore, the occurrence of HAIs is influenced by factors other than hand hygiene, such as outbreaks that may be occurring, antimicrobial use, and environmental cleanliness, so it is difficult to isolate the contribution of hand hygiene interventions to changing infection rates. Despite these limitations, several recent hand hygiene intervention studies deserve closer examination, whether for their exemplary methods or for the impact that they have had in the infection control field.

One of the more high-profile hand hygiene intervention studies of recent times was a negative study that provided several important insights despite its negative outcome. The study by Rupp and colleagues[82] was a controlled, crossover trial examining the impact of the introduction of an alcohol-based hand rub into one of two ICUs in a US hospital. Both units demonstrated improved hand hygiene adherence with the introduction of the alcohol-based hand rub (37% to 68% and 38% to 69%, $P<.001$), yet there was no reduction in the outcomes of device-associated infection, infection due to multidrug-resistant organisms, or C difficile infection. The investigators noted that baseline infection rates were low; thus, the study was likely underpowered to demonstrate a reduction in infection rates. Subsequent commentators raised the possibility that the intervention failed to reduce infections because an alcohol gel, rather than a rinse, was used.[83,84] Additionally, the fact that active surveillance cultures were not performed during the study raised the possibility that the measured outcomes presented an incomplete picture of the total extent of ongoing infections and transmissions.[85] The lively debate provoked by this study within the infection control community has furthered understanding about what an optimal study design would be and helped level expectations regarding the impact that hand hygiene can have given the multifactorial problem of HAI.

An older study that has been extremely influential is the work by Pittet and colleagues,[67] which demonstrated the success of a multicomponent campaign to promote the use of an alcohol-based hand rub at a large hospital in Geneva, Switzerland. The program encouraged hand hygiene through increased accessibility of alcohol-based hand rub at the patient bedside and in individual pocket-sized bottles; a poster campaign that was developed by collaborative groups of health care workers; and strong institutional commitment to the program. Hospital-wide hand hygiene adherence increased from 48% in 1994 to 66% in 1997 ($P<.001$). Over the same time period there was a significant reduction in prevalence of nosocomial infections and MRSA transmission. In follow-up studies these investigators have reported sustained hand hygiene and infection outcomes out to 7 years.[86] The success of this program has inspired others to attempt similar campaigns.

Table 3
Studies demonstrating that interventions to improve hand hygiene performance effectively reduce HAIs

Reference, Year Published	Setting	Metric of Hand Hygiene Performance (and Reported Improvement)	Infection Outcome	Comments
Doebbeling et al,[92] 1992	3 ICUs in a US hospital	HH adherence	Nosocomial infections	Improvement in HH rates and nosocomial infections occurred during period when CHG soap used (vs ABHR)
Larson et al,[93] 2000	4 ICUs in 2 US hospitals	Soap usage	Nosocomial VRE infections	No difference in nosocomial MRSA infection rates between intervention and control hospitals
Pittet et al,[67] 2000	Hospital-wide in a hospital in Switzerland	HH adherence (from 48% to 66%)	Prevalence of nosocomial infection; MRSA transmission rates	Selected patients decolonized with mupirocin and CHG; results sustained over at least 7 years[86]
Swoboda et al,[94] 2004	1 Intermediate care unit in a US hospital	HH adherence (from 19.1% to 27.3%)	Nosocomial infections	Nosocomial infections reduced when combining phase with voice prompt and subsequent phase, but not when phases considered independently; short follow-up
Won et al,[95] 2004	1 NICU in Taiwan	HH adherence (from 48% to 80%)	Nosocomial infections; respiratory infection	2 Years of follow-up
Zerr et al,[96] 2005	2 Wards in a US hospital	HH adherence (from 62% to 81%)	Hospital-associated rotavirus infections	Hospital-wide intervention, 4 years of follow-up

Study	Setting	HH outcome	Nosocomial infection rates	Follow-up/Results
Rosenthal et al,[97] 2005	2 ICUs in a hospital in Argentina	HH adherence (from 23.1% to 64.5%)	Nosocomial infection rates	21-Month follow-up
Johnson et al,[98] 2005	1 Hospital with 3 campuses in Australia	HH adherence (from 21% to 42%)	MRSA infection; MRSA bacteremia; ESBL infection	MRSA-infected or colonized patients decolonized with mupirocin and triclosan; 36-month follow-up
Pessoa-Silva et al,[99] 2007	1 NICU in a hospital in Switzerland	HH adherence (from 42% to 55%)	Bacteremia due to clonally related pathogens	Improved HH adherence independently associated with reduction of infection risk in VLBW
Harrington et al,[100] 2007	1 Hospital in Australia	ABHR usage	New-onset MRSA infection; MRSA bacteremia; MRSA CLABSI in the ICU	Time series analysis; product usage not collected after the first 9 months of the study; overall ICU CLABSI not significantly improved
Trick et al,[101] 2007	4 US hospitals	HH adherence or glove use (HH rates improved from 23% to 46% at hospital with improved infection outcomes)	Incidence of clinical isolates of antimicrobial-resistant bacteria	Improvement in infection outcomes only observed at a single intervention hospital that had the greatest improvement in HH performance
Grayson et al,[102] 2008	6 Pilot hospitals in Australia; 75 Australian hospitals for the state-wide rollout	HH adherence (from 21% to 48% in pilot; from 20% to 53% statewide)	MRSA bacteremia; MRSA clinical infection	Very large study; 2 years of follow-up; HH evaluated only on pilot wards
Nguyen et al,[103] 2008	1 Urology ward in a hospital in Vietnam	HH adherence (from 0% to 28.2%)	Nosocomial infections	Investigators state that virtually no hand hygiene occurred before introduction of ABHR; no change in ESBL infections

(continued on next page)

Table 3
(continued)

Reference, Year Published	Setting	Metric of Hand Hygiene Performance (and Reported Improvement)	Infection Outcome	Comments
Cromer et al,[104] 2008	1 US hospital	HH adherence (from 63.8% to 70.8% before patient contact; from 83.6% to 89.2% after patient contact)	Hospital-onset MRSA infections	Intervention also incorporated feedback of HH adherence to hospital wards
Herud et al,[105] 2009	1 Hospital in Norway	HH product usage	HAI	Did not see a significant decline in HAIs but did see a significant association between HAI reduction and increased use of HH product
Kaier et al,[22] 2009	1 Hospital in Germany	AHBR usage	Incidence of nosocomial MRSA infection	Time series analysis; multivariable analysis also identified AHBR use as a negative predictor for MRSA infection; no relationship between AHBR use and *C difficile* infection

Abbreviations: ABHR, alcohol-based hand rub; CHG, chlorhexidine; CLABSI, central line–associated blood stream infection; ESBL, extended-spectrum β-lactamase; HAI, health care–associated infection; HH, hand hygiene; NICU, neonatal intensive care unit; VLBW, very low birth weight; VRE, vancomycin-resistant enterococci.

Data from Allegranzi B, Pittet D. Role of hand hygiene in healthcare-associated infection prevention. J Hosp Infect 2009;73:305–15.

Additionally, lessons from the Geneva experience have been incorporated into the WHO programs.[13]

The time-series analysis has been identified as a model experimental design for isolating the contribution of an uncontrolled intervention on an outcome with multiple influences.[87] A recent time-series analysis performed at a German medical center elegantly demonstrated an association between the consumption of alcohol-based hand rub and the monthly incidence of nosocomial MRSA infections.[22] Consumption of certain antimicrobial agents was also found associated with MRSA infection. Conversely, there was no association between alcohol-based hand rub use and C difficile infection, although there was an association between antimicrobial use and C difficile infection. Future studies examining the impact of hand hygiene interventions on HAIs would do well to use this methodology.

Despite the abundance of hand hygiene literature, there remain many unanswered questions that should engage future researchers, for example, What is the optimal level of hand hygiene adherence necessary to effect change in infectious outcomes? Several modeling studies have explored this issue and seem to reach consensus that there exists a level of adherence beyond which incremental improvements will achieve no further reduction in the transmission of infection, yet it is not clear what the threshold adherence might be and whether or not it might vary for different organisms or different levels of colonization pressure.[88,89] A further question is, What is the most appropriate metric of infection to use as the outcome for hand hygiene intervention studies? And lastly, What is the relative contribution of hand hygiene adherence and the product used for hand hygiene on infectious outcomes?

SUMMARY

The toll of HAIs on patients and the seeming ease of the procedure thought best able to prevent them have focused a spotlight on hand hygiene performance within the health care environment. Knowledge of poor performance of hand hygiene by health care workers inspires incredulity and outrage by the general public. Much is now understood regarding the barriers and motivators of hand hygiene performance. Changes in national guidelines to encourage the use of alcohol-based hand hygiene agents have facilitated hand hygiene improvement efforts. These efforts and a preponderance of evidence in the literature demonstrating that improved hand hygiene performance is associated with a reduction in HAIs should encourage those in the trenches of hand hygiene campaigns.

REFERENCES

1. Boyce JM, Pittet D. Guideline for hand hygiene in health-care settings. Recommendations of the Healthcare Infection Control Practices Advisory Committee and the HICPAC/SHEA/APIC/IDSA hand hygiene task force. MMWR Recomm Rep 2002;51(RR–16):1–45 [quiz: CE1–4].
2. Rotter ML. Semmelweis' sesquicentennial: a little-noted anniversary of handwashing. Curr Opin Infect Dis 1998;11(4):457–60.
3. Mortimer EA Jr, Lipsitz PJ, Wolinsky E, et al. Transmission of staphylococci between newborns. Importance of the hands to personnel. Am J Dis Child 1962;104:289–95.
4. Larson EL. APIC guideline for handwashing and hand antisepsis in health care settings. Am J Infect Control 1995;23(4):251–69.
5. Larson E. Hygiene of the skin: when is clean too clean? Emerg Infect Dis 2001;7(2):225–30.

6. Rocha LA, Ferreira de Almeida EBL, Gontijo Filho PP. Changes in hands micro-biota associated with skin damage because of hand hygiene procedures on the health care workers. Am J Infect Control 2009;37(2):155–9.

7. Widmer AF. Replace hand washing with use of a waterless alcohol hand rub? Clin Infect Dis 2000;31(1):136–43.

8. Kampf G, Kramer A. Epidemiologic background of hand hygiene and evaluation of the most important agents for scrubs and rubs. Clin Microbiol Rev 2004;17(4): 863–93.

9. Garner JS, Favero MS. CDC guidelines for the prevention and control of noso-comial infections. Guideline for handwashing and hospital environmental control, 1985. Supersedes guideline for hospital environmental control pub-lished in 1981. Am J Infect Control 1986;14(3):110–29.

10. Hospital Infection Control Practices Advisory Committee (HICPAC). Recommen-dations for preventing the spread of vancomycin resistance. Infect Control Hosp Epidemiol 1995;16(2):105–13.

11. Garner JS. Guideline for isolation precautions in hospitals. The Hospital Infection Control Practices Advisory Committee. Infect Control Hosp Epidemiol 1996; 17(1):53–80.

12. Mody L, Saint S, Kaufman SR, et al. Adoption of alcohol-based handrub by United States hospitals: a national survey. Infect Control Hosp Epidemiol 2008;29(12):1177–80.

13. Pittet D, Allegranzi B, Boyce J. The World Health Organization guidelines on hand hygiene in health care and their consensus recommendations. Infect Control Hosp Epidemiol 2009;30(7):611–22.

14. Sax H, Allegranzi B, Uckay I, et al. 'My five moments for hand hygiene': a user-centred design approach to understand, train, monitor and report hand hygiene. J Hosp Infect 2007;67(1):9–21.

15. Rotter ML. Arguments for alcoholic hand disinfection. J Hosp Infect 2001; 48(Suppl A):S4–8.

16. Loffler H, Kampf G. Hand disinfection: how irritant are alcohols? J Hosp Infect 2008;70(Suppl 1):44–8.

17. Voss A, Widmer AF. No time for handwashing!? Handwashing versus alcoholic rub: can we afford 100% compliance? Infect Control Hosp Epidemiol 1997; 18(3):205–8.

18. Boyce JM, Pearson ML. Low frequency of fires from alcohol-based hand rub dispensers in healthcare facilities. Infect Control Hosp Epidemiol 2003;24(8): 618–9.

19. Bryant KA, Pearce J, Stover B. Flash fire associated with the use of alcohol-based antiseptic agent. Am J Infect Control 2002;30(4):256–7.

20. Kramer A, Kampf G. Hand rub-associated fire incidents during 25,038 hospital-years in germany. Infect Control Hosp Epidemiol 2007;28(6):745–6.

21. Boyce JM, Ligi C, Kohan C, et al. Lack of association between the increased incidence of Clostridium difficile-associated disease and the increasing use of alcohol-based hand rubs. Infect Control Hosp Epidemiol 2006;27(5):479–83.

22. Kaier K, Hagist C, Frank U, et al. Two time-series analyses of the impact of anti-biotic consumption and alcohol-based hand disinfection on the incidences of nosocomial methicillin-resistant Staphylococcus aureus infection and Clos-tridium difficile infection. Infect Control Hosp Epidemiol 2009;30(4):346–53.

23. Dubberke ER, Gerding DN, Classen D, et al. Strategies to prevent Clostridium difficile infections in acute care hospitals. Infect Control Hosp Epidemiol 2008; 29(Suppl 1):S81–92.

24. Muto CA, Blank MK, Marsh JW, et al. Control of an outbreak of infection with the hypervirulent *Clostridium difficile* bi strain in a university hospital using a comprehensive "Bundle" approach. Clin Infect Dis 2007;45(10):1266–73.
25. Food and Drug Administration. Tentative Final Monograph for healthcare antiseptic drug products; proposed rule. Fed Regist 1994;59:31441–52.
26. Guilhermetti M, Hernandes SE, Fukushigue Y, et al. Effectiveness of handcleansing agents for removing methicillin-resistant *Staphylococcus aureus* from contaminated hands. Infect Control Hosp Epidemiol 2001;22(2):105–8.
27. Oughton MT, Loo VG, Dendukuri N, et al. Hand hygiene with soap and water is superior to alcohol rub and antiseptic wipes for removal of *Clostridium difficile*. Infect Control Hosp Epidemiol 2009;30(10):939–44.
28. Girou E, Loyeau S, Legrand P, et al. Efficacy of handrubbing with alcohol based solution versus standard handwashing with antiseptic soap: randomised clinical trial. BMJ 2002;325(7360):362.
29. Pietsch H. Hand antiseptics: rubs versus scrubs, alcoholic solutions versus alcoholic gels. J Hosp Infect 2001;48(Suppl A):S33–6.
30. Laustsen S, Lund E, Bibby BM, et al. Effect of correctly using alcohol-based hand rub in a clinical setting. Infect Control Hosp Epidemiol 2008;29(10):954–6.
31. Tvedt C, Bukholm G. Alcohol-based hand disinfection: a more robust handhygiene method in an intensive care unit. J Hosp Infect 2005;59(3):229–34.
32. Widmer AE, Dangel M. Alcohol-based handrub: evaluation of technique and microbiological efficacy with international infection control professionals. Infect Control Hosp Epidemiol 2004;25(3):207–9.
33. Widmer AF, Conzelmann M, Tomic M, et al. Introducing alcohol-based hand rub for hand hygiene: the critical need for training. Infect Control Hosp Epidemiol 2007;28(1):50–4.
34. European Committee for Standardization. Chemical disinfectants and antiseptics–hygienic hand rub–test method and requirements (phase2/step2) [European standard EN 1500]. Brussels (Belgium): Central Secretariat; 1997.
35. Kampf G, Ostermeyer C. Efficacy of alcohol-based gels compared with simple hand wash and hygienic hand disinfection. J Hosp Infect 2004;56(Suppl 2):S13–5.
36. Kramer A, Rudolph P, Kampf G, et al. Limited efficacy of alcohol-based hand gels. Lancet 2002;359(9316):1489–90.
37. Traore O, Hugonnet S, Lubbe J, et al. Liquid versus gel handrub formulation: a prospective intervention study. Crit Care 2007;11(3):R52.
38. McDonald LC. Hand hygiene in the new millennium: drawing the distinction between efficacy and effectiveness. Infect Control Hosp Epidemiol 2003;24(3):157–9.
39. Pittet D. Compliance with hand disinfection and its impact on hospital-acquired infections. J Hosp Infect 2001;48(Suppl A):S40–6.
40. Raboud J, Saskin R, Wong K, et al. Patterns of handwashing behavior and visits to patients on a general medical ward of healthcare workers. Infect Control Hosp Epidemiol 2004;25(3):198–202.
41. Boyce JM. Hand hygiene compliance monitoring: current perspectives from the USA. J Hosp Infect 2008;70(Suppl 1):2–7.
42. Haas JP, Larson EL. Measurement of compliance with hand hygiene. J Hosp Infect 2007;66(1):6–14.
43. Eckmanns T, Bessert J, Behnke M, et al. Compliance with antiseptic hand rub use in intensive care units: the Hawthorne effect. Infect Control Hosp Epidemiol 2006;27(9):931–4.

44. Jenner EA, Fletcher BC, Watson P, et al. Discrepancy between self-reported and observed hand hygiene behaviour in healthcare professionals. J Hosp Infect 2006;63(4):418–22.

45. Moret L, Tequi B, Lombrail P. Should self-assessment methods be used to measure compliance with handwashing recommendations? A study carried out in a French university hospital. Am J Infect Control 2004;32(7):384–90.

46. Muller A, Denizot V, Mouillet S, et al. Lack of correlation between consumption of alcohol-based solutions and adherence to guidelines for hand hygiene. J Hosp Infect 2005;59(2):163–4.

47. van de Mortel T, Murgo M. An examination of covert observation and solution audit as tools to measure the success of hand hygiene interventions. Am J Infect Control 2006;34(3):95–9.

48. Braun BI, Kusek L, Larson E. Measuring adherence to hand hygiene guidelines: a field survey for examples of effective practices. Am J Infect Control 2009; 37(4):282–8.

49. McArdle FI, Lee RJ, Gibb AP, et al. How much time is needed for hand hygiene in intensive care? A prospective trained observer study of rates of contact between healthcare workers and intensive care patients. J Hosp Infect 2006; 62(3):304–10.

50. Lankford MG, Zembower TR, Trick WE, et al. Influence of role models and hospital design on hand hygiene of healthcare workers. Emerg Infect Dis 2003;9(2):217–23.

51. Whitby M, McLaws ML. Handwashing in healthcare workers: accessibility of sink location does not improve compliance. J Hosp Infect 2004;58(4):247–53.

52. Graham M, Nixon R, Burrell LJ, et al. Low rates of cutaneous adverse reactions to alcohol-based hand hygiene solution during prolonged use in a large teaching hospital. Antimicrob Agents Chemother 2005;49(10):4404–5.

53. Heeg P. Does hand care ruin hand disinfection? J Hosp Infect 2001;48(Suppl A): S37–9.

54. Kim PW, Roghmann MC, Perencevich EN, et al. Rates of hand disinfection associated with glove use, patient isolation, and changes between exposure to various body sites. Am J Infect Control 2003;31(2):97–103.

55. Golan Y, Doron S, Griffith J, et al. The impact of gown-use requirement on hand hygiene compliance. Clin Infect Dis 2006;42(3):370–6.

56. Duggan JM, Hensley S, Khuder S, et al. Inverse correlation between level of professional education and rate of handwashing compliance in a teaching hospital. Infect Control Hosp Epidemiol 2008;29(6):534–8.

57. Wendt C, Knautz D, von Baum H. Differences in hand hygiene behavior related to the contamination risk of healthcare activities in different groups of healthcare workers. Infect Control Hosp Epidemiol 2004;25(3):203–6.

58. Rome M, Sabel A, Price CS, et al. Hand hygiene compliance. J Hosp Infect 2007;65(2):173.

59. Erasmus V, Brouwer W, van Beeck EF, et al. A qualitative exploration of reasons for poor hand hygiene among hospital workers: lack of positive role models and of convincing evidence that hand hygiene prevents cross-infection. Infect Control Hosp Epidemiol 2009;30(5):415–9.

60. Pittet D, Simon A, Hugonnet S, et al. Hand hygiene among physicians: performance, beliefs, and perceptions. Ann Intern Med 2004;141(1):1–8.

61. Wisniewski MF, Kim S, Trick WE, et al. Effect of education on hand hygiene beliefs and practices: a 5-year program. Infect Control Hosp Epidemiol 2007; 28(1):88–91.

62. Whitby M, McLaws ML. Methodological difficulties in hand hygiene research. J Hosp Infect 2007;67(2):194–5.

63. Whitby M, Pessoa-Silva CL, McLaws ML, et al. Behavioural considerations for hand hygiene practices: the basic building blocks. J Hosp Infect 2007;65(1):1–8.

64. Sax H, Uckay I, Richet H, et al. Determinants of good adherence to hand hygiene among healthcare workers who have extensive exposure to hand hygiene campaigns. Infect Control Hosp Epidemiol 2007;28(11):1267–74.

65. Nicol PW, Watkins RE, Donovan RJ, et al. The power of vivid experience in hand hygiene compliance. J Hosp Infect 2009;72(1):36–42.

66. Girou E, Oppein F. Handwashing compliance in a French university hospital: new perspective with the introduction of hand-rubbing with a waterless alcohol-based solution. J Hosp Infect 2001;48(Suppl A):S55–7.

67. Pittet D, Hugonnet S, Harbarth S, et al. Effectiveness of a hospital-wide programme to improve compliance with hand hygiene. Lancet 2000;356(9238): 1307–12.

68. Randle J, Clarke M, Storr J. Hand hygiene compliance in healthcare workers. J Hosp Infect 2006;64(3):205–9.

69. Souweine B, Lautrette A, Aumeran C, et al. Comparison of acceptability, skin tolerance, and compliance between handwashing and alcohol-based handrub in icus: results of a multicentric study. Intensive Care Med 2009;35(7):1216–24.

70. Harbarth S, Pittet D, Grady L, et al. Interventional study to evaluate the impact of an alcohol-based hand gel in improving hand hygiene compliance. Pediatr Infect Dis J 2002;21(6):489–95.

71. Santana SL, Furtado GH, Coutinho AP, et al. Assessment of healthcare professionals' adherence to hand hygiene after alcohol-based hand rub introduction at an intensive care unit in Sao Paulo, Brazil. Infect Control Hosp Epidemiol 2007; 28(3):365–7.

72. Whitby M, McLaws ML, Slater K, et al. Three successful interventions in health care workers that improve compliance with hand hygiene: is sustained replication possible? Am J Infect Control 2008;36(5):349–55.

73. McGuckin M, Waterman R, Govednik J. Hand hygiene compliance rates in the United States–a one-year multicenter collaboration using product/volume usage measurement and feedback. Am J Med Qual 2009;24(3):205–13.

74. McGuckin M, Shubin A, McBride P, et al. The effect of random voice hand hygiene messages delivered by medical, nursing, and infection control staff on hand hygiene compliance in intensive care. Am J Infect Control 2006; 34(10):673–5.

75. Swoboda SM, Earsing K, Strauss K, et al. Isolation status and voice prompts improve hand hygiene. Am J Infect Control 2007;35(7):470–6.

76. Venkatesh AK, Lankford MG, Rooney DM, et al. Use of electronic alerts to enhance hand hygiene compliance and decrease transmission of vancomycin-resistant enterococcus in a hematology unit. Am J Infect Control 2008; 36(3):199–205.

77. McGuckin M, Waterman R, Shubin A. Consumer attitudes about health care-acquired infections and hand hygiene. Am J Med Qual 2006;21(5):342–6.

78. Julian KG, Subramanian K, Brumbach A, et al. Attitudes of healthcare workers and patients toward individualized hand hygiene reminders. Infect Control Hosp Epidemiol 2008;29(8):781–2.

79. Lent V, Eckstein EC, Cameron AS, et al. Evaluation of patient participation in a patient empowerment initiative to improve hand hygiene practices in a Veterans Affairs medical center. Am J Infect Control 2009;37(2):117–20.

80. Longtin Y, Sax H, Allegranzi B, et al. Patients' beliefs and perceptions of their participation to increase healthcare worker compliance with hand hygiene. Infect Control Hosp Epidemiol 2009;30(9):830–9.
81. Gould DJ, Chudleigh JH, Moralejo D, et al. Interventions to improve hand hygiene compliance in patient care. Cochrane Database Syst Rev 2007;2: CD005186.
82. Rupp ME, Fitzgerald T, Puumala S, et al. Prospective, controlled, cross-over trial of alcohol-based hand gel in critical care units. Infect Control Hosp Epidemiol 2008;29(1):8–15.
83. Maiwald M. Alcohol-based hand hygiene and nosocomial infection rates. Infect Control Hosp Epidemiol 2008;29(6):579–80 [author reply: 80–2].
84. Widmer AF, Rotter M. Effectiveness of alcohol-based hand hygiene gels in reducing nosocomial infection rates. Infect Control Hosp Epidemiol 2008; 29(6):576 [author reply: 80–2].
85. Mermel LA, Boyce JM, Voss A, et al. Trial of alcohol-based hand gel in critical care units. Infect Control Hosp Epidemiol 2008;29(6):577–9 [author reply 80–2].
86. Pittet D, Sax H, Hugonnet S, et al. Cost implications of successful hand hygiene promotion. Infect Control Hosp Epidemiol 2004;25(3):264–6.
87. Harbarth S, Samore MH. Interventions to control MRSA: high time for time-series analysis? J Antimicrob Chemother 2008;62(3):431–3.
88. Austin DJ, Bonten MJ, Weinstein RA, et al. Vancomycin-resistant enterococci in intensive-care hospital settings: transmission dynamics, persistence, and the impact of infection control programs. Proc Natl Acad Sci U S A 1999;96(12): 6908–13.
89. Beggs CB, Shepherd SJ, Kerr KG. How does healthcare worker hand hygiene behaviour impact upon the transmission of MRSA between patients? An analysis using a Monte Carlo model. BMC Infect Dis 2009;9:64.
90. Lam BC, Lee J, Lau YL. Hand hygiene practices in a neonatal intensive care unit: a multimodal intervention and impact on nosocomial infection. Pediatrics 2004;114(5):e565–71.
91. Picheansathian W, Pearson A, Suchaxaya P. The effectiveness of a promotion programme on hand hygiene compliance and nosocomial infections in a neonatal intensive care unit. Int J Nurs Pract 2008;14(4):315–21.
92. Doebbeling BN, Stanley GL, Sheetz CT, et al. Comparative efficacy of alternative hand-washing agents in reducing nosocomial infections in intensive care units. N Engl J Med 1992;327(2):88–93.
93. Larson EL, Early E, Cloonan P, et al. An organizational climate intervention associated with increased handwashing and decreased nosocomial infections. Behav Med 2000;26(1):14–22.
94. Swoboda SM, Earsing K, Strauss K, et al. Electronic monitoring and voice prompts improve hand hygiene and decrease nosocomial infections in an intermediate care unit. Crit Care Med 2004;32(2):358–63.
95. Won SP, Chou HC, Hsieh WS, et al. Handwashing program for the prevention of nosocomial infections in a neonatal intensive care unit. Infect Control Hosp Epidemiol 2004;25(9):742–6.
96. Zerr DM, Allpress AL, Heath J, et al. Decreasing hospital-associated rotavirus infection: a multidisciplinary hand hygiene campaign in a children's hospital. Pediatr Infect Dis J 2005;24(5):397–403.
97. Rosenthal VD, Guzman S, Safdar N. Reduction in nosocomial infection with improved hand hygiene in intensive care units of a tertiary care hospital in Argentina. Am J Infect Control 2005;33(7):392–7.

98. Johnson PD, Martin R, Burrell LJ, et al. Efficacy of an alcohol/chlorhexidine hand hygiene program in a hospital with high rates of nosocomial methicillin-resistant *Staphylococcus aureus* (MRSA) infection. Med J Aust 2005;183(10):509–14.

99. Pessoa-Silva CL, Hugonnet S, Pfister R, et al. Reduction of health care associated infection risk in neonates by successful hand hygiene promotion. Pediatrics 2007;120(2):e382–90.

100. Harrington G, Watson K, Bailey M, et al. Reduction in hospitalwide incidence of infection or colonization with methicillin-resistant *Staphylococcus aureus* with use of antimicrobial hand-hygiene gel and statistical process control charts. Infect Control Hosp Epidemiol 2007;28(7):837–44.

101. Trick WE, Vernon MO, Welbel SF, et al. Multicenter intervention program to increase adherence to hand hygiene recommendations and glove use and to reduce the incidence of antimicrobial resistance. Infect Control Hosp Epidemiol 2007;28(1):42–9.

102. Grayson ML, Jarvie LJ, Martin R, et al. Significant reductions in methicillin-resistant *Staphylococcus aureus* bacteraemia and clinical isolates associated with a multisite, hand hygiene culture-change program and subsequent successful statewide roll-out. Med J Aust 2008;188(11):633–40.

103. Nguyen KV, Nguyen PT, Jones SL. Effectiveness of an alcohol-based hand hygiene programme in reducing nosocomial infections in the Urology Ward of Binh Dan Hospital, Vietnam. Trop Med Int Health 2008;13(10):1297–302.

104. Cromer AL, Latham SC, Bryant KG, et al. Monitoring and feedback of hand hygiene compliance and the impact on facility-acquired methicillin-resistant *Staphylococcus aureus*. Am J Infect Control 2008;36(9):672–7.

105. Herud T, Nilsen RM, Svendheim K, et al. Association between use of hand hygiene products and rates of health care-associated infections in a large university hospital in Norway. Am J Infect Control 2009;37(4):311–7.

Sterilization, High-Level Disinfection, and Environmental Cleaning

William A. Rutala, PhD, MPH[a,b,]*, David J. Weber, MD, MPH[a,b]

KEYWORDS

- Sterilization • High-level disinfection
- Environmental cleaning • Healthcare-associated infection

Failure to perform proper disinfection and sterilization of medical devices may lead to introduction of pathogens, resulting in infection. The method of disinfection and sterilization depends on the intended use of the medical device: critical items (contact sterile tissue) must be sterilized before use; semicritical items (contact mucous membranes or nonintact skin) must be high-level disinfected; and noncritical items (contact intact skin) should receive low-level disinfection. Cleaning should always precede high-level disinfection and sterilization. Current disinfection and sterilization guidelines must be strictly followed.

New technologies have been developed for achieving high-level disinfection (ie, accelerated hydrogen peroxide) and sterilization (ie, hydrogen peroxide vapor or ozone). Automated endoscope reprocessors (AERs) are increasingly used because they offer several advantages, including reducing the likelihood that any essential reprocessing steps will be skipped, decreasing personnel exposure to germicides, providing significant microbial reduction, and retarding biofilm generation.

Environmental contamination has been linked to transmission of methicillin-resistant *Staphylococcus aureus* (MRSA), vancomycin-resistant enterococcus (VRE), norovirus, *Clostridium difficile*, and *Acinetobacter* spp. Unfortunately, recent studies have demonstrated that potentially contaminated environmental surfaces are often not adequately cleaned. Improved surface disinfection can be achieved by improved training and use of checklists by environmental services. Alternatively, a "no-touch" method of room decontamination can be used, such as hydrogen peroxide vapor or ultraviolet light.

[a] Department of Hospital Epidemiology, University of North Carolina Health Care, Chapel Hill, 101 Manning Drive, NC 27514, USA
[b] Division of Infectious Diseases, University of North Carolina School of Medicine, 2163 Bioinformatics, 130 Mason Farm Road, Chapel Hill, NC 27599-7030, USA
* Corresponding author. Division of Infectious Diseases, University of North Carolina School of Medicine, 2163 Bioinformatics, 130 Mason Farm Road, Chapel Hill, NC 27599-7030.
E-mail address: brutala@unch.unc.edu

Infect Dis Clin N Am 25 (2011) 45–76
doi:10.1016/j.idc.2010.11.009
0891-5520/11/$ – see front matter © 2011 Published by Elsevier Inc.

All invasive procedures involve contact by a medical device or surgical instrument with a patient's sterile tissue or mucous membranes. A major risk of all such procedures is the introduction of pathogenic microbes, leading to infection. Failure to properly disinfect or sterilize reusable medical equipment carries a risk associated with breach of the host barriers.

Multiple studies in many countries have documented lack of compliance with established guidelines for disinfection and sterilization.[1,2] Failure to comply with scientifically based guidelines has led to numerous outbreaks.[2–6] This article, which is updated and modified from previous articles,[7,8] examines new technologies for sterilization and high-level disinfection of critical and semicritical items, respectively, and because semicritical items carry the greatest risk of infection, the authors discuss reprocessing semicritical items such as endoscopes and AERs, endocavitary probes, prostate biopsy probes, tonometers, laryngoscopes, and infrared coagulation devices. In addition, current issues and practices associated with environmental cleaning are reviewed.

A RATIONAL APPROACH TO DISINFECTION AND STERILIZATION

More than 40 years ago, Earle H. Spaulding[9] devised a rational approach to disinfection and sterilization of patient-care items or equipment. This classification scheme is so clear and logical that it has been retained, refined, and successfully used by infection control professionals and others when planning methods for disinfection or sterilization.[10–13] Spaulding believed that the nature of disinfection could be understood more readily if instruments and items for patient care were divided into 3 categories based on the degree of risk of infection involved in the use of the items. The 3 categories he described were critical, semicritical, and noncritical. This terminology is employed by the Centers for Disease Control and Prevention (CDC) *Guidelines for Environmental Infection Control in Healthcare Facilities*[14] and the CDC *Guideline for Disinfection and Sterilization in Healthcare Facilities*.[10]

Critical Items

Critical items are so called because of the high risk of infection if such an item is contaminated with any microorganism, including bacterial spores. Thus, it is critical that objects that enter sterile tissue or the vascular system be sterile because any microbial contamination could result in disease transmission. This category includes surgical instruments, cardiac and urinary catheters, implants, and ultrasound probes used in sterile body cavities. The items in this category should be purchased as sterile or be sterilized by steam sterilization if possible. If heat-sensitive, the object may be treated with ethylene oxide (ETO), hydrogen peroxide gas plasma, ozone, vaporized hydrogen peroxide, or liquid chemical sterilants if other methods are unsuitable. **Table 1** lists sterilization processes and liquid chemical sterilants. With the exception of 0.2% peracetic acid (12 minutes at 50–56°C), the indicated exposure times range from 3 to 12 hours.[15] Liquid chemical sterilants can be relied on to produce sterility only if cleaning, which eliminates organic and inorganic material, precedes treatment, and if proper guidelines as to concentration, contact time, temperature, and pH are met. Another limitation to sterilization of devices with liquid chemical sterilants is that the devices cannot be wrapped during processing in a liquid chemical sterilant, thus it is impossible to maintain sterility following processing and during storage. Furthermore, devices may require rinsing following exposure to the liquid chemical sterilant with water that generally is not sterile. Therefore, due to the inherent limitations of using liquid chemical sterilants in a nonautomated reprocessor, their use should be restricted to reprocessing critical devices that are heat-sensitive and incompatible with other sterilization methods.

Semicritical Items

Semicritical items are those that come in contact with mucous membranes or nonintact skin. Respiratory therapy and anesthesia equipment, gastrointestinal endoscopes, bronchoscopes, laryngoscopes, esophageal manometry probes, anorectal manometry catheters, endocavitary probes, prostate biopsy probes, infrared coagulation devices, and diaphragm fitting rings are included in this category. These medical devices should be free of all microorganisms (ie, mycobacteria, fungi, viruses, bacteria), although small numbers of bacterial spores may be present. Intact mucous membranes, such as those of the lungs or the gastrointestinal tract, generally are resistant to infection by common bacterial spores but are susceptible to other organisms such as bacteria, mycobacteria, and viruses. Semicritical items minimally require high-level disinfection using chemical disinfectants. Glutaraldehyde, hydrogen peroxide, *ortho*-phthalaldehyde, and peracetic acid with hydrogen peroxide, and chlorine are cleared by the Food and Drug Administration (FDA)[15] and are dependable high-level disinfectants provided the factors influencing germicidal procedures are met (see **Table 1**). The exposure time for most high-level disinfectants varies from 8 to 45 minutes at 20°C to 25°C. Outbreaks continue to occur when ineffective disinfectants, including iodophor, alcohol, and overdiluted glutaraldehyde,[4] are used for high-level disinfection. When a disinfectant is selected for use with certain patient-care items, the chemical compatibility after extended use with the items to be disinfected must also be considered. For example, compatibility testing by Olympus America of the 7.5% hydrogen peroxide found cosmetic and functional changes with the tested endoscopes (Olympus, October 15, 1999, written communication). Similarly, Olympus does not endorse the use of the hydrogen peroxide with peracetic acid products because of cosmetic and functional damage (Olympus America, April 15, 1998 and September 13, 2000, written communications).

Semicritical items that will have contact with the mucous membranes of the respiratory tract or gastrointestinal tract should be rinsed with sterile water, filtered water, or tap water followed by an alcohol rinse.[10,16] An alcohol rinse and forced-air drying markedly reduces the likelihood of contamination of the instrument (eg, endoscope), most likely by removing the wet environment favorable for bacterial growth.[17] After rinsing, items should be dried and stored in a manner that protects them from damage or contamination. There is no recommendation to use sterile or filtered water rather than tap water for rinsing semicritical equipment that will have contact with the mucous membranes of the rectum (eg, rectal probes, anoscope) or vagina (eg, vaginal probes).[10]

Semicritical items represent the greatest risk of disease transmission, as far more health care–associated infections have been caused by semicritical items than by critical or noncritical items.[10] There is virtually no documented risk of transmitting infectious agents to patients via noncritical items[18] when they are used as noncritical items and do not contact nonintact skin and/or mucous membranes. Critical items have a high risk of infection if such an item is contaminated with any microorganism; however, sterilization cycles that are designed for hospitals are usually based on the "overkill" approach. The time required for a 6-$\log_{10}$ reduction of highly resistant spores by the process is considered a half cycle, and the full-cycle exposure time is the time for the half cycle doubled. Thus, a sterilization processes can achieve a 12-$\log_{10}$ reduction of highly resistant spores while medical/surgical devices are contaminated with low numbers of microorganisms (85% of instruments <100 bacteria)

Table 1
Methods for disinfection and sterilization of patient-care items and environmental surfaces

Process	Level of Microbial Inactivation	Method	Examples (with Processing Times [Exposure Times for HLD and CS are Temperature Dependent])	Health Care Application (Examples)
Sterilization	Destroys all microorganisms, including bacterial spores	High temperature	Steam (~40 min), dry heat (1–6 h depending on temperature)	Heat-tolerant critical (surgical instruments) and semicritical patient-care items
		Low temperature	Ethylene oxide gas (~15 h), hydrogen peroxide gas plasma (~40 min), ozone, vaporized hydrogen peroxide (~55 min)	Heat-sensitive critical and semicritical patient-care items
		Liquid immersion	Chemical sterilants[a]: >2% glut (~10 h); 1.12% glut and 1.93% phenol (12 h); 7.35% HP and 0.23% PA (3 h); 7.5% HP (6 h); 1.0% HP and 0.08% PA (8 h); ≥0.2% PA (~50 min [12 min CS time] at 50–56°C); 8.3% HP and 7.0% PA (5 h)	Heat-sensitive critical and semicritical patient-care items that can be immersed
High-level disinfection	Destroys all microorganisms except high numbers of bacterial spores	Heat-automated	Pasteurization (~50 min)	Heat-sensitive semicritical items (respiratory therapy equipment)
		Liquid immersion	Chemical sterilants/HLDs[a]: >2% glut (20–45 min); 0.55% OPA (12 min); 1.12% glut and 1.93% phenol (20 min); 7.35% HP and 0.23% PA (15 min); 7.5% HP (30 min); 1.0% HP and 0.08% PA (25 min); 650–675 ppm chlorine (10 min); 8.3% HP and 7.0% PA (5 min); accelerated HP (8 min)	Heat-sensitive semicritical items (GI endoscopes, bronchoscopes)

Intermediate-level disinfection	Destroys vegetative bacteria, mycobacteria, most viruses, most fungi, but not bacterial spores	Liquid contact	EPA-registered hospital disinfectant with label claim regarding tuberculocidal activity (eg, chlorine-based products, phenolics—exposure times at least 1 min)	Noncritical patient care item (blood pressure cuff) or surface with visible blood
Low-level disinfection	Destroys vegetative bacteria, some fungi and viruses, but not mycobacteria or spores	Liquid contact	EPA-registered hospital disinfectant with no tuberculocidal claim (eg, chlorine-based products, phenolics, quaternary ammonium compounds—exposure times at least 1 min) or 70%–90% alcohol	Noncritical patient care item (blood pressure cuff) or surface (bedside table) with no visible blood

Abbreviations: CS, chemical sterilant; EPA, Environmental Protection Agency; FDA, Food and Drug Administration; GI, gastrointestinal; glut, glutaraldehyde; HLD, high-level disinfectant; HP, hydrogen peroxide; OPA, *ortho*-phthalaldehyde; PA, peracetic acid; ppm, parts per million.

[a] Consult the FDA cleared package insert for information about the cleared contact time and temperature, and see text for discussion why one product is used at a reduced exposure time (2% glutaraldehyde at 20 min, 20°C). Increasing the temperature using an automated endoscope reprocess (AER) will reduce the contact time (eg, OPA 12 min at 20°C but 5 min at 25°C in AER). Tubing must be completely filled for high-level disinfection and liquid chemical sterilization. Material compatibility should be investigated when appropriate (eg, HP and HP with PA will cause functional damage to endoscopes).

Data from Rutala WA, Weber DJ. Disinfection and sterilization in health care facilities: what clinicians need to know. Clin Infect Dis 2004;39:702–9; and Kohn WG, Collins AS, Cleveland JL, et al. Guidelines for infection control in dental health-care settings—2003. MMWR Recomm Rep 2003;52(no RR–17):1–67.

after use in surgery.[19] This process results in a huge margin of safety and a sterility assurance level of 10^{-6}, which means there is less than 1 chance in 1 million that a contaminant will survive on a medical product after the sterilization process. In contrast, semicritical items (eg, gastrointestinal endoscopes), by virtue of the body cavities they enter, may be contaminated with 1 billion bacteria.[20] A further complication is that many of these devices are constructed in a way that makes it very difficult to properly clean them (eg, long, narrow lumens) before the high-level disinfection procedure. Thus, the result is a device with a sterility assurance level of 10^0 to 10^{-3}, which means there is a greater chance that a contaminant will survive on a medical device after the high-level disinfection procedure than after sterilization (ie, greater than 1 in 1000 chance that a contaminant will survive after the high-level disinfection procedure).[21] Thus, reprocessing semicritical items has a narrower margin of safety, and any deviation from the reprocessing protocol can lead to the survival of microorganisms and an increased risk of infection.

Noncritical Items

Noncritical items are those that come in contact with intact skin but not mucous membranes. Intact skin acts as an effective barrier to most microorganisms; therefore, the sterility of items coming into contact with intact skin is "not critical." Examples of noncritical items are bedpans, blood pressure cuffs, crutches, bed rails, linens, bedside tables, patient furniture, and floors. In contrast to critical and some semicritical items, most noncritical reusable items may be decontaminated where they are used and do not need to be transported to a central processing area. There is virtually no documented risk of transmitting infectious agents to patients via noncritical items[18] when they are used as noncritical items and do not contact nonintact skin and/or mucous membranes. However, these items (eg, bedside tables, bed rails) could potentially contribute to secondary transmission by contaminating the hands of health care workers or by contact with medical equipment that will subsequently come into contact with patients.[22] **Table 1** lists several low-level disinfectants that may be used for noncritical items. The exposure time for low-level disinfection of noncritical items is at least 1 minute.

NEW TECHNOLOGIES FOR STERILIZATION AND HIGH-LEVEL DISINFECTION
Hydrogen Peroxide Vapor Low-Temperature Sterilization

A new low-temperature sterilization system (V-Pro) uses vaporized hydrogen peroxide to sterilize reusable metal and nonmetal devices used in health care facilities. The system is compatible with a wide range of medical instruments and materials (eg, polypropylene, brass, polyethylene). There are nontoxic by-products, as only water vapor and oxygen are produced. The system is not intended to process liquids, linens, powders, or any cellulose materials. The system can sterilize: instruments with diffusion-restricted spaces (eg, scissors) and medical devices with single stainless steel lumens based on lumen internal diameter and length (eg, an inside diameter of 1 mm or larger and a length of 125 mm or shorter; see manufacturer's recommendations). Thus, gastrointestinal (GI) endoscopes and bronchoscopes cannot be sterilized in this system at present. Although this system has not been comparatively evaluated with other sterilization processes, vaporized hydrogen peroxide has been shown to be effective in killing spores, viruses, mycobacteria, fungi, and bacteria (Technical Data Monograph, Steris, 2008). **Table 2** lists the advantages and disadvantages of this and other processes.

Table 2
Summary of advantages and disadvantages of new sterilization processes and high-level disinfectants

Sterilization Method	Advantages	Disadvantages
Accelerated hydrogen peroxide (2.0%); high-level disinfectant	• No activation required • No odor • Nonstaining • No special venting requirements • Manual or automated applications • 12-month shelf life, 14-day reuse • 8 min at 20°C high-level disinfectant claim	• Material compatibility concerns due to limited clinical experience • Antimicrobial claims not independently verified • Organic material resistance concerns due to limited data
Vaporized hydrogen peroxide; sterilization process	• Safe for the environment and health care worker • Leaves no toxic residue; no aeration necessary • Fast cycle time, 55 min • Used for heat- and moisture-sensitive items (metal and nonmetal devices)	• Sterilization chamber is small, about 4.8 ft³ (1.5 m³) • Medical devices restrictions based on lumen internal diameter and length—see manufacturer's recommendations, eg, stainless steel lumen 1 mm diameter, 125 mm length • Not used for liquid, linens, powders, or any cellulose materials • Requires synthetic packaging (polypropylene) • Limited materials compatibility data • Limited comparative microbicidal efficacy data
Ozone; sterilization process	• Used for moisture- and heat-sensitive items • Ozone generated from oxygen and water (nontoxic) • No aeration needed due to no toxic by-products • FDA cleared for metal and plastic instruments including some instruments with lumens	• Sterilization chamber is small, 4 ft³ (1.3 m³) • Limited use (material compatibility/penetrability/organic material resistance?) and limited microbicidal efficacy data

Ozone Sterilization

Ozone has been used for years as a drinking water disinfectant. Ozone is produced when O_2 is energized and split into 2 monatomic (O_1) molecules. The monatomic oxygen molecules then collide with O_2 molecules to form ozone, which is O_3. Thus, ozone consists of O_2 with a loosely bonded third oxygen atom that is readily available to attach to, and oxidize, other molecules. This additional oxygen atom makes ozone a powerful oxidant that destroys microorganisms but is highly unstable (ie, half-life of 22 minutes at room temperature).

A new sterilization process, which uses ozone as the sterilant, was cleared by the FDA in August 2003 for processing reusable medical devices. The sterilizer creates its own sterilant internally from United States Pharmacopeia grade oxygen, steam-quality water, and electricity; the sterilant is converted back to oxygen and water vapor at the end of the cycle by passing through a catalyst before being exhausted into the room. The duration of the sterilization cycle is about 4 hours 15 minutes, and occurs at 30°C to 35°C. Microbial efficacy has been demonstrated by achieving a sterility assurance level (SAL) of 10^{-6} with a variety of microorganisms to include the most resistant microorganism, Geobacillus stearothermophilus.[23] The SAL is defined as the probability of a single unit being nonsterile after it has been subject to the sterilization process. **Table 2** lists the advantages and disadvantages of this and other processes.

Automated Endoscope Reprocessors

AERs offer several advantages over manual reprocessing: they automate and standardize several important reprocessing steps[24–26]; reduce the likelihood that an essential reprocessing step will be skipped; reduce personnel exposure to high-level disinfectants or chemical sterilants; provide significant microbial reduction[27] and filtered tap water; and remove established biofilms and retard biofilm generation.[28] Disadvantages associated with some AERs include: generally they do not eliminate cleaning; failure and outbreaks have been linked to poorly designed reprocessors; and they do not monitor high-level disinfectant concentration. Failure of AERs has been linked to outbreaks of infections[29] or colonization,[3,30] and the AER water filtration system may not be able to reliably provide "sterile" or bacteria-free rinse water.[31,32] It is critical that correct connectors between the AER and the device are established to ensure complete flow of disinfectants and rinse water.[3,33] In addition, some endoscopes such as the duodenoscopes (eg, for endoscopic retrograde cholangiopancreatography) contain features (eg, elevator-wire channel) that require a flushing pressure that is not achieved by some AERs and must be reprocessed manually using a 2- to 5-mL syringe. There is a need for further development and redesign of AERs[3,34] and endoscopes[35,36] to decrease the likelihood that they might serve as a potential source of infectious agents. The potential for transmission of infection during endoscopy remains a concern for health care workers and patients.[10]

A variety of capabilities has been incorporated into the available AERs, which have been recently summarized.[37] All models have disinfection and rinsing cycles, and some have detergent cleaning, alcohol flush, and/or extended forced-air-drying cycles. Additional features may include: variable cycle times; printed documentation of the process; low-intensity ultrasound waves; high-level disinfectant vapor recovery systems; heating to optimize the high-level disinfectant's efficacy; a variable number of endoscopes processed per cycle; automated leak testing; automated detection of channel obstructions; and table-top, floor-standing, and cart-mounted models.[37]

Not all reprocessors are compatible with all high-level disinfectants or with endoscopes from all manufacturers. Newer AERs should offer benefits over older models.

One AER integrates cleaning and has achieved an FDA-cleared cleaning claim (Evotech; Advanced Sterilization Products, Irvine, CA). The users must continue to do the "bedside" cleaning (wipe external surfaces and flush each lumen with a detergent solution) and then place the scope directly (within 1 hour) into the Evotech machine. This process eliminates the labor-intensive manual cleaning. It also automatically detects leaks, flushes alcohol through the channels before cycle completion to promote drying, and integrates minimum effective concentration (MEC) monitoring. In addition, the printer provides complete monitoring of critical cycle parameters including MEC of the high-level disinfectant (*ortho*-phthalaldehyde), disinfection time, channel blockage detection, temperature, pressure, and time to ensure compliance throughout the process. Data provided by the manufacturer demonstrated that residual protein levels following cleaning of the internal channels as well as external insertion tube surfaces were below the limit of less than 8.5 $\mu g/cm^2$. Another AER (Reliance; Steris Canada Corp, Beauport, QC, Canada) requires a minimal number of connections to the endoscope channels and uses a control boot (a housing apparatus that creates pressure differentials to ensure connector-less fluid flow through all channels that are accessible through the endoscope's control handle channel ports). Data demonstrate that the soil and microbial removal effected by the Reliance washing phase was equivalent to that achieved by optimal manual cleaning. For example, there was greater than 99% reduction in protein and hemoglobin, and both methods reduced the level of residual organic material to less than 6.4 $\mu g/cm^2$.[38] Olympus has informed customers of reports indicating degradation of flexible endoscope adhesives after use with the Reliance endoscope processing system (Olympus, December 8, 2009).

Accelerated Hydrogen Peroxide

Accelerated hydrogen peroxide (AHP) is a newer disinfectant that contains very low levels of anionic and nonionic surfactants, which act with hydrogen peroxide to produce microbicidal activity. These ingredients are considered safe for humans and are benign for the environment. AHP is prepared and marketed in several concentrations from 0.5% to 7%.

A high-level disinfectant based on AHP (Resert; Steris Canada Corp), which contains 2% hydrogen peroxide, is available for heat-sensitive semicritical medical devices, and can be used for the manual and automatic reprocessing of flexible endoscopes. Resert is odorless, nonstaining, ready to use, and has a 12-month shelf life and 14-day reuse life. This product has demonstrated sporicidal activity, with a reduction in viability titer of greater than 6-$\log_{10}$ in 6 hours at 20°C but also mycobactericidal, fungicidal, and virucidal activity with a contact time of 8 minutes. It is reported to be a relatively mild solution for end users and is considered to be compatible with flexible endoscopes. Resert is slightly irritating to skin and mildly irritating to the eyes according to accepted standard test methods (same as 3% topical hydrogen peroxide).[39]

REPROCESSING SEMICRITICAL ITEMS
Reprocessing of Endoscopes

Physicians use endoscopes to diagnose and treat numerous medical disorders. Although endoscopes represent a valuable diagnostic and therapeutic tool in modern medicine and the incidence of infection associated with use has been reported as very low (about 1 in 1.8 million procedures),[40] more health care–associated outbreaks have been linked to contaminated endoscopes than to any other medical device.[2–4,41,42] To prevent the spread of health care–associated infections, all heat-sensitive endoscopes (eg, gastrointestinal endoscopes, bronchoscopes, nasopharygoscopes) must be properly cleaned and at a minimum subjected to high-level disinfection following each use. High-level disinfection can be expected to destroy all microorganisms, although when high numbers of bacterial spores are present a few spores may survive.

Flexible endoscopes, by virtue of the types of body cavities they enter, acquire high levels of microbial contamination (bioburden) during each use.[43] For example, the bioburden found on flexible gastrointestinal endoscopes following use has ranged from 10^5 colony-forming units (CFU)/mL to 10^{10} CFU/mL, with the highest levels being found in the suction channels.[43–46] The average load on bronchoscopes before cleaning was 6.4×10^4 CFU/mL. Cleaning reduces the level of microbial contamination by 4 to 6 $\log_{10}$.[47,48] Using human immunodeficiency virus (HIV)-contaminated endoscopes, several investigators have shown that cleaning completely eliminates the microbial contamination on the scopes.[49,50] Similarly, other investigators found that ETO sterilization or high-level disinfection (soaking in 2% glutaraldehyde for 20 minutes) was effective only when the device was first properly cleaned.[51]

The FDA maintains a list of cleared liquid chemical sterilants and high-level disinfectants that can be used to reprocess heat-sensitive medical devices, such as flexible endoscopes. Users can access and view the list at http://www.fda.gov/cdrh/ode/germlab.html.[15] At this time, the FDA-cleared and marketed formulations include: 2.4% or more glutaraldehyde; 0.55% ortho-phthalaldehyde; 1.12% glutaraldehyde with 1.93% phenol/phenate; 7.35% hydrogen peroxide with 0.23% peracetic acid; 1.0% hydrogen peroxide with 0.08% peracetic acid; 2.0% AHP; 3.4% glutaraldehyde with 26% isopropanol; 8.3% hydrogen peroxide with 7.0% peracetic acid; and 7.5% hydrogen peroxide.[15] These products have excellent antimicrobial activity; however, some oxidizing chemicals (eg, 7.5% hydrogen peroxide, and 1.0% hydrogen peroxide with 0.08% peracetic acid) have been reported to cause cosmetic and functional damage to endoscopes.[52] Users should check with device manufacturers for information on germicide compatibility with their device. If the germicide is FDA cleared then it is safe when used according to the label directions; however, professionals should review the scientific literature as new data may become available regarding human safety or materials compatibility. ETO sterilization of flexible endoscopes is infrequent because it requires a lengthy processing and aeration time (eg, 12–15 hours) and is a potential hazard to staff and patients. Three products that are commonly used for reprocessing endoscopes in the United States are ortho-phthalaldehyde, glutaraldehyde, and an automated, liquid chemical sterilization process that uses peracetic acid.[53] In December 2009, the FDA disseminated a notice to health care facilities stating that the latter process (Steris System 1) had been significantly modified, and the FDA has not approved or cleared this modified product. Thus, the FDA has not determined whether this processor is safe or effective for its labeled claims, including claims that it sterilizes medical devices. The FDA recommends that users find an acceptable alternative to the product within 3 to 6 months to ensure continued patient safety.

ortho-phalaldehyde has replaced glutaraldehyde in many health care facilities, as it possesses several potential advantages over glutaraldehyde: it causes no known irritation to the eyes and nasal passages, does not require activation or exposure monitoring, and has a 12-minute high-level disinfection claim in the United States.[52] Disinfectants that are not FDA cleared and should not be used for reprocessing endoscopes include iodophors, chlorine solutions, alcohols, quaternary ammonium compounds, and phenolics. These solutions may still be in use outside the United States, but their use should be strongly discouraged because of lack of proven efficacy against all microorganisms or material incompatibility.

The FDA's clearance of the contact conditions listed on germicide labeling is based on the manufacturer's test results. The manufacturers conduct the testing under worst-case conditions for germicide formulation (ie, minimum recommended concentration of the active ingredient), and include organic soil. Typically, manufacturers use 5% serum as the organic soil and hard water as examples of organic and inorganic challenges. The soil is used to represent the organic loading to which the device is exposed during actual use and that would remain on the device in the absence of cleaning. This method assures that the contact conditions provide complete elimination of the test mycobacteria (eg, 10^5–10^6 *Mycobacterium tuberculosis* in organic soil and dried on a scope) if inoculated in the most difficult areas for the disinfectant to penetrate and contact in the absence of cleaning, and thus provides a margin of safety.[54] For 2.4% glutaraldehyde that requires a 45-minute immersion at 25°C to achieve high-level disinfection (ie, 100% kill of *M tuberculosis*). The FDA itself does not conduct testing, but relies solely on the disinfectant manufacturer's data. Users can find the contact conditions for cleared high-level disinfectants and chemical sterilants at http://www.fda.gov/cdrh/ode/germlab.html. It must be noted that data suggest that *M tuberculosis* levels can be reduced by at least 8 $\log_{10}$ with cleaning (4 $\log_{10}$)[45–47,55] followed by chemical disinfection for 20 minutes at 20°C (4–6 $\log_{10}$).[47,56–58] Based on these data, the Association for Professionals in Infection Control,[59] the Society of Gastroenterology Nurses and Associates,[60–62] the American Society for Gastrointestinal Endoscopy,[63] the American College of Chest Physicians,[42] and a multi-society guideline[16] recommend alternative contact conditions with 2% glutaraldehyde to achieve high-level disinfection based on articles in the literature (eg, that equipment be immersed in 2% glutaraldehyde at 20°C for at least 20 minutes for high-level disinfection).[47,56,63–71] It is the FDA's position that if the user chooses to use alternative contact conditions, the user assumes liability. In the absence of several well-designed experimental scientific studies regarding alternative exposure times of high-level disinfectants, the manufacturers' recommendations to achieve high-level disinfection should be followed. At present, such data are available only for 2% glutaraldehyde solutions.

Dilution of glutaraldehyde during use commonly occurs, and studies show a glutaraldehyde concentration decline after a few days of use in an automatic endoscope washer.[72,73] This situation occurs because instruments are not thoroughly dried and water is carried in with the instrument, which increases the solution's volume and dilutes its effective concentration.[74] This outcome emphasizes the need to ensure that semicritical equipment is disinfected with an acceptable concentration of glutaraldehyde. Data suggest that when used as a high-level disinfectant, 1.0% to 1.5% glutaraldehyde is the MEC for glutaraldehyde solutions above 2%.[73,75–77] Chemical test strips or liquid chemical monitors[74,78] are available for determining whether an effective concentration of glutaraldehyde is present despite repeated use and dilution. The frequency of testing should be based on how frequently the solutions are used (eg, used daily, test daily; used weekly, test before use; used 30 times per day, test each tenth use), but the strips should not be used to extend the use life beyond the expiration date. Data suggest that the chemicals in the test strip deteriorate with time,[79] so a manufacturer's expiration date should be placed on the bottles. The bottle of test strips should be dated when opened and used for the period of time indicated on the bottle (eg, 120 days). The results of test strip monitoring should be documented in a written log. The glutaraldehyde test kits have been preliminarily evaluated for accuracy and range[79] but their reliability has been questioned.[80] Manufacturers of some, but not all, chemical test strips, for ensuring that the MEC of the high-level disinfectant is present, recommend the use of quality control procedures to ensure the strips perform properly. If the manufacturer of the chemical test strip recommends a quality control procedure, the manufacturer's recommendations should be complied with. The concentration should be considered unacceptable or unsafe when the test indicates a dilution below the product's MEC (generally to 1.0%–1.5% glutaraldehyde or lower) by the indicator not changing color.

Flexible endoscopes are particularly difficult to disinfect[81] and are easy to damage because of their intricate design and delicate materials.[36] Meticulous cleaning must precede any sterilization or high-level disinfection of these instruments. Failure to perform thorough cleaning may result in a sterilization or disinfection failure, and outbreaks of infection may occur. Several studies have demonstrated the importance of cleaning in experimental studies with the duck hepatitis B virus (HBV),[51,82] HIV,[83] and *Helicobacter pylori*.[84]

Recommendations for the cleaning and disinfection of endoscopic equipment have been published and should be strictly followed.[16,42,59–63,85–88] Unfortunately, audits have shown that personnel do not consistently adhere to guidelines on reprocessing,[89–91] and outbreaks of infection continue to occur.[92–95] To ensure that reprocessing personnel are properly trained, there should be initial and annual competency testing for each individual who reprocesses endoscopic instruments.[62,96]

In general, endoscope disinfection or sterilization with a liquid chemical sterilant involves 5 steps after leak testing: (1) clean: mechanically clean internal and external surfaces, including brushing internal channels and flushing each internal channel with water and a detergent or enzymatic cleaners (leak testing is recommended for endoscopes before immersion); (2) disinfect: immerse endoscope in high-level disinfectant (or chemical sterilant) and perfuse (eliminates air pockets and ensures contact of the germicide with the internal channels) disinfectant into all accessible channels such as the suction/biopsy channel and air/water channel, and expose for a time recommended for specific products; (3) rinse: rinse the endoscope and all channels with sterile water, filtered water (commonly used with AERs), or tap water (ie, high-quality potable water that meets federal clean water standards at the point of use); (4) dry: rinse the insertion tube and inner channels with alcohol and dry with forced air after disinfection and before storage; and (5) store: store the endoscope in a way that prevents recontamination and promotes drying (eg, hung vertically). Drying the endoscope (steps 3 and 4) is essential to greatly reduce the chance of recontamination of the endoscope by microorganisms that may be present in the rinse water.[16,97] Because tap water may contain low levels of microorganisms,[98] some have suggested that only sterile water (which may be prohibitively expensive)[99] or AER-filtered water be used. The suggestion to use only sterile water or filtered water is not consistent with published guidelines that allow tap water with an alcohol rinse and forced air-drying[59,62,63] or the scientific literature.[17,57] In addition, there has been no evidence of disease transmission when tap water followed by an alcohol rinse and forced air-drying has been used. AERs produce filtered water via passage through a bacterial filter (eg, 0.2 μm). In addition to the endoscope reprocessing steps, a protocol should be developed that assures the user knows whether an endoscope has been appropriately cleaned and disinfected (eg, using a room or cabinet for processed endoscopes only) or has not been reprocessed. Confusion can result when users leave endoscopes on movable carts whereby it is unclear whether the endoscope has been processed or not. Whereas one guideline has recommended that an endoscope (eg, a duodenoscope) should be reprocessed immediately before its use,[87] other guidelines do not require this activity[61–63] and with the exception of the Association of Perioperative Registered Nurses, professional organizations do not recommended that reprocessing be repeated so long as the original processing is done correctly. Based on studies that have assessed the microbiological stability of endoscopes after high-level disinfection, it appears that reprocessing after storage for a week or 2 weeks is unnecessary.[100–102] As part of a quality assurance program, health care facility personnel may consider random bacterial surveillance cultures of processed endoscopes to ensure high-level disinfection or sterilization,[3,103–106] although some investigators have suggested it is too time-consuming and costly and that process controls are preferable.[107] Reprocessed endoscopes should be free of microbial pathogens except for small numbers of relatively avirulent microbes that represent exogenous environmental contamination (eg, coagulase-negative *Staphylococcus*, *Bacillus* spp, diphtheroids). It has also been suggested that the final rinse water used during endoscope reprocessing be microbiologically cultured at least monthly.[108] The microbiologic standard that should be met has not been set and the value of routine endoscope cultures has not been shown.[109] In addition, neither the routine culture of reprocessed endoscopes nor the final rinse water has been validated by correlating viable counts on an endoscope to infection following an endoscopic procedure. If culturing of reprocessed endoscopes were done, sampling the endoscope would assess water quality as well as other important steps (eg, disinfectant effectiveness, exposure time, cleaning) in the reprocessing procedure. Several methods for sampling endoscopes and water have been described.[101,104,110–114] Novel approaches (eg, adenosine triphosphate) to evaluate the effectiveness of endoscope cleaning[115,116] or endoscope reprocessing[117] have also been evaluated, but there is no accepted method for assessing the outcome of endoscope reprocessing.

The carrying case used to transport clean and reprocessed endoscopes outside of the health care environment should not be used to store an endoscope or to transport the instrument within the health care facility. A contaminated endoscope should never be placed in the carrying case, as the case can also become contaminated. When the endoscope is removed from the case and properly reprocessed and put back in the case, the endoscope can become recontaminated by the case. If the carrying case becomes contaminated, it should be discarded (Olympus America, June 2002, written communication).

Infection control professionals should ensure that institutional policies are consistent with national guidelines, and conduct infection control rounds periodically (eg, at least annually) in areas where endoscopes are reprocessed to make certain there is compliance with policy. Breaches in policy should be documented and corrective action instituted. Some studies suggest the assurance of quality for endoscopic use could be achieved through process control (eg, MEC, training) as opposed to product control (ie, microbiological monitoring).[107] In incidents in which endoscopes were not exposed to a high-level disinfection process, all patients exposed to the endoscopes were assessed for possible acquisition of HIV, HBV, and hepatitis C virus. A 14-step method for managing a failure incident associated with high-level disinfection or sterilization has been described.[118] The possible transmission of blood-borne pathogens and other infectious agents highlights the importance of rigorous infection control.[119,120]

Tonometers

Disinfection strategies for other semicritical items (eg, applanation tonometers, rectal/vaginal probes, cryosurgical instruments, and diaphragm fitting rings) are highly variable. At present, the FDA requests that the device manufacturers include at least one validated cleaning and disinfection/sterilization protocol in the labeling for their device. As with all medications and devices, users should be familiar with the label instructions. One study revealed that no uniform technique was in use for disinfection of applanation tonometers, with disinfectant contact times varying from less than 15 seconds to 20 minutes.[121] In view of the potential for transmission of viruses (eg, herpes simplex virus [HSV], adenovirus type 8, or HIV)[122] by tonometer tips, the CDC has recommended[123] that the tonometer tips be wiped clean and disinfected for 5 to 10 minutes with either 3% hydrogen peroxide, 5000 ppm chlorine, 70% ethyl alcohol, or 70% isopropyl alcohol. However, more recent data suggest that 3% hydrogen peroxide and 70% isopropyl alcohol are not effective against adenovirus capable of causing epidemic keratoconjunctivitis and similar viruses, and should not be used for disinfecting applanation tonometers.[124–126] For this reason the CDC guideline recommends to wipe clean tonometer tips and then disinfect them by immersing for 5 to 10 minutes in either 5000 ppm chlorine or 70% ethyl alcohol.[10,123–127] Structural damage to Schiotz tonometers has been observed with 1:10 sodium hypochlorite (5000 ppm chlorine) and 3% hydrogen peroxide.[128] After disinfection, the tonometer should be thoroughly rinsed in tap water and air dried before use.

Because a short and simple decontamination procedure is desirable in the clinical setting, swabbing the tonometer tip with a 70% isopropyl alcohol wipe is sometimes practiced.[129] Preliminary reports suggest that wiping the tonometer tip with an alcohol swab and then allowing the alcohol to evaporate may be an effective means of eliminating HSV, HIV, and adenovirus.[129–131] However, because these studies involved only a few replicates and were conducted in a controlled laboratory setting, further studies are needed before this technique can be recommended. In addition, 2 reports have found that disinfection of pneumotonometer tips between uses with a 70% isopropyl alcohol wipe contributed to outbreaks of epidemic keratoconjunctivitis caused by adenovirus type 8.[132,133]

Endocavitary Probes

Vaginal probes are used in sonographic scanning. A vaginal probe and all endocavitary probes without a probe cover are semicritical devices, as they have direct contact with mucous membranes (eg, vagina, rectum, pharynx). While one could argue that the use of the probe cover changes the category, the CDC guideline proposes that a new condom/probe cover should be used to cover the probe for each patient and because condoms/probe covers may fail,[134–137] high-level disinfection of the probe also should be performed.[10] The relevance of this recommendation is reinforced with the findings that sterile transvaginal ultrasound probe covers have a very high rate of perforation even before use (0%, 25%, and 65% perforations from 3 suppliers).[137] After oocyte retrieval use, Hignett and Claman[137] found a very high rate of perforations in used endovaginal probe covers from 2 suppliers (75% and 81%), whereas Amis and colleagues[138] and Milki and Fisch[134] demonstrated a lower rate of perforations after use of condoms (0.9% and 2.0%, respectively). Rooks and colleagues[139] found that condoms were superior to commercially available probe covers for covering the ultrasound probe (1.7% for condoms vs 8.3% leakage for probe covers). These studies underscore the need for routine probe disinfection between examinations. Although most ultrasound manufacturers recommend the use of 2% glutaraldehyde for high-level disinfection of contaminated transvaginal transducers, the use of this agent has been questioned[140] because it may shorten the life of the transducer and may have toxic effects on the gametes and embryos.[141] An alternative procedure for disinfecting the vaginal transducer has been offered by Garland and de Crespigny.[142] This method involves the mechanical removal of the gel from the transducer, cleaning the transducer in soap and water, wiping the transducer with 70% alcohol or soaking it for 2 minutes in 500 ppm chlorine, and rinsing with tap water and air drying. The effectiveness of this and other methods[138] has not been validated in either rigorous laboratory experiments or in clinical use. High-level disinfection with a product (eg, hydrogen peroxide) that is not toxic to staff, patients, probes, and retrieved cells should be used until such time as the effectiveness of alternative procedures against microbes of importance at the cavitary site is demonstrated by well-designed experimental scientific studies. Other probes such as rectal, cryosurgical, and transesophageal probes or devices should also be subjected to high-level disinfection between patients.

Ultrasound probes may also be used during surgical procedures, and have contact with sterile body sites. These probes may be covered with a sterile sheath to reduce the level of contamination on the probe and reduce the risk of infection. However, because the sheath does not provide complete protection of the probe, the probes should be sterilized between each patient use, as with other critical items. If this is not possible, at a minimum the probe should be covered with a sterile probe cover and undergo high-level disinfection following use.

Some cryosurgical probes are not fully immersible. When reprocessing these probes, the tip of the probe should be immersed in a high-level disinfectant for the appropriate time (eg, 20 minutes exposure with 2% glutaraldehyde) and any other portion of the probe that could have mucous membrane contact could be disinfected by immersion or wrapping with a cloth soaked in a high-level disinfectant to allow the recommended contact time. After disinfection, the probe should be rinsed with tap water and dried before use. Health care facilities that use nonimmersible probes should replace them as soon as possible with fully immersible probes.

As with other high-level disinfection procedures, proper cleaning of probes is necessary to ensure the success of the subsequent disinfection.[143] Muradali and colleagues[144] demonstrated a reduction of vegetative bacteria inoculated on vaginal ultrasound probes when the probes were cleaned with a towel. No information is available on either the level of contamination of such probes by potential viral pathogens such as HBV and human papilloma virus or their removal by cleaning (such as with a towel). Because these pathogens may be present in vaginal and rectal secretions and contaminate probes during use, high-level disinfection of the probes after such use is recommended.

One study showed that the use of a high-quality, snugly fitting, sterile, disposable polyurethane sheath on a nasopharyngoscope during a clinical examination, combined with enzymatic detergent cleaning and disinfection with 70% ethanol, can provide a reliably decontaminated, patient-ready instrument that eliminates the need for high-level disinfection of nasopharyngoscopes.[145] If other studies corroborate the integrity of the sterile polyurethane sheaths used in nasopharyngoscopy (or other procedures), this practice may be an option to high-level disinfection.

The CDC guideline[10] states that even if probe covers have been used, clean and high-level disinfect other semicritical devices such as rectal probes, vaginal probes, and cryosurgical probes with a product that is not toxic to staff, patients, probes, and retrieved germ cells (if applicable). Use a high-level disinfectant at the FDA-cleared exposure time. When probe covers are available, use a probe cover or condom to reduce the level of microbial contamination. Do not use a lower category of disinfection or cease to follow the appropriate disinfectant recommendations when using probe covers because these sheaths and condoms may fail. Following high-level disinfection, rinse all items. Use sterile water, filtered water, or tap water followed by an alcohol rinse for semicritical equipment that will have contact with the mucous membranes of the upper respiratory tract (eg, nose, pharynx, esophagus).

Prostate Biopsy Probes

Transrectal ultrasound–guided prostate biopsies are among the most common outpatient diagnostic procedures performed in urology practice to evaluate patients for prostate cancer after an elevated prostate-specific antigen level or abnormal digital rectal examination findings.[146] This type of biopsy involves obtaining multiple prostate tissue cores by passing a disposable biopsy needle through a needle guide under ultrasound guidance. All prostatic biopsy procedures likely result in contamination of the probe with blood or feces. During this procedure, the transducer assembly is generally covered with a barrier sheath.[147] Breaches in the reprocessing of prostate biopsy probes can pose a risk of disease transmission.[146,148]

Disinfection or sterilization of ultrasound transducer components is based on the function or use of each component. Because the biopsy needle penetrates sterile tissue for biopsy, it should be sterile. Ideally, the needle guide should be sterilized between patient uses. However, if this is not possible (ie, the clinic does not have a sterilizer because biopsy needles are likely purchased as single-use sterile devices) then high-level disinfection after disassembly and cleaning is acceptable, as the needle guide has contact with mucous membranes but not sterile tissue. The FDA alert[147] and a CDC article[146] recommend that the needle guide be sterilized, as the biopsy needle makes contact with the needle guide before it penetrates sterile tissue. This recommendation is inconsistent with the current recommendation for the disinfection of endoscopes. It is currently recommended that gastrointestinal endoscopes be high-level disinfected minimally, but that medical devices that pass through the endoscope and enter sterile tissue (biopsy forceps) be sterilized. There is no recommendation that the lumen or channel through which they pass should also be sterilized. One possible explanation for the inconsistency in this FDA recommendation is that the gastrointestinal endoscopes are high-level disinfected because there is no practical way to sterilize them, whereas the reusable needle guide for prostate probes can be sterilized (MJ Arduino, August 2006, written communication). While a barrier sheath is used on the transducer assembly during the biopsy procedure, this sheath is compromised by the penetration of the needle.[147] Although prostate probes and other endocavitary probes are often covered with a disposable sheath or condom[147] such covers do not adequately protect the probe from microbial contamination due to leakage (9%),[149] and thus the use of a cover does not alter the minimal requirement for high-level disinfection.[10] The FDA specifies the use of a sterile barrier sheath in their recommendation for reprocessing reusable ultrasound transducer assemblies.[147] It is appropriate to use a sterile barrier sheath when an ultrasound probe is entering a sterile body cavity, but when the probe is entering the rectum the need for a sterile barrier sheath is unclear.

All semicritical and critical medical devices must be thoroughly cleaned with enzymatic or nonenzymatic detergents before they are subjected to a high-level disinfection or sterilization process, respectively. Brushes should be used, when possible, to effectively clean the transducer assemblies, especially the lumens. The authors' investigation shows that the needle guide and prostate probe can be effectively disinfected with glutaraldehyde, but the needle guide must be disassembled from the transducer assembly.[150]

The FDA issued a Public Health Notification in June 2006 as a result of follow-up to the Department of Veterans Affairs, Veterans Health Administration Patient Safety Alert related to a particular company's ultrasound transducer assemblies. During patient safety rounds, the lumen of a needle guide of an ultrasound transducer assembly was found to be soiled. The FDA guidance consisted of several steps (see http://www.fda.gov/MedicalDevices/Safety/AlertsandNotices/PublicHealthNotifications/ucm062086.htm for complete guidance recommend by the FDA). The authors have evaluated the FDA steps and suggest some modifications (**Box 1**). These recommendations are consistent with the CDC Guideline on Disinfection and Sterilization in Health Care Facilities and, if followed, scientific evidence suggests would eliminate transmission of infection. Do not reuse items labeled for single use (eg, single-use biopsy needles). Additional recommendations may be available in the operator manuals or user guides. It is important that these recommendations be consistent with disinfection and sterilization guidelines/principles or that these recommendations have been validated by appropriate scientific studies. Do not use any disinfectant that can cause irreparable damage to the materials used to construct the probe. For example, if an alcohol rinse is not compatible with the probe, rinse with sterile water (not filtered water or tap water) and do not rinse with alcohol. These recommendations could be adapted to all ultrasonic prostate probes to include those with an external needle-guide attachment.

Box 1
Recommendation for reprocessing transrectal ultrasound prostate biopsy probes[a]

Cleaning

- Clean immediately after use
- Disassemble the transducer (remove needle guide from the probe)
- Brush clean (if possible) or flush each lumen and thoroughly clean all surfaces of reusable components with enzymatic or nonenzymatic detergent
- Rinse with tap water
- Dry with disposable cloth/towel or air dry
- Visibly inspect the entire device to ensure it is clean

High-Level Disinfection or Sterilization

- Steam sterilize all heat stable reusable components
- Alternatively, high-level disinfect the probe and the needle guide separately following disassembly
- High-level disinfect all heat sensitive components (ensure disinfectants reaches all areas inside the lumens and the MEC of the high-level disinfectant is monitored)
- Rinse with sterile water, filtered water or tap water (FDA specifies sterile water for rinsing)
- If filtered water or tap water is used, follow with an alcohol rinse (not immersion of the probe in alcohol) to enhance drying and prevent the device remaining wet, which would promote microbial growth
- Dry the device
- Appropriately store the device to ensure the device is not recontaminated

[a] Users should be familiar with the manufacturer's recommendations for use and disinfection of the specific device used by the facility.
Data from Rutala WA, Gergen MF, Weber DJ. Disinfection of a probe used in ultrasound-guided prostate biopsy. Infect Control Hosp Epidemiol 2007;28(8):916–9.

Infrared Coagulation

Infrared coagulation is a widely used method for treating hemorrhoids. The procedure involves applying infrared light to compress and seal hemorrhoid veins. The manufacturer of the device sells a sterile disposable sheath and states that removing and soaking lightguides between procedures is no longer required. The manufacturer also states that the lightguide is damaged by immersion in a disinfectant, as the lightguide is not sealed at the end and the disinfectant gets between the quartz glass and the covering.

As mentioned, the CDC guideline recommends immersion for reprocessing endocavitary probes with covers because integrity of the cover is compromised. Because the lightguide cannot be immersed, the authors investigated an alternative procedure. This method involved wiping the probe for 2 minutes with a 1:10 bleach (5000 ppm) and after that is completed, wiping the probe with sterile water and letting the probe air dry. This procedure has been found to be effective in eliminating approximately 7 $\log_{10}$ reduction (7.8×10^6) of *Mycobacterium terrae* and is used at the authors' hospital for decontamination of the sheathed device after use.

Laryngoscopes

Laryngoscopes are routinely used to view the vocal cords and larynx and for airway management. A laryngoscope typically consists of a blade that connects to a handle, which usually contains 2 batteries that power the light source. Limited guidelines are available for reprocessing laryngoscope blades and handles, and hospital practices vary.[151,152] For example, some guidelines and hospitals low-level disinfect the handle as it does not have direct contact with a mucous membrane, and others recommend that the handle be high-level disinfected to prevent disease transmission. While blades have been linked to health care–associated infections, handles have not been directly linked to such infections but contamination with blood and other potentially infected materials during clinical use suggest a possible potential risk,[153] and the blade and handle function together. For this reason, it is ideal that the blades and handles be high-level disinfected or sterilized even if a protective barrier or sheath is used during the procedure.

ENVIRONMENTAL CLEANING

Surfaces may contribute to transmission of epidemiologically important microbes such as MRSA, VRE, *C difficile*, and viruses (norovirus, rotavirus, rhinovirus). Several investigators have demonstrated that inanimate surfaces near infected patients commonly become contaminated with MRSA and VRE,[22,154–156] and that the contamination can persist for hours to weeks on dry surfaces.[22,156] The fact that personnel may contaminate their gloves (or their hands in the absence of glove use)[154] by touching such surfaces suggests that contaminated environmental surfaces may serve as a reservoir or source of MRSA and VRE in hospitals. Although the precise role of the environment in the transmission of diseases has not been fully delineated, environmental surface contamination may contribute to endemic or epidemic spread, as the surfaces may act as a reservoir or source from which personnel contaminate their hands.[155,157] An aggressive environmental decontamination program has been credited with eradicating VRE from a burn unit[158] and *Acinetobacter* on a neurosurgical intensive care unit.[159] Similarly, environmental contamination associated with *C difficile* outbreaks is well described.[160–163] Of importance in a prospective study, transmission to personnel or patient contacts of the strain cultured from the corresponding index case correlated strongly with the intensity of environmental contamination.[162] Because bacterial spores are relatively resistant to quaternary ammonium compounds and phenolics, several investigators have studied the efficacy of environmental decontamination with chlorine. For example, Mayfield and colleagues[160] showed a marked reduction in *C difficile*–associated diarrhea rates in the bone marrow transplant unit (from 8.6 to 3.3 cases per 1000 patient-days) during the period of bleach disinfection (1:10 dilution) of environmental surfaces compared with cleaning with a quaternary ammonium compound.

Viruses can be acquired from environmental surfaces either directly from surface to finger to mouth, or directly from surface to mouth.[164–166] Chemical disinfection of contaminated environmental surfaces has been shown to interrupt transfer of rhinovirus from these surfaces to hands.[167] In experimental studies, the use of disinfectants has been shown to be an efficient method of inhibiting the transmission of rotavirus to human subjects.[168]

Surface disinfection of noncritical surfaces and equipment is normally performed by manually applying a liquid disinfectant to the surface with a cloth, wipe, or mop. Process noncritical patient-care equipment using an EPA-registered hospital disinfectant, following the label's safety precautions and directions (see **Table 1**).[13,22,167–176] Most EPA-registered hospital disinfectants have a label contact time of 10 minutes. However, multiple scientific studies have demonstrated the efficacy of hospital disinfectants against pathogens with a contact time of at least 1 minute.[13,22,71,167–169,172,174,177–186] Ensure that the frequency for disinfecting noncritical patient-care surfaces be done minimally when visibly soiled, and on a regular basis (such as after use on each patient or once daily or once weekly).[169,187,188] If dedicated, disposable equipment is not available, disinfect noncritical patient-care equipment after using it on a patient who is on contact precautions before using this equipment on another patient.[22,154,176,189]

Clean housekeeping surfaces (eg, floors, tabletops) on a regular basis, when spills occur, and when these surfaces are visibly soiled.[111,169,172,187,188,190] Disinfect (or clean) environmental surfaces on a regular basis (eg, daily, 3 times per week) and when surfaces are visibly soiled.[169,187,188,191] Follow manufacturers' instructions for proper use of disinfecting (or detergent) products, such as recommended-use dilution, material compatibility, storage, shelf-life, and safe use and disposal.[192–194] Clean walls, blinds, and window curtains in patient-care areas when these surfaces are visibly contaminated or soiled.[195] Prepare disinfecting (or detergent) solutions as needed, and replace these with fresh solution frequently (eg, replacing floor-mopping solution every 3 patient rooms, changing no less often than at 60-minute intervals), according to the facility's policy.[170,196] Decontaminate mop heads and cleaning cloths regularly to prevent contamination (eg, launder and dry at least daily).[170,191,197] Do not use high-level disinfectants/liquid chemical sterilants for disinfection of noncritical surfaces.[52,111,198] Wet-dust horizontal surfaces regularly (eg, daily, 3 times per week) using clean cloths moistened with an EPA-registered hospital disinfectant (or detergent). Prepare the disinfectant (or detergent) as recommended by the manufacturer.[169,170,187,188,191,197] Disinfect noncritical surfaces with an EPA-registered hospital disinfectant using the label's safety precautions and use directions. Most EPA-registered hospital disinfectants have a label contact time of 10 minutes. Many scientific studies have demonstrated the efficacy of hospital disinfectants against pathogens with a contact time of at least 1 minute.[13,22,71,167–169,172,174,177–186] Do not use disinfectants to clean infant bassinets and incubators while these items are occupied. If disinfectants (eg, phenolics) are used for the terminal cleaning of infant bassinets and incubators, the surfaces of these items should be rinsed thoroughly with water and dried before these items are reused.[13,199,200]

Promptly clean and decontaminate spills of blood and other potentially infectious materials. Discard blood-contaminated items in compliance with federal regulations.[201] Disinfect areas contaminated with blood spills using an EPA-registered tuberculocidal agent, or a solution of 5.25% to 6.15% sodium hypochlorite (household bleach) diluted between 1:10 and 1:100 with water, or a registered germicide on the EPA Lists D and E (ie, products with specific label claims for HIV or HBV).[201–204] For site decontamination of spills of blood or other potentially infectious materials (OPIM), implement the following procedures. Use protective gloves and other personal protective equipment (PPE) (eg, when sharps are involved use forceps to pick up sharps, and discard these items in a puncture-resistant container) appropriate for this task. If sodium hypochlorite solutions are selected, use a 1:100 dilution (eg, 1:100 dilution of a 5.25%–6.15% sodium hypochlorite provides 525–615 ppm available chlorine) to decontaminate nonporous surfaces after a small spill (eg, <10 mL) of either blood or OPIM. If a spill involves large amounts (eg, >10 mL) of blood or OPIM, or involves a culture spill in the laboratory, use a 1:10 dilution for the first application of hypochlorite solution before cleaning to reduce the risk during the cleaning process in the event of a sharp injury. Follow this decontamination process with a terminal disinfection, using a 1:100 dilution of sodium hypochlorite.[184,202,204] If the spill contains large amounts of blood or body fluids, clean the visible matter with disposable absorbent material, and discard the contaminated materials in appropriate, labeled containment.[14,201] Use protective gloves and other PPE appropriate for this task.[14,201] In units with high endemic *C difficile* infection rates or in an outbreak setting, use dilute solutions of 5.25% to 6.15% sodium hypochlorite (eg, 1:10 dilution of bleach) for routine environmental disinfection.[10] At present, only one chlorine-containing product has an EPA-registered claim for inactivating *C difficile* spores.[160,161,163]

Recent studies have identified significant opportunities in hospitals to improve the cleaning of frequently touched objects in the patient's immediate environment.[205–207] For example, of 20,646 standardized environmental surfaces (14 types of objects), only 9910 (48%) were cleaned at terminal room cleaning.[206] Epidemiologic studies have shown that patients admitted to rooms previously occupied by individuals infected or colonized with MRSA,[208] VRE,[209] or *C difficile*[210] are at significant risk of acquiring these organisms from contaminated environmental surfaces. These data have led to the development of room decontamination units that avoid the problems associated with the thoroughness of terminal cleaning activities in patient rooms.

Hydrogen peroxide vapor (HPV) has been used increasingly for the decontamination of biologic safety cabinets and rooms in health care.[211–220] These studies found that HPV is a highly effective method for eradicating various pathogens (eg, MRSA, *M tuberculosis*, *Serratia*, *C difficile* spores, *Clostridium botulinum* spores) from rooms, furniture, and equipment. This room decontamination system has been found not only to be effective in eradicating pathogens from contaminated surfaces but also to significantly reduce the incidence of *C difficile* infection rates.[211]

Ultraviolet C light units have also been proposed for room decontamination. One unit (Tru-D) uses an array of UV sensors, which determines and targets shadowed areas to deliver a measured dose of UV energy that destroys microorganisms. This unit is fully automated, activated by a hand-held remote, and the room ventilation does not need to be modified; it uses UV-C (254 nm range) to decontaminate surfaces. The unit measures UV reflected from walls, ceiling, floors, or other treated areas and calculates the operation time to deliver the programmed lethal dose for pathogens.[221] After the UV dose is delivered, it powers down and an audible alarm notifies the operator. In preliminary studies it has reduced colony counts of MRSA, VRE, and

Acinetobacter by approximately 3.5 $\log_{10}$ in about 15 minutes. Sixty minutes is needed to achieve a 2.7-$\log_{10}$ reduction of *C difficile* spores (Rutala, Weber, and Gergen, unpublished results, 2009).

SUMMARY

When properly used, disinfection and sterilization can ensure the safe use of invasive and noninvasive medical devices. The method of disinfection and sterilization depends on the intended use of the medical device: critical items (contact sterile tissue) must be sterilized before use; semicritical items (contact mucous membranes or nonintact skin) must be high-level disinfected; and noncritical items (contact intact skin) should receive low-level disinfection. Cleaning should always precede high-level disinfection and sterilization. Current disinfection and sterilization guidelines must be strictly followed.

Because semicritical equipment has been associated with reprocessing errors that result in patient lookback and patient notifications, it is essential that control measures be instituted to prevent patient exposures.[118] Before new equipment (especially semicritical equipment, as the margin of safety is less than that for sterilization)[21] is used for patient care on more than one patient, reprocessing procedures for that equipment should be developed. Staff should receive training on the safe use and reprocessing of the equipment and be competency tested. Infection control rounds or audits should be conducted annually in all clinical areas that reprocess semicritical devices to ensure adherence to the reprocessing standards and policies. Results of infection control rounds should be provided to the unit managers, and deficiencies in reprocessing should be corrected and the corrective measures documented to infection control within 2 weeks.

REFERENCES

1. McCarthy GM, Koval JJ, John MA, et al. Infection control practices across Canada: do dentists follow the recommendations? J Can Dent Assoc 1999;65: 506–11.
2. Spach DH, Silverstein FE, Stamm WE. Transmission of infection by gastrointestinal endoscopy and bronchoscopy. Ann Intern Med 1993;118:117–28.
3. Weber DJ, Rutala WA. Lessons from outbreaks associated with bronchoscopy. Infect Control Hosp Epidemiol 2001;22:403–8.
4. Weber DJ, Rutala WA, DiMarino AJ Jr. The prevention of infection following gastrointestinal endoscopy: the importance of prophylaxis and reprocessing. In: DiMarino AJ Jr, Benjamin SB, editors. Gastrointestinal diseases: an endoscopic approach. Thorofare (NJ): Slack Inc; 2002. p. 87–106.
5. Meyers H, Brown-Elliott BA, Moore D, et al. An outbreak of *Mycobacterium chelonae* infection following liposuction. Clin Infect Dis 2002;34:1500–7.
6. Lowry PW, Jarvis WR, Oberle AD, et al. *Mycobacterium chelonae* causing otitis media in an ear-nose-and-throat practice. N Engl J Med 1988;319:978–82.
7. Rutala WA, Weber DJ. Cleaning, disinfection and sterilization. In: Carrico R, editor. APIC text of infection control and epidemiology. Washington, DC: Association for Professionals in Infection Control and Epidemiology, Inc; 2009. p. 21:1–21:27.
8. Rutala WA, Weber DJ. Disinfection and sterilization in healthcare facilities. In: Lautenbach E, Woeltje K, Malani PN, editors. Practical handbook for healthcare epidemiologists. Chicago: The University of Chicago Press; 2010. p. 61–80.

9. Spaulding EH. Chemical disinfection of medical and surgical materials. In: Lawrence C, Block SS, editors. Disinfection, sterilization, and preservation. Philadelphia: Lea & Febiger; 1968. p. 517–31.

10. Rutala WA, Weber DJ, Healthcare Infection Control Practices Advisory Committee. Guideline for disinfection and sterilization in healthcare facilities, 2008. Available at: http://www.cdc.gov/ncidod/dhqp/pdf/guidelines/Disinfection_Nov_2008.pdf. Accessed December, 2010.

11. Simmons BP. CDC guidelines for the prevention and control of nosocomial infections. Guideline for hospital environmental control. Am J Infect Control 1983;11: 97–120.

12. Rutala WA, Weber DJ. Disinfection and sterilization in health care facilities: what clinicians need to know. Clin Infect Dis 2004;39:702–9.

13. Rutala WA. 1994, 1995, and 1996 APIC Guidelines Committee. APIC guideline for selection and use of disinfectants. Association for Professionals in Infection Control and Epidemiology, Inc. Am J Infect Control 1996;24:313–42.

14. Sehulster L, Chinn RY. Healthcare Infection Control Practices Advisory Committee. Guidelines for environmental infection control in health-care facilities. MMWR Recomm Rep 2003;52:1–44.

15. Food and Drug Administration. FDA-cleared sterilant and high-level disinfectants with general claims for processing reusable medical and dental devices—March 2009. Available at: http://www.fda.gov/cdrh/ode/germlab.html. Accessed December, 2010.

16. Nelson DB, Jarvis WR, Rutala WA, et al. Multi-society guideline for reprocessing flexible gastrointestinal endoscopes. Infect Control Hosp Epidemiol 2003;24: 532–7.

17. Gerding DN, Peterson LR, Vennes JA. Cleaning and disinfection of fiberoptic endoscopes: evaluation of glutaraldehyde exposure time and forced-air drying. Gastroenterology 1982;83:613–8.

18. Weber DJ, Rutala WA. Environmental issues and nosocomial infections. In: Wenzel RP, editor. Prevention and control of nosocomial infections. Baltimore (MD): Williams and Wilkins; 1997. p. 491–514.

19. Rutala WA, Gergen MF, Jones JF, et al. Levels of microbial contamination on surgical instruments. Am J Infect Control 1998;26:143–5.

20. Chu NS, Chan-Myers H, Ghazanfari N, et al. Levels of naturally occurring microorganisms on surgical instruments after clinical use and after washing. Am J Infect Control 1999;27:315–9.

21. Favero MS. Sterility assurance: concepts for patient safety. In: Rutala WA, editor. Disinfection, sterilization and antisepsis: principles and practices in healthcare facilities. Washington, DC: Association for Professional in Infection Control and Epidemiology; 2001. p. 110–9.

22. Weber DJ, Rutala WA. Role of environmental contamination in the transmission of vancomycin-resistant enterococci. Infect Control Hosp Epidemiol 1997;18: 306–9.

23. Dufresne S, Leblond H, Chaunet M. Relationship between lumen diameter and length sterilized in the 125L ozone sterilizer. Am J Infect Control 2008;36:291–7.

24. Bradley CR, Babb JR. Endoscope decontamination: automated vs. manual. J Hosp Infect 1995;30:537–42.

25. Muscarella LF. Advantages and limitations of automatic flexible endoscope reprocessors. Am J Infect Control 1996;24:304–9.

26. Muscarella LF. Automatic flexible endoscope reprocessors. Gastrointest Endosc Clin N Am 2000;10:245–57.

27. Kircheis U, Martiny H. Comparison of the cleaning and disinfecting efficacy of four washer-disinfectors for flexible endoscopes. J Hosp Infect 2007;66:255–61.

28. Vickery K, Ngo QD, Zou J, et al. The effect of multiple cycles of contamination, detergent washing, and disinfection on the development of biofilm in endoscope tubing. Am J Infect Control 2009;37:470–5.

29. Alvarado CJ, Stolz SM, Maki DG. Nosocomial infections from contaminated endoscopes: a flawed automated endoscope washer. An investigation using molecular epidemiology. Am J Med 1991;91:272S–80S.

30. Fraser VJ, Jones M, Murray PR, et al. Contamination of flexible fiberoptic bronchoscopes with *Mycobacterium chelonae* linked to an automated bronchoscope disinfection machine. Am Rev Respir Dis 1992;145:853–5.

31. Cooke RP, Whymant-Morris A, Umasankar RS, et al. Bacteria-free water for automatic washer-disinfectors: an impossible dream? J Hosp Infect 1998;39: 63–5.

32. Muscarella LF. Deja vu. All over again? The importance of instrument drying. Infect Control Hosp Epidemiol 2000;21:628–9.

33. Rutala WA, Weber DJ. Importance of lumen flow in liquid chemical sterilization. Am J Infect Control 1999;20:458–9.

34. Lynch DA, Porter C, Murphy L, et al. Evaluation of four commercial automatic endoscope washing machines. Endoscopy 1992;24:766–70.

35. Bond WW. Disinfection and endoscopy: microbial considerations. J Gastroenterol Hepatol 1991;6:31–6.

36. Bond WW. Endoscope reprocessing: problems and solutions. In: Rutala WA, editor. Disinfection, sterilization, and antisepsis in healthcare. Champlain (NY): Polyscience Publications; 1998. p. 151–63.

37. Petersen BT, Adler DG, Chand B, et al, American Society of Gastrointestinal Endoscopists Technology Committee. Automated endoscope reprocessors. Gastrointest Endosc 2009;69:771–6.

38. Alfa MJ, Olson N, Degagne P. Automated washing with the Reliance endoscope processing system and its equivalence to optimal manual cleaning. Am J Infect Control 2006;34:561–70.

39. Omidbakhsh N. A new peroxide-based flexible endoscope-compatible high-level disinfectant. Am J Infect Control 2006;34:571–7.

40. Schembre DB. Infectious complications associated with gastrointestinal endoscopy. Gastrointest Endosc Clin N Am 2000;10:215–32.

41. Nelson DB. Infectious disease complications of GI endoscopy: part II, exogenous infections. Gastrointest Endosc 2003;57:695–711.

42. Mehta AC, Prakash UB, Garland R, et al. Prevention of flexible bronchoscopy-associated infection. Chest 2006;128:1742–55.

43. Chu NS, Favero M. The microbial flora of the gastrointestinal tract and the cleaning of flexible endoscopes. Gastrointest Endosc Clin N Am 2000;10:233–44.

44. Alfa MJ, Sitter DL. In-hospital evaluation of orthophthalaldehyde as a high level disinfectant for flexible endoscopes. J Hosp Infect 1994;26:15–26.

45. Vesley D, Melson J, Stanley P. Microbial bioburden in endoscope reprocessing and an in-use evaluation of the high-level disinfection capabilities of Cidex PA. Gastroenterol Nurs 1999;22:63–8.

46. Chu NS, McAlister D, Antonoplos PA. Natural bioburden levels detected on flexible gastrointestinal endoscopes after clinical use and manual cleaning. Gastrointest Endosc 1998;48:137–42.

47. Rutala WA, Weber DJ. FDA labeling requirements for disinfection of endoscopes: a counterpoint. Infect Control Hosp Epidemiol 1995;16:231–5.

48. Rutala WA, Weber DJ. Reprocessing endoscopes: United States perspective. J Hosp Infect 2004;56:S27–39.
49. Hanson PJ, Gor D, Clarke JR, et al. Contamination of endoscopes used in AIDS patients. Lancet 1989;2:86–8.
50. Hanson PJ, Gor D, Clarke JR, et al. Recovery of the human immunodeficiency virus from fibreoptic bronchoscopes. Thorax 1991;46:410–2.
51. Chaufour X, Deva AK, Vickery K, et al. Evaluation of disinfection and sterilization of reusable angioscopes with the duck hepatitis B model. J Vasc Surg 1999;30: 277–82.
52. Rutala WA, Weber DJ. Disinfection of endoscopes: review of new chemical sterilants used for high-level disinfection. Infect Control Hosp Epidemiol 1999;20:69–76.
53. Cheung RJ, Ortiz D, DiMarino AJ Jr. GI endoscopic reprocessing practices in the United States. Gastrointest Endosc 1999;50:362–8.
54. Food and Drug Administration. Content and format of premarket notification [510 (k)]·submissions for liquid chemical sterilants/high level disinfectants. 2000. Available at: http://www.fda.gov/cdrh/ode/397. Accessed December, 2010.
55. Urayama S, Kozarek RA, Sumida S, et al. Mycobacteria and glutaraldehyde: is high-level disinfection of endoscopes possible? Gastrointest Endosc 1996;43:451–6.
56. Jackson J, Leggett JE, Wilson DA, et al. *Mycobacterium gordonae* in fiberoptic bronchoscopes. Am J Infect Control 1996;24:19–23.
57. Lee RM, Kozarek RA, Sumida SE, et al. Risk of contamination of sterile biopsy forceps in disinfected endoscopes. Gastrointest Endosc 1998;47:377–81.
58. Martiny H, Floss H, Zuhlsdorf B. The importance of cleaning for the overall results of processing endoscopes. J Hosp Infect 2004;56:S16–22.
59. Alvarado CJ, Reichelderfer M. APIC guideline for infection prevention and control in flexible endoscopy. Association for Professionals in Infection Control. Am J Infect Control 2000;28:138–55.
60. Society of Gastroenterology Nurses and Associates. Guideline for the use of high-level disinfectants and sterilants for reprocessing of flexible gastrointestinal endoscopes. Gastroenterol Nurs 2000;23:180–7.
61. Society of Gastroenterology Nurses and Associates. Standards of infection control in reprocessing of flexible gastrointestinal endoscopes. Gastroenterol Nurs 2006;29:142–8.
62. Society of Gastroenterology Nurses and Associates. Standards for infection control and reprocessing of flexible gastrointestinal endoscopes. Gastroenterol Nurs 2000;23:172–9.
63. American Society for Gastrointestinal Endoscopy. Position statement: reprocessing of flexible gastrointestinal endoscopes. Gastrointest Endosc 1996;43:541–6.
64. Rutala WA. APIC guideline for selection and use of disinfectants. Am J Infect Control 1990;18:99–117.
65. Martin MA, Reichelderfer M. 1991, and 1993 APIC Guidelines Committee. APIC guidelines for infection prevention and control in flexible endoscopy. Am J Infect Control 1994;22:19–38.
66. Rey JF, Halfon P, Feryn JM, et al. Risk of transmission of hepatitis C virus by digestive endoscopy. Gastroenterol Clin Biol 1995;19:346–9.
67. Cronmiller JR, Nelson DK, Jackson DK, et al. Efficacy of conventional endoscopic disinfection and sterilization methods against *Helicobacter pylori* contamination. Helicobacter 1999;4:198–203.
68. Sartor C, Charrel RN, de Lamballerie X, et al. Evaluation of a disinfection procedure for hysteroscopes contaminated by hepatitis C virus. Infect Control Hosp Epidemiol 1999;20:434–6.

69. Hanson PJ, Chadwick MV, Gaya H, et al. A study of glutaraldehyde disinfection of fibreoptic bronchoscopes experimentally contaminated with *Mycobacterium tuberculosis*. J Hosp Infect 1992;22:137–42.

70. Kinney TP, Kozarek RA, Raltz S, et al. Contamination of single-use biopsy forceps: a prospective in vitro analysis. Gastrointest Endosc 2002;56: 209–12.

71. Best M, Springthorpe VS, Sattar SA. Feasibility of a combined carrier test for disinfectants: studies with a mixture of five types of microorganisms. Am J Infect Control 1994;22:152–62.

72. Leong D, Dorsey G, Klapp M. Dilution of glutaraldehyde by automatic endoscope machine washers: the need for a quality control program. Abstracts of the 14th Annual Educational Conference of Association for Practitioners in Infection Control. Washington, DC: Association for Professionals in Infection Control and Epidemiology; 1987:108. p.130.

73. Mbithi JN, Springthorpe VS, Sattar SA, et al. Bactericidal, virucidal, and mycobactericidal activities of reused alkaline glutaraldehyde in an endoscopy unit. J Clin Microbiol 1993;31:2988–95.

74. Kleier DJ, Averbach RE. Glutaraldehyde nonbiologic monitors. Infect Control Hosp Epidemiol 1990;11:439–41.

75. Cole EC, Rutala WA, Nessen L, et al. Effect of methodology, dilution, and exposure time on the tuberculocidal activity of glutaraldehyde-based disinfectants. Appl Environ Microbiol 1990;56:1813–7.

76. Collins FM, Montalbine V. Mycobactericidal activity of glutaraldehyde solutions. J Clin Microbiol 1976;4:408–12.

77. Masferrer R, Marquez R. Comparison of two activated glutaraldehyde solutions: Cidex Solution and Sonacide. Respir Care 1977;22:257–62.

78. Kleier DJ, Tucker JE, Averbach RE. Clinical evaluation of glutaraldehyde nonbiologic monitors. Quintessence Int 1989;20:271–7.

79. Overton D, Burgess JO, Beck B, et al. Glutaraldehyde test kits: evaluation for accuracy and range. Gen Dent 1989;37:126 128.

80. Cooke RP, Goddard SV, Chatterley R, et al. Monitoring glutaraldehyde dilution in automated washer/disinfectors. J Hosp Infect 2001;48:242–6.

81. Merighi A, Contato E, Scagliarini R, et al. Quality improvement in gastrointestinal endoscopy: microbiologic surveillance of disinfection. Gastrointest Endosc 1996;43:457–62.

82. Deva AK, Vickery K, Zou J, et al. Establishment of an in-use testing method for evaluating disinfection of surgical instruments using the duck hepatitis B model. J Hosp Infect 1996;33:119–30.

83. Hanson PJ, Gor D, Jeffries DJ, et al. Elimination of high titre HIV from fibreoptic endoscopes. Gut 1990;31:657–9.

84. Wu MS, Wang JT, Yang JC, et al. Effective reduction of *Helicobacter pylori* infection after upper gastrointestinal endoscopy by mechanical washing of the endoscope. Hepatogastroenterology 1996;43:1660–4.

85. Kruse A, Rey JF. Guidelines on cleaning and disinfection in GI endoscopy. Update 1999. The European Society of Gastrointestinal Endoscopy. Endoscopy 2000;32:77–80.

86. British Thoracic Society. British Thoracic Society guidelines on diagnostic flexible bronchoscopy. Thorax 2001;56:1–21.

87. Association of Operating Room Nurses. Recommended practices for use and care of endoscopes. 2000 standards, recommended practices, and guidelines. Denver (CO): AORN; 2000. p. 243–7.

88. British Society of Gastroenterology. Cleaning and disinfection of equipment for gastrointestinal endoscopy. Report of a working party of the British Society of Gastroenterology Endoscope Committee. Gut 1998;42:585–93.

89. Jackson FW, Ball MD. Correction of deficiencies in flexible fiberoptic sigmoidoscope cleaning and disinfection technique in family practice and internal medicine offices. Arch Fam Med 1997;6:578–82.

90. Orsi GB, Filocamo A, Di Stefano L, et al. Italian National Survey of Digestive Endoscopy Disinfection Procedures. Endoscopy 1997;29:732–8 [quiz: 739–40].

91. Honeybourne D, Neumann CS. An audit of bronchoscopy practice in the United Kingdom: a survey of adherence to national guidelines. Thorax 1997;52:709–13.

92. Michele TM, Cronin WA, Graham NM, et al. Transmission of *Mycobacterium tuberculosis* by a fiberoptic bronchoscope. Identification by DNA fingerprinting. JAMA 1997;278:1093–5.

93. Bronowicki JP, Venard V, Botte C, et al. Patient-to-patient transmission of hepatitis C virus during colonoscopy. N Engl J Med 1997;337:237–40.

94. Agerton T, Valway S, Gore B, et al. Transmission of a highly drug-resistant strain (strain W1) of *Mycobacterium tuberculosis*. Community outbreak and nosocomial transmission via a contaminated bronchoscope. JAMA 1997;278:1073–7.

95. Srinivasan A, Wolfenden LL, Song X, et al. An outbreak of *Pseudomonas aeruginosa* infections associated with flexible bronchoscopes. N Engl J Med 2003; 348:221–7.

96. Food and Drug Administration, Centers for Disease Control and Prevention. FDA and CDC public health advisory: infections from endoscopes inadequately reprocessed by an automated endoscope reprocessing system. Rockville (MD): Food and Drug Administration; 1999.

97. Nelson DB, Muscarella LF. Current issues in endoscope reprocessing and infection control during gastrointestinal endoscopy. World J Gastroenterol 2006;12: 3953–64.

98. Willis C. Bacteria-free endoscopy rinse water—a realistic aim? Epidemiol Infect 2005;134:279–84.

99. Humphreys H, McGrath H, McCormick PA, et al. Quality of final rinse water used in washer-disinfectors for endoscopes. J Hosp Infect 2002;51:151–3.

100. Vergis AS, Thomson D, Pieroni P, et al. Reprocessing flexible gastrointestinal endoscopes after a period of disuse: is it necessary? Endoscopy 2007;39: 737–9.

101. Riley R, Beanland C, Bos H. Establishing the shelf life of flexible colonoscopes. Gastroenterol Nurs 2002;25:114–9.

102. Rejchrt S, Cermak P, Pavlatova L, et al. Bacteriologic testing of endoscopes after high-level disinfection. Gastrointest Endosc 2004;60:76–8.

103. Leung J, Vallero R, Wilson R. Surveillance cultures to monitor quality of gastrointestinal endoscope reprocessing. Am J Gastroenterol 2003;98(1):3–5.

104. Moses FM, Lee J. Surveillance cultures to monitor quality of gastrointestinal endoscope reprocessing. Am J Gastroenterol 2003;98:77–81.

105. Tunuguntla A, Sullivan MJ. Monitoring quality of flexible endoscopic disinfection by microbiologic surveillance cultures. Tenn Med 2004;97(10):453–6.

106. Beilenhoff U, Neumann CS, Rey JF, et al. ESGE-ESGENA guideline for quality assurance in reprocessing: microbiological surveillance testing in endoscopy. Endoscopy 2007;39:175–81.

107. Gillespie EE, Kotsanas D, Stuart RL. Microbiological monitoring of endoscopes: 5-year review. J Gastroenterol Hepatol 2008;23:1069–74.

108. Muscarella LF. Application of environmental sampling to flexible endoscope reprocessing: the importance of monitoring the rinse water. Infect Control Hosp Epidemiol 2002;23:285–9.
109. Fraser TG, Reiner S, Malcznski M, et al. Multidrug-resistant *Pseudomonas aeruginosa* cholangiopancreatography: failure of routine endoscope cultures to prevent an outbreak. Infect Control Hosp Epidemiol 2004;25:856–9.
110. Bond WW, Hedrick ER. Microbiological culturing of environmental and medical-device surfaces. In: Isenberg HD, Gilchrist MJR, editors. Clinical microbiology procedures handbook, section 11, epidemiologic and infection control microbiology. Washington, DC: American Society for Microbiology; 1992. p. 11.10.1–11.10.9.
111. Centers for Disease Control. Guidelines for environmental infection control in health-care facilities, 2003. MMWR Recomm Rep 2003;52(No RR–10):1–44.
112. Pang J, Perry P, Ross A, et al. Bacteria-free rinse water for endoscope disinfection. Gastrointest Endosc 2002;56:402–6.
113. Widmer AF, Frei R. Decontamination, disinfection and sterilization. In: Murray PR, Baron EJ, Pfaller MA, et al, editors. Manual of clinical microbiology. Washington, DC: American Society of Microbiology; 2003. p. 77–108.
114. Buss AJ, Been MH, Borgers RP, et al. Endoscope disinfection and its pitfalls-requirement for retrograde surveillance cultures. Endoscopy 2008;40:327–32.
115. Blob R, Kampf G. Test models to determine cleaning efficacy with different types of bioburden and its clinical correlation. J Hosp Infect 2004;56(Suppl):S44–8.
116. Obee PC, Griffith CJ, Cooper RA, et al. Real-time monitoring in managing the decontamination of flexible gastrointestinal endoscopes. Am J Infect Control 2005;33:202–6.
117. Sciortino CV, Xia EL, Mozee A. Assessment of a novel approach to evaluate the outcome of endoscope reprocessing. Infect Control Hosp Epidemiol 2004;25:284–90.
118. Rutala WA, Weber DJ. How to assess disease transmission when there is a failure to follow recommended disinfection and sterilization principles. Infect Control Hosp Epidemiol 2007;28:519–24.
119. Murphy C. Inactivated glutaraldehyde: Lessons for infection control. Am J Infect Control 1998;26:159–60.
120. Carsauw H, Debacker N. Recall of patients after use of inactive batch of Cidex disinfection solution in Belgian hospitals, Fifth International Conference of the Hospital Infection Society. Edinburgh, September 15–18, 2002. Hospital Infections Society.
121. Rutala WA, Clontz EP, Weber DJ, et al. Disinfection practices for endoscopes and other semicritical items. Infect Control Hosp Epidemiol 1991;12:282–8.
122. Weber DJ, Rutala WA. Nosocomial ocular infections. In: Mayhall CG, editor. Hospital epidemiology and infection control. Philadelphia: Lippincott Williams & Wilkins; 1999. p. 287–99.
123. Centers for Disease Control. Recommendations for preventing possible transmission of human T-lymphotropic virus type III/lymphadenopathy-associated virus from tears. MMWR Morb Mortal Wkly Rep 1985;34:533–4.
124. Rutala WA, Peacock JE, Gergen MF, et al. Efficacy of hospital germicides against adenovirus 8, a common cause of epidemic keratoconjunctivitis in health care facilities. Antimicrob Agents Chemother 2006;50:1419–24.
125. Tyler R, Ayliffe GA, Bradley C. Virucidal activity of disinfectants: studies with the poliovirus. J Hosp Infect 1990;15:339–45.

126. Sattar SA, Springthorpe VS, Karim Y, et al. Chemical disinfection of non-porous inanimate surfaces experimentally contaminated with four human pathogenic viruses. Epidemiol Infect 1989;102:493–505.

127. Nagington J, Sutehall GM, Whipp P. Tonometer disinfection and viruses. Br J Ophthalmol 1983;67:674–6.

128. Chronister CL. Structural damage to Schiotz tonometers after disinfection with solutions. Optom Vis Sci 1997;74:164–6.

129. Craven ER, Butler SL, McCulley JP, et al. Applanation tonometer tip sterilization for adenovirus type 8. Ophthalmology 1987;94:1538–40.

130. Pepose JS, Linette G, Lee SF, et al. Disinfection of Goldmann tonometers against human immunodeficiency virus type 1. Arch Ophthalmol 1989;107:983–5.

131. Ventura LM, Dix RD. Viability of herpes simplex virus type 1 on the applanation tonometer. Am J Ophthalmol 1987;103:48–52.

132. Koo D, Bouvier B, Wesley M, et al. Epidemic keratoconjunctivitis in a university medical center ophthalmology clinic; need for re-evaluation of the design and disinfection of instruments. Infect Control Hosp Epidemiol 1989;10:547–52.

133. Jernigan JA, Lowry BS, Hayden FG, et al. Adenovirus type 8 epidemic kerato-conjunctivitis in an eye clinic: risk factors and control. J Infect Dis 1993;167:1307–13.

134. Milki AA, Fisch JD. Vaginal ultrasound probe cover leakage: implications for patient care. Fertil Steril 1998;69:409–11.

135. Storment JM, Monga M, Blanco JD. Ineffectiveness of latex condoms in preventing contamination of the transvaginal ultrasound transducer head. South Med J 1997;90:206–8.

136. Fritz S, Hust MH, Ochs C, et al. Use of a latex cover sheath for transesophageal echocardiography (TEE) instead of regular disinfection of the echoscope? Clin Cardiol 1993;16:737–40.

137. Hignett M, Claman P. High rates of perforation are found in endovaginal ultrasound probe covers before and after oocyte retrieval for *in vitro* fertilization-embryo transfer. J Assist Reprod Genet 1995;12:606–9.

138. Amis S, Ruddy M, Kibbler CC, et al. Assessment of condoms as probe covers for transvaginal sonography. J Clin Ultrasound 2000;28:295–8.

139. Rooks VJ, Yancey MK, Elg SA, et al. Comparison of probe sheaths for endovaginal sonography. Obstet Gynecol 1996;87:27–9.

140. Odwin CS, Fleischer AC, Kepple DM, et al. Probe covers and disinfectants for transvaginal transducers. J Diagnostic Med Sonography 1990;6:130–5.

141. Benson WG. Exposure to glutaraldehyde. J Soc Occup Med 1984;34:63–4.

142. Garland SM, de Crespigny L. Prevention of infection in obstetrical and gynaecological ultrasound practice. Aust N Z J Obstet Gynaecol 1996;36:392–5.

143. Fowler C, McCracken D. US probes: risk of cross infection and ways to reduce it–comparison of cleaning methods. Radiology 1999;213:299–300.

144. Muradali D, Gold WL, Phillips A, et al. Can ultrasound probes and coupling gel be a source of nosocomial infection in patients undergoing sonography? An in vivo and in vitro study. AJR Am J Roentgenol 1995;164:1521–4.

145. Alvarado CJ, Anderson AG, Maki DG. Microbiologic assessment of disposable sterile endoscopic sheaths to replace high-level disinfection in reprocessing: a prospective clinical trial with nasopharygoscopes. Am J Infect Control 2009;37:408–13.

146. Gillespie JL, Arnold KE, Noble-Wang J, et al. Outbreak of *Pseudomonas aeruginosa* infections after transrectal ultrasound-guided prostate biopsy. Urology 2007;69:912–4.

147. Food and Drug Administration. FDA Public Health Notification: reprocessing of reusable ultrasound transducer assemblies used for biopsy procedures. Available at: http://www.fda.gov/MedicalDevices/Safety/AlertsandNotices/PublicHealthNotification/ucm062086.htm. Accessed November 1, 2009.
148. Lessa F, Tak S, DeVader SR, et al. Risk of infections associated with improperly reprocessed transrectal ultrasound-guided prostate biopsy equipment. Infect Control Hosp Epidemiol 2008;29:289–93.
149. Masood J, Voulgaris S, Awogu O, et al. Condom perforation during transrectal ultrasound guided (TRUS) prostate biopsies: a potential risk. Int Urol Nephrol 2007;39:1121–4.
150. Rutala WA, Gergen MF, Weber DJ. Disinfection of a probe used in ultrasound-guided prostate biopsy. Infect Control Hosp Epidemiol 2007;28(8):916–9.
151. Muscarella LF. Prevention of disease transmission during flexible laryngoscopy. Am J Infect Control 2007;35:536–44.
152. Muscarella LF. Recommendations to resolve inconsistent guidelines for the reprocessing of sheathed and unsheathed rigid laryngoscopes. Infect Control Hosp Epidemiol 2007;28:504–7.
153. Call TR, Auerbach FG, Riddell SW, et al. Nosocomial contamination of laryngoscope handles: challenging current guidelines. Anesth Analg 2009;109:479–83.
154. Boyce JM, Potter-Bynoe G, Chenevert C, et al. Environmental contamination due to methicillin-resistant Staphylococcus aureus: possible infection control implications. Infect Control Hosp Epidemiol 1997;18:622–7.
155. Bonten MJ, Hayden MJ, Nathan C, et al. Epidemiology of colonisation of patients and environment with vancomycin-resistant enterococci. Lancet 1996;348:1615–9.
156. Muto CA, Jernigan JA, Ostrowsky BE, et al. SHEA guideline for preventing nosocomial transmission of multidrug-resistant strains of Staphylococcus aureus and Enterococcus. Infect Control Hosp Epidemiol 2003;24:362–86.
157. Griffith CJ, Cooper RA, Gilmore J, et al. An evaluation of hospital cleaning regimes and standards. J Hosp Infect 2000;45:19–28.
158. Falk PS, Winnike J, Woodmansee C, et al. Outbreak of vancomycin-resistant enterococci in a burn unit. Infect Control Hosp Epidemiol 2000;21:575–82.
159. Denton M, Wilcox MH, Parnell P, et al. Role of environmental cleaning in controlling an outbreak of Acinetobacter baumannii on a neurosurgical intensive care unit. J Hosp Infect 2004;56:106–10.
160. Mayfield JL, Leet T, Miller J, et al. Environmental control to reduce transmission of Clostridium difficile. Clin Infect Dis 2000;31:995–1000.
161. Kaatz GW, Gitlin SD, Schaberg DR, et al. Acquisition of Clostridium difficile from the hospital environment. Am J Epidemiol 1988;127:1289–94.
162. Samore MH, Venkataraman L, DeGirolami PC, et al. Clinical and molecular epidemiology of sporadic and clustered cases of nosocomial Clostridium difficile diarrhea. Am J Med 1996;100:32–40.
163. Wilcox MH, Fawley WN, Wigglesworth N, et al. Comparison of the effect of detergent versus hypochlorite cleaning on environmental contamination and incidence of Clostridium difficile infection. J Hosp Infect 2003;54:109–14.
164. Evans MR, Meldrum R, Lane W, et al. An outbreak of viral gastroenteritis following environmental contamination at a concert hall. Epidemiol Infect 2002;129:355–60.
165. Wilde J, Van R, Pickering L, et al. Detection of rotaviruses in the day care environment by reverse transcriptase polymerase chain reaction. J Infect Dis 1992; 166:507–11.

166. Akhter J, al-Hajjar S, Myint S, et al. Viral contamination of environmental surfaces on a general paediatric ward and playroom in a major referral centre in Riyadh. Eur J Epidemiol 1995;11:587–90.
167. Sattar SA, Jacobsen H, Springthorpe VS, et al. Chemical disinfection to interrupt transfer of rhinovirus type 14 from environmental surfaces to hands. Appl Environ Microbiol 1993;59:1579–85.
168. Ward RL, Bernstein DI, Knowlton DR, et al. Prevention of surface-to-human transmission of rotaviruses by treatment with disinfectant spray. J Clin Microbiol 1991;29:1991–6.
169. Rutala WA, Weber DJ. Surface disinfection: should we do it? J Hosp Infect 2001; 48(Suppl A):S64–8.
170. Westwood JC, Mitchell MA, Legace S. Hospital sanitation: the massive bacterial contamination of the wet mop. Appl Microbiol 1971;21:693–7.
171. Whitby JL, Rampling A. *Pseudomonas aeruginosa* contamination in domestic and hospital environments. Lancet 1972;1:15–7.
172. Dharan S, Mourouga P, Copin P, et al. Routine disinfection of patients' environmental surfaces. Myth or reality? J Hosp Infect 1999;42:113–7.
173. Sattar SA, Lloyd-Evans N, Springthorpe VS, et al. Institutional outbreaks of rotavirus diarrhoea: potential role of fomites and environmental surfaces as vehicles for virus transmission. J Hyg (Lond) 1986;96:277–89.
174. Gwaltney JM Jr, Hendley JO. Transmission of experimental rhinovirus infection by contaminated surfaces. Am J Epidemiol 1982;116:828–33.
175. Sattar SA, Jacobsen H, Rahman H, et al. Interruption of rotavirus spread through chemical disinfection. Infect Control Hosp Epidemiol 1994;15:751–6.
176. Ray AJ, Hoyen CK, Taub TF, et al. Nosocomial transmission of vancomycin-resistant enterococci from surfaces. JAMA 2002;287:1400–1.
177. Rutala WA, Barbee SL, Aguiar NC, et al. Antimicrobial activity of home disinfectants and natural products against potential human pathogens. Infect Control Hosp Epidemiol 2000;21:33–8.
178. Silverman J, Vazquez JA, Sobel JD, et al. Comparative in vitro activity of antiseptics and disinfectants versus clinical isolates of *Candida* species. Infect Control Hosp Epidemiol 1999;20:676–84.
179. Best M, Sattar SA, Springthorpe VS, et al. Efficacies of selected disinfectants against *Mycobacterium tuberculosis*. J Clin Microbiol 1990;28:2234–9.
180. Best M, Kennedy ME, Coates F. Efficacy of a variety of disinfectants against *Listeria* spp. Appl Environ Microbiol 1990;56:377–80.
181. Springthorpe VS, Grenier JL, Lloyd-Evans N, et al. Chemical disinfection of human rotaviruses: efficacy of commercially-available products in suspension tests. J Hyg (Lond) 1986;97:139–61.
182. Akamatsu T, Tabata K, Hironga M, et al. Transmission of *Helicobacter pylori* infection via flexible fiberoptic endoscopy. Am J Infect Control 1996;24:396–401.
183. Resnick L, Veren K, Salahuddin SZ, et al. Stability and inactivation of HTLV-III/LAV under clinical and laboratory environments. JAMA 1986;255:1887–91.
184. Weber DJ, Barbee SL, Sobsey MD, et al. The effect of blood on the antiviral activity of sodium hypochlorite, a phenolic, and a quaternary ammonium compound. Infect Control Hosp Epidemiol 1999;20:821–7.
185. Rice EW, Clark RM, Johnson CH. Chlorine inactivation of *Escherichia coli* O157:H7. Emerg Infect Dis 1999;5:461–3.
186. Anderson RL, Carr JH, Bond WW, et al. Susceptibility of vancomycin-resistant enterococci to environmental disinfectants. Infect Control Hosp Epidemiol 1997;18:195–9.

187. Ayliffe GA, Collins BJ, Lowbury EJ, et al. Ward floors and other surfaces as reservoirs of hospital infection. J Hyg (Lond) 1967;65:515–36.
188. Palmer PH, Yeoman DM. A study to assess the value of disinfectants when washing ward floors. Med J Aust 1972;2:1237–9.
189. Centers for Disease Control and Prevention. Preventing the spread of vancomycin resistance—report from the Hospital Infection Control Practices Advisory Committee. Fed Regist 1994;59:25758–63.
190. Ayliffe GA, Collins BJ, Lowbury EJ. Cleaning and disinfection of hospital floors. BMJ 1966;5511:442–5.
191. Scott E, Bloomfield SF. The survival and transfer of microbial contamination via cloths, hand and utensils. J Appl Bacteriol 1990;68:271–8.
192. Rutala WA, Cole EC. Antiseptics and disinfectants—safe and effective? Infect Control 1984;5:215–8.
193. Rutala WA, Cole EC, Thomann CA, et al. Stability and bactericidal activity of chlorine solutions. Infect Control Hosp Epidemiol 1998;19:323–7.
194. Russell AD, McDonnell G. Concentration: a major factor in studying biocidal action. J Hosp Infect 2000;44:1–3.
195. Neely AN. A survey of gram-negative bacteria survival on hospital fabrics and plastics. J Burn Care Rehabil 2000;21:523–7.
196. Ayliffe GA, Collins DM, Lowbury EJ. Cleaning and disinfection of hospital floors. Br Med J 1966;2:442–5.
197. Scott E, Bloomfield SF. Investigations of the effectiveness of detergent washing, drying and chemical disinfection on contamination of cleaning cloths. J Appl Bacteriol 1990;68:279–83.
198. Weber DJ, Rutala WA. Occupational risks associated with the use of selected disinfectants and sterilants. In: Rutala WA, editor. Disinfection, sterilization, and antisepsis in healthcare. Champlain (NY): Polyscience Publications; 1998. p. 211–26.
199. Wysowski DK, Flynt JW Jr, Goldfield M, et al. Epidemic neonatal hyperbilirubinemia and use of a phenolic disinfectant detergent. Pediatrics 1978;61:165–70.
200. Doan HM, Keith L, Shennan AT. Phenol and neonatal jaundice. Pediatrics 1979; 64:324–5.
201. Occupational Safety and Health Administration. Occupational exposure to bloodborne pathogens; final rule. Fed Regist 1991;56:64003–182.
202. Occupational Safety and Health Administration. OSHA Memorandum from Stephen Mallinger. EPA-registered disinfectants for HIV/HBV. Washington, DC: Occupational Health and Safety Administration; 1997.
203. Environmental Protection Agency. Pesticides: regulating pesticides. 2003. Available at: http://www.epa.gov/oppad001/chemregindex.htm. Accessed December, 2010.
204. Chitnis V, Chitnis S, Patil S, et al. Practical limitations of disinfection of body fluid spills with 10,000 ppm sodium hypochlorite (NaOCl). Am J Infect Control 2004; 32:306–8.
205. Carling PC, Briggs JL, Perkins J, et al. Improved cleaning of patient rooms using a new targeting method. Clin Infect Dis 2006;42:385–8.
206. Carling PC, Parry MF, Rupp ME, et al. Improving cleaning of the environment surrounding patients in 36 acute care hospitals. Infect Control Hosp Epidemiol 2008;29:1035–41.
207. Carling PC, Parry MF, Von Beheren SM, et al. Identifying opportunities to enhance environmental cleaning in 23 acute care hospitals. Infect Control Hosp Epidemiol 2008;29:1–7.

208. Huang SS, Datta R, Platt R. Risk of acquiring antibiotic-resistant bacteria from prior room occupants. Arch Intern Med 2006;166:1945–51.

209. Drees M, Snydman DR, Schmid CH, et al. Prior environmental contamination increases the risk of acquisition of vancomycin-resistant enterococci. Clin Infect Dis 2008;46:678–85.

210. Shaughnessy M, Micielli R, Depestel D, et al. Evaluation of hospital room assignment and acquisition of Clostridium difficile associated diarrhea (CDAD), 48th Annual Interscience Conference on Antimicrobial Agents and Chemotherapy and the Infections Disease Society of America. Washington, DC, Abstract K-4194, 2008.

211. Boyce JM, Havill NL, Otter JA, et al. Impact of hydrogen peroxide vapor room decontamination on Clostridium difficile environmental contamination and transmission in a healthcare setting. Infect Control Hosp Epidemiol 2008;29:723–9.

212. French GL, Otter JA, Shannon KP, et al. Tackling contamination of the hospital environment by methicillin-resistant Staphylococcus aureus (MRSA): a comparison between conventional terminal cleaning and hydrogen peroxide vapour decontamination. J Hosp Infect 2004;57:31–7.

213. Bartels MD, Kristofferson K, Slotsbjerg T, et al. Environmental methicillin-resistant Staphylococcus aureus (MRSA) disinfection using dry-mist-generated hydrogen peroxide. J Hosp Infect 2008;70:35–41.

214. Hall L, Otter JA, Chewins J, et al. Use of hydrogen peroxide vapor for deactivation of Mycobacterium tuberculosis in a biological safety cabinet and a room. J Clin Microbiol 2007;45:810–5.

215. Hardy KJ, Gossain S, Henderson N, et al. Rapid recontamination with MRSA of the environment of an intensive care unit after decontamination with hydrogen peroxide vapour. J Hosp Infect 2007;66:360–8.

216. Johnston MD, Lawson S, Otter JA. Evaluation of hydrogen peroxide vapour as a method for the decontamination of surfaces contaminated with Clostridium botulinum spores. J Microbiol Methods 2005;60:403–11.

217. Heckert RA, Best M, Jordan LT, et al. Efficacy of vaporized hydrogen peroxide against exotic animal viruses. Appl Environ Microbiol 1997;63:3916–8.

218. Klapes NA, Vesley D. Vapor-phase hydrogen peroxide as a surface decontaminant and sterilant. Appl Environ Microbiol 1990;56:503–6.

219. Bates CJ, Pearse R. Use of hydrogen peroxide vapour for environmental control during a Serratia outbreak in a neonatal intensive care unit. J Hosp Infect 2005; 61:364–6.

220. Shapey S, Machin K, Levi K, et al. Activity of a dry mist hydrogen peroxide system against environmental Clostridium difficile contamination in elderly care wards. J Hosp Infect 2008;70:136–41.

221. Owens MU, Deal DR, Shoemaker MO, et al. High-dose ultraviolet C light inactivates spores of Bacillus subtilis var. niger and Bacillus anthracis Sterne on non-reflective surfaces. Appl Biosaf 2005;November:1–6 J Am Biological Safety Assoc.

Central Line–Associated Bloodstream Infections: Prevention and Management

David J. Weber, MD, MPH[a,b,]*, William A. Rutala, PhD, MPH[a,b]

KEYWORDS

- Central line catheters • Bloodstream infection • Antibiotics
- Antiseptics

Each year in the United States it is estimated that there are 1.7 million health care–associated infections (HAIs) resulting in approximately 99,000 deaths.[1] Of these deaths, approximately 31,000 are caused by bloodstream infections. Wenzel and Edmond[2] calculated that nosocomial bloodstream infections represented the eighth leading cause of death in the United States.

Overall, there are an estimated 249,000 bloodstream infections in United States hospitals each year.[1] These bloodstream infections have been estimated to increase the duration of hospitalization by 7 to 21 days.[3] Following a systematic review of literature, Stone and colleagues[4] estimated the attributable cost of a bloodstream infection as being between \$36,441 and \$37,078 (2002 dollars). More recently, Anderson and colleagues[5] calculated the cost of nosocomial bloodstream infections as \$23,242 ± \$5184 (2005 dollars).

DEFINITIONS

To understand the literature one must understand the terminology used to describe different types of catheters. A catheter can be defined by the type of vessel cannulated (eg, peripheral vein, central vein, artery); its planned duration (eg, short-term vs permanent); its site of insertion (eg, for central venous catheters: subclavian, femoral, internal jugular, or peripherally inserted central catheter [PICC]); the catheter's pathway from skin to vessel (eg, tunneled vs nontunneled); and special features (eg, germicide impregnated, presence or absence of a cuff). This article focuses on the prevention

[a] Division of Infectious Diseases, University of North Carolina School of Medicine, 2163 Bioinformatics, 130 Mason Farm Road, Chapel Hill, NC 27599-7030, USA
[b] Department of Hospital Epidemiology, University of North Carolina Health Care, 101 Manning Drive, Chapel Hill, NC 27514, USA
* Corresponding author. 2163 Bioinformatics, CB #7030, Chapel Hill, NC 27599–7030.
E-mail address: dweber@unch.unc.edu

Infect Dis Clin N Am 25 (2011) 77–102
doi:10.1016/j.idc.2010.11.012
0891-5520/11/\$ – see front matter © 2011 Elsevier Inc. All rights reserved.

id.theclinics.com

and management of central line–associated bloodstream infections (CLA-BSIs), as the greatest risk factor for nosocomial bloodstream infections is the presence of a central vascular catheter.[6]

PREVALENCE, INCIDENCE, AND IMPACT OF CLA-BSIS

In a 1-day point prevalence study during 1992 of 10,038 patients in 1417 European intensive care units (ICUs), Vincent and colleagues[7] reported that 12% had a bloodstream infection. A follow-up 1-day point prevalence study during 2007 of 13,796 adult patients in 1265 ICUs from 75 countries revealed that 15.1% had a bloodstream infection.[8] The prevalence of CLA-BSIs has not been determined but in the United States, it has been estimated that there are approximately 80,000 CLA-BSIs per year in ICUs.[9]

The premier surveillance systems for HAIs in the United States have been the National Nosocomial Infection Surveillance (NNIS) system and more recently the National Healthcare Safety Network (NHSN), managed by the Centers for Disease Control and Prevention (CDC). A major advantage of these systems is the use of strict definitions for reporting of CLA-BSIs.[10,11] Limitations of the data include that the hospitals in the surveillance systems are not randomly selected and that the participating hospitals vary from year to year. Hence, strictly speaking, data provided by these systems should not be compared across years. The rate of CLA-BSIs (primary bloodstream infections per 1000 central line-days) reported by NNIS from 2002 to 2004[12] has declined from the more recently reported data, 2006 to 2007, by NHSN (**Fig. 1**).[13] In the NHSN data the range of the pooled mean CLA-BSI rate varies approximately 5.5-fold among ICUs from 1.0 in pediatric medical ICUs to 5.6 in burn ICUs. However, the rate of CLA-BSIs among individual ICUs can vary more than 100-fold between the rates reported by the 10th- and 90th-percentile hospitals. Thus, there is much greater variation among reporting hospitals than among ICU types. The reason for this wide disparity in rates of CLA-BSIs in unknown but possibilities include: patient mix (ie, differences in the underlying risk factors among the ICUs), reporting

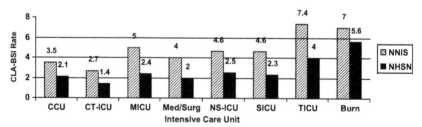

Fig. 1. CLA-BSI rates for NNIS (2002–2004) compared with NHSN (2006–2007). Rates are calculated as {(number of central line–associated bloodstream infections/number of central line-days)×1000}. Burn, burn ICU; CCU, coronary care unit; CLA-BSI, central line-associated bloodstream infection; CT-ICU, cardiothoracic ICU; ICU, intensive care unit; Med/Surg, Medical-Surgical (major teaching) ICU; MICU, medical ICU; NHSN, National Healthcare Safety Network; NNIS, National Nosocomial Infection Surveillance system; NS-ICU, neurosurgical ICU; SICU, surgical ICU; TICU, thoracic ICU. (*Adapted from* Centers for Disease Control and Prevention. National Nosocomial Infection Surveillance (NNIS) system report, data summary from January 1992 through June 2004, issued October 2004. Am J Infect Control 2004;32:470–85; and Edwards JR, Peterson KD, Andrus ML, et al. National Healthcare Safety Network (NHSN) report, data summary for 2006 through 2007, issued November 2008. Am J Infect Control 2008;36:609–26.)

bias (failure to count all cases or imprecision in applying NHSN definitions), or differences in adherence to recommended prevention guidelines.

Only limited data are available on the rate of CLA-BSIs outside of ICUs. Weber and colleagues[14] reported that rates of CLA-BSIs decreased from both surgical and medical ICUs compared with step-down units to floors (**Fig. 2**). Data from the NHSN system also showed lower rates among floor patients compared with ICU patients.[13]

The average attributable cost per patient of a CLA-BSI has been estimated to range between $14,806 and $27,520 using the Consumer Price Index for all urban consumers and between $19,633 and $28,508 using the Consumer Price Index for inpatient hospital services (2007 dollars).[15] Using these cost estimates and estimated number of CLA-BSIs provided by Klevens and colleagues,[1] the total cost of CLA-BSIs per year in the United States has been estimated at between $0.59 and $2.38 billion using the Consumer Price Index for all urban consumers, and between $0.67 and $2.68 billion using the Consumer Price Index for inpatient hospital services (2007 dollars).[15]

PATHOGENS

The pathogens causing nosocomial bloodstream infections and their associated mortality have been described in an analysis of 49 United States hospitals in the SCOPE surveillance system (**Fig. 3**).[16] The top 3 pathogens were all gram-positive cocci (ie, coagulase-negative *Staphylococcus*, *Staphylococcus aureus*, and *Enterococcus* spp). The SENTRY system monitored both health care- and community-acquired bloodstream infections from a sample of hospitals worldwide. Their data revealed that *S aureus* was the most frequent bloodstream pathogen in both hospital-acquired (23.6%) and community-acquired (23.7%) infections.[17] *Enterococcus* spp (11.0%), *Pseudomonas aeruginosa* (7.2%), *Acinetobacter* spp (2.9%), and *Serratia* spp (2.2%) were approximately 2-fold more common among nosocomial bacteremia than community-acquired bloodstream infections.[17] Conversely, *Escherichia coli* (12.2%) was approximately 2-fold and streptococci (3.6%) were approximately 4-fold less common as a cause of nosocomial bacteremia compared with community-acquired bloodstream infections.[17] *S aureus* and coagulase-negative strains causing nosocomial as opposed to community-acquired bacteremia have been reported to be more likely to be methicillin resistant, and *Enterococcus* spp causing nosocomial bacteremia were more likely to be vancomycin resistant.[18] The investigators attributed the higher frequency of coagulase-negative staphylococci

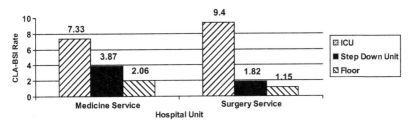

Fig. 2. CLA-BSI rates by hospital unit type. CLA-BSI, central line–associated bloodstream infection; ICU, intensive care unit. (*Data from* Weber DJ, Sickbert-Bennett EE, Brown V, et al. Comparison of hospitalwide surveillance and targeted intensive care unit surveillance of healthcare-associated infections. Infect Control Hosp Epidemiol 2007;28:1361–6.)

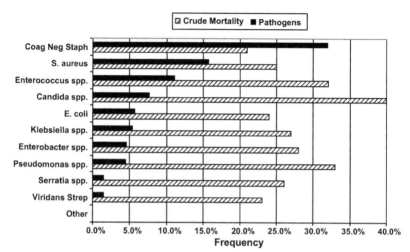

Fig. 3. Distribution of nosocomial bloodstream pathogens, 1995 to 1998. (*Data from* Edmond MB, Wallace SE, McClish DK, et al. Nosocomial bloodstream infections in United States hospitals: a three-year analysis. Clin Infect Dis 1999;29:239–44.)

found in the SCOPE surveillance system as compared with the SENTRY surveillance system to differences in the definitions of bacteremia, especially the use of a single positive culture of coagulase-negative staphylococci as defining the pathogen responsible for a bloodstream infection.[18]

The pathogens associated with CLA-BSIs in the United States have been ascertained for 2006 to 2007 by the NHSN system (**Fig. 4**).[19] Three of the top 5 pathogens

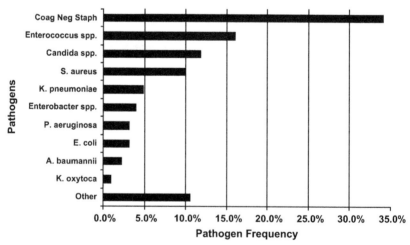

Fig. 4. Distribution of pathogens reported by NHSN for CLA-BSI, 2006 to 2007. CLA-BSI, central line–associated bloodstream infection; NHSN, National Healthcare Safety Network. (*Data from* Hidron AI, Edwards JR, Patel J, et al. Antimicrobial-resistant pathogens associated with healthcare-associated infections: annual summary of data reported to the National Healthcare Safety Network at the Centers for Disease Control and Prevention, 2006–2007. Infect Control Hosp Epidemiol 2008;29:996–1011.)

were gram-positive cocci (ie, coagulase-negative *Staphylococcus*, *S aureus*, and *Enterococcus* spp). The NHSN network has also reported the resistance of these pathogens to key antibiotics as follows: *S aureus*, oxacillin-66.8%; *Enterococcus faecium*, vancomyin-78.9%, ampicillin-90.5%; *Enterococcus faecalis*, vancomycin-7.5%, ampicillin-4.2%; *P aeruginosa*, fluoroquinoles-30.5%, piperacillin or piperacillin/tazobactam-20.2%, imipenem or meropenem-23.0%, ceftazidime-18.7%, cefepime-12.6%; *Klebsiella pneumoniae*, ceftriaxone or ceftazidime-27.1%, imipenem or meropenem or ertapenem-10.8%; *Klebsiella oxytoca*, ceftriaxone or ceftazidime-15.9%, imipenem or meropenem or ertapenem-29.2%; *Acinetobacter baumannii*, imipenem or meropenem-29.2%; and, *E coli*, fluoroquinoles-30.8%, ceftriaxome or ceftazidime-8.1%, imipenem or meropenem or ertapenem-30.8%.[19] A key determinant of the likelihood of isolating a resistant organism as the cause of a CLA-BSI has been shown to be duration of hospitalization. Patients hospitalized more than 7 days had on average a 2- to 3-fold increased risk of having an infection due to a pathogen resistant to a key antibiotic as compared with patients hospitalized for 7 days or less.[20]

PATHOGENESIS

Colonization of a central venous catheter is a prerequisite for infection.[21] Colonization most commonly occurs via migration of bacteria along the skin-catheter interface (extraluminal route) or via contamination of a hub (endoluminal route). For short-term use central venous catheters (ie, duration less than 7–10 days), the skin around the catheter insertion site is the most common source of organisms.[21,22] For long-term use central venous catheters, the most common source of organisms are contaminated hubs that are used to access the catheter.[23,24] Colonization less commonly occurs due to bacteremia from a secondary site (eg, urinary tract infection with bacteremia) or from a contaminated infusate.[21] Instilled fluids may in turn be contaminated either by the manufacturer (intrinsic contamination) or during manipulation by the facility (extrinsic contamination). Although bacteremia/fungemia from contaminated infusate has been considered to be rare, this problem may have been underestimated because infusates are rarely cultured. In a recent study, a contaminated infusate was responsible for 7% of CLA-BSI.[25]

RISK FACTORS FOR CLA-BSI

Independent risk factors for CLA-BSI reported in 2 or more published studies have included the following: (1) prolonged hospitalization before catheterization, (2) prolonged duration of catheterization, (3) heavy microbial colonization at the insertion site, (4) heavy microbial colonization of the catheter hub, (5) internal jugular catheterization, (6) neutropenia, (7) premature birth, (8) total parenteral nutrition through the catheter, and (9) substandard care of the catheter (eg, excessive manipulation of the catheter or reduced nurse-to-patient ratio).[26–28]

Female gender has been associated with a reduced risk of infection. A systematic review of the literature provided evidence that the subclavian site was associated with a lower risk of major infectious complications (sepsis with or without bacteremia) than the femoral site.[29] In addition, an extensive systematic review by Maki and colleagues[30] reported that the infection risk for implanted catheters using a subcutaneous venous port was substantially lower than for short-term noncuffed central venous catheters. For this reason, catheters with a subcutaneous venous port are preferred when patients require long-term central venous access.

PREVENTION
Basic Recommendations

Several guidelines and reviews have provided recommendations for the prevention of CLA-BSIs.[31–36] These recommendations are based on studies demonstrating a risk with failure to follow the recommendations as well as studies demonstrating effectiveness of the recommended procedures to reduce the risk of CLA-BSI. Recommendations of the most current guidelines from the Society of Healthcare Epidemiologists of America (SHEA) and the Infectious Disease Society of America (IDSA) are summarized in **Box 1**.

Key recommendations to prevent CLA-BSI at the time of insertion CLA-BSI include the following at the time of insertion[35]: (1) perform hand hygiene before catheter insertion[37–39]; (2) use an all-inclusive catheter cart or kit[40]; (3) use maximal sterile barrier precautions during central venous catheter insertion including a full-body drape over the patient[41–44]; (4) use a 2% chlorhexidine-based antiseptic for skin preparation in patients older than 2 months[45–49]; and (5) preferentially use the subclavian vein for placement of the central venous catheter (unless contraindicated).[29,41,50] In contrast to adults, studies in children have demonstrated that femoral catheters have a low incidence of mechanical complications and might have an infection rate similar to that of nonfemoral catheters.[51–53] The type of catheter selected should depend on its intended purpose and duration of use, risks and benefits of the particular catheter, and experience of the catheter operators. The use of dynamic 2-dimensional ultrasound for the placement of central venous catheters has been shown in 2 meta-analyses to substantially reduce mechanical complications and decrease the number of attempts required to successfully cannulate the vein.[54,55] Maximal sterile barrier precautions should also be used when exchanging a catheter over a guidewire.

Key recommendations to prevent CLA-BSI after insertion include the following[35]: (1) disinfect catheter hubs, needleless connectors, and injection ports before accessing the catheter[56–58]; (2) remove nonessential catheters[59,60]; and, (3) replace administration sets not used for blood, blood products, or lipids at intervals not longer than 96 hours.[61] Topical antibiotic ointment or creams should not be used on the insertion site, except for dialysis catheters, because of their potential to promote fungal infection and antimicrobial resistance.[62,63] Systemic antibiotics should not be administered as prophylaxis either before insertion or during use on an intravascular catheter to prevent catheter colonization or CLA-BSI.[64]

Several other interventions have demonstrated value in reducing CLA-BSIs and should be considered for use in locations and/or populations within hospitals that have unacceptably high CLA-BSI rates despite implementation of the basic CLA-BSI prevention strategies listed above.

Antibiotic- or Antiseptic-Impregnated Central Venous Catheters

Background

More than 20 randomized clinical trials have evaluated the use of antiseptic or antibiotic impregnated central venous catheters to reduce the rate of CLA-BSIs. These studies have been summarized in several recent systematic reviews, which also included a meta-analysis.[65–69] The most common germicides used to impregnate catheters have been chlorhexidine-silver sulfadiazine and minocycline-rifampin. Other agents studied have included heparin, benzalkonium chloride, silver, silver-platinum-carbon, and miconazole-rifampin. First-generation catheters were coated only on the exterior surface whereas current second-generation catheters are coated on both internal and external surfaces with the germicide(s).

Efficacy of antibiotic- or antiseptic-impregnated central venous catheters
The several recent systematic reviews[65–69] provide excellent analyses of the many randomized clinical trials of anti-infective impregnated catheters. However, it must be noted that the different reviews may have chosen different time periods for reviewing the literature, chosen different patient populations, used different methods for abstracting and analyzing different studies, and chosen different methods for performing a meta-analysis. Thus, the number of articles used in the analysis differed as follows: Niel-Weise and colleagues,[65] 21 trials; Niel-Weise and colleagues,[66] 9 trials; Casey and colleagues,[67] 34 trials, Ramitu and colleagues,[68] 34 trials, and Hockenhull and colleagues,[69] 38 trials.

Consistent conclusions among the systematic reviews were as follows. First, the methodologic quality of most of the studies was judged to be generally poor.[65–67,69] Second, differences in the type of impregnated catheter used (ie, specific agents incorporated into the catheter), the generation of the catheter used (ie, first or second generation), and the comparator (ie, a control catheter without an anti-infective or a different anti-infective catheter) resulted in small numbers of similar studies for comparison and hence limited the power of the meta-analyses. Third, the use of an anti-infective catheter versus a standard catheter reduced the risk of CLA-BSI.[65,67–69] The studies suggested a decreased risk of approximately 1.5- to 3.0-fold. Fourth, catheters coated with both chlorhexidine-silver sulfadiazine and minocycline-rifampin were effective in reducing both colonization and CLA-BSIs. Fifth, trials comparing minocycline-rifampin–impregnated catheters with chlorhexidine-silver sulfadiazine–impregnated catheters have shown inconsistent results and therefore neither catheter has demonstrated superiority for preventing CLS-BSIs. Sixth, catheters coated with other agents such as benzalkonium chloride, miconazole-rifampin, or platinum-silver have not demonstrated benefit.

Risks that impregnated catheters will precipitate microbial resistance
Clinical resistance associated with chlorhexidine-silver sulfadiazine has not been reported. Given the multiple mechanisms of action of antiseptics, the development of resistance would seem to be unlikely.[70]

Although in vitro studies have shown that resistance to either rifampin or minocycline may occur if either antibiotic (especially rifampin) is used alone, they have demonstrated that resistance to the combination is very unlikely.[71,72] To date, at least 4 prospective randomized trials have evaluated the skin at the catheter insertion site before and after the insertion of the minocycline-rifampin catheter and have failed to detect any emergence of resistance.[73–76]

Guideline recommendations
The number needed to treat (NNT) to prevent a single CLA-BSI has ranged from 12 to 182, with baseline risks ranging from 1% to 10%.[65] The higher the facilities baseline rate of CLA-BSI, the more useful it would seem to use an anti-infective catheter. The value of these catheters when used as part of a "bundle" to reduce the risk of CLA-BSIs has not been evaluated. Based on these data, the recent SHEA/IDSA Guideline recommends the use of an antiseptic-impregnated (eg, chlorhexidine-silver sulfadiazine) or antimicrobial (eg, minocycline-rifampin) coated catheter in the following circumstances.[35] First, the hospital units or patient populations have a CLA-BSI rate higher than the institutional goal, despite compliance with base CLA-BSI prevention practices. Second, patients have limited venous access and a history of recurrent CLA-BSI. Third, patients are at heightened risk for severe

Box 1
Summary of SHEA/IDSA guidelines for the prevention of CLA-BSIs

Basic practices for prevention and monitoring of CLA-BSI: recommended for all acute care hospitals

Before insertion

1. Educate health care personnel involved in the insertion and maintenance of central venous catheters (CVCs) about CLA-BSI prevention (A-II).

At insertion

1. Use a catheter checklist to ensure adherence to infection prevention practices at the time of CVC insertion (B-II).

   Use a checklist to ensure and document compliance with aseptic technique.

   CVC insertion should be observed by a nurse, physician, or other health care personnel who has received appropriate education, to ensure that the aseptic technique is maintained.

   These health care personnel should be empowered to stop the procedure if breaches in aseptic technique are observed.

2. Perform hand hygiene before catheter insertion or manipulation (B-II).

   Use an alcohol-based waterless product or antiseptic soap and water.

   Use of gloves does not obviate hand hygiene.

3. Avoid using the femoral vein for central venous access in adult patients (A-I).

   Use of the femoral access site is associated with greater risk of infection and deep venous thrombosis in adults.

   Increased risk of infection with femoral catheters may be limited to overweight adult patients with a body mass index greater than 24.8.

   Femoral vein catheterization can be done without general anesthesia in children and has not been associated with an increased risk of infection in children.

   Several nonrandomized studies show that the subclavian vein is associated with a lower risk of CLA-BSI than is the jugular vein, but the risks and benefits in light of potential infectious and noninfectious complications must be considered on an individual basis when determining which insertion site to use.

   The use of peripherally inserted central venous catheters is not an evidence-based strategy to reduce the risk of CLA-BSI.

4. Use an all-inclusive catheter cart or kit (B-II).

5. Use maximum sterile barrier precautions during central venous catheter insertion (A-I).

   Use maximal sterile barrier precautions.

   A mask, cap, sterile gown, and sterile gloves are to be worn by all health care personnel involved in the catheter insertion procedure.

   The patient is to be covered with a large sterile drape during catheter insertion.

   These measures must also be followed when exchanging a catheter over a guidewire.

6. Use a chlorhexidine-based antiseptic for skin preparation in patients older than 2 months (A-I).

   Before catheter insertion, apply an alcohol chlorhexidine solution containing 0.5% chlorhexidine to the insertion site.

   The antiseptic solution must be allowed to dry before making the skin puncture.

   For children younger than 2 months use a povidone-iodine solution.

After insertion

1. Disinfect catheter hubs, needleless connectors, and injection ports before accessing the catheter (B-II).

   Before accessing the catheter hubs or injection ports, clean them with an alcohol chlorhexidine preparation or 70% alcohol to reduce contamination.

2. Remove nonessential catheters (A-II).

   Assess the need for continued intravascular access on a daily basis during multidisciplinary rounds. Remove catheters not required for patient care.

3. For nontunneled central venous catheters in adults and adolescents, change transparent dressings and perform site care with a chlorhexidine-based antiseptic every 5–7 days or more frequently if the dressing is soiled, loose, or damp; change gauze dressings every 2 days or more frequently if the dressing is soiled, loose, or damp (A-I).

4. Replace administration sets not used for blood, blood products, or lipids at intervals not longer than 96 hours (A-II).

5. Use antimicrobial ointments for hemodialysis catheter insertion sites (A-I).

   Povidone-iodine or polysporin ointment should be applied to hemodialysis catheter insertion sites in patients with a history of recurrent *S aureus* CLA-BSI.

   Mupirocin ointment should not be applied to the catheter insertion site due to the risks of mupirocin resistance and damage to the polyurethane catheters.

---

sequelae from a CLA-BSI (eg, patients with recently implanted intravascular access devices, such as a prosthetic heart valve or aortic graft).

At present, anti-infective catheters are not approved by the Food and Drug Administration (FDA) for use in children. However, preliminary data suggest that they appear to be safe and may be effective in pediatric patients.[77,78]

Chlorhexidine Washes

Chlorhexidine is widely used as an antiseptic in health care because of its excellent antimicrobial activity, prolonged residual effect, and rapidity of action.[37,79,80] It has good activity against gram-positive bacteremia but somewhat less activity against gram-negative bacilli and fungi. Several studies have demonstrated a reduction in CLA-BSI rates in an intensive care setting with daily bathing with a chlorhexidine solution[81,82] or daily washing with a 2% chlorhexidine-impregnated washcloth.[83] For example, daily washing with a 2% chlorhexidine-impregnated washcloth was shown in a cross-over study conducted in a medical ICU to significantly reduce primary bloodstream infections (4.3/1000 patient-days in the intervention arm vs 10.4/1000 patient-days in the control arm, $P<.05$).[83] Using a before-after study design, Munoz-Price and colleagues[81] showed that daily baths with 2% chlorhexidine resulted in a net reduction of 99% in CLA-BSIs in a long-term acute care hospital. Using a similar design, Climo and colleagues[82] demonstrated a reduction in the incidence of vancomycin-resistant *Enterococcus* spp bacteremia in ICUs.

Antiseptic-Impregnated Sponge Dressing Placed at the Catheter Exit Site

A chlorhexidine-impregnated sponge ($\sim$2.5 cm in diameter) that is used to cover the exit site of a central venous catheter has been demonstrated to reduce bloodstream infections in several studies.[84–86] A meta-analysis of studies using this chlorhexidine-impregnated sponge showed its use was associated with a trend toward reduction of CLA-BSIs.[87] More recently, in a very large randomized, controlled trial of the chlorhexidine-impregnated sponge versus standard dressings, Timsit and colleagues[86] reported that the impregnated sponge significantly reduced the incidence of CLA-BSI (per 1000 catheter-days) from 1.3 to 0.4. Severe chlorhexidine-related contact dermatitis occurred in 8 patients (5.3 per 1000 catheter-days). Based on the earlier data, the SHEA/IDSA guideline recommends considering the addition of this dressing in several circumstances including: (1) hospital units or patient populations have a CLA-BSI rate higher than the institutional goal, despite compliance with an evidence-based prevention bundle; (2) patients have limited venous access and a history of recurrent CLA-BSI; or (3) patients are at heightened risk for severe sequelae from CLA-BSI (eg, patients with a recently implanted intravascular device, such as prosthetic heart valve or aortic graft).

Anti-Infective "Locks" to Prevent CLA-BSIs

Anti-infective locks are created by filling the lumen of the catheter with a supraphysiologic concentration of an antimicrobial solution or a germicide, and leaving the solution in place until the catheter hub is reaccessed.[35] Antibiotics used to prophylactically flush or lock central venous catheters have included vancomycin, cefazolin, cefotaxime, ceftazidime, gentamicin, amikacin ciprofloxacin, and minocycline. Antiseptics have included alcohol, taurolidine, and trisodium citrate (the latter 2 agents are not approved for this use in the United States). These agents have usually been combined with a compound acting as an anticoagulant, such as heparin or EDTA (ethylenediaminetetraacetic acid). Assessing the value of lock "prophylaxis" is difficult, as most studies have been relatively small and have focused only on a high-risk population (eg, hemodialysis, neutropenic patients, neonates). The potential benefits of lock prophylaxis must be weighed against potential risks such as toxicity (eg, ethanol), allergic reactions, and emergence of bacterial resistance. At present there are no FDA-approved formulations for use in lock prophylaxis.

Systematic reviews of the literature have been published focusing on either specific anti-infectives used as the lock solution such as urokinase-heparin,[88] vancomycin,[89] or ethanol,[90] or focusing on specific patient populations and catheters such as hemodialysis catheters.[91–95] In a meta-analysis, vancomycin used as a lock solution in high-risk patient populations being treated with long-term central venous catheters was demonstrated to confer a benefit with a risk ratio of 0.34 ($P = .04$).[89] However, most studies included in the meta-analysis used total implantable catheters or tunneled catheters. Similarly, ethanol has been assessed in several small studies with a variety of tunneled or implantable catheters and has showed promise.[90] Although several randomized studies have shown a benefit in using a anti-infective instilled as a lock solution, it is difficult to make specific recommendations because of differences among the studies, including type of catheter (indwelling or percutaneous), germicide used, and patient population.[95–98] The recent SHEA/IDSA guideline recommends that anti-infective locks be used as part of a preventive strategy only in the following circumstances.[35] First, prophylaxis for patients with limited venous access and a history of recurrent CLA-BSIs; second, patients who are at heightened risk for severe sequelae from a CLA-BSI.

Approaches that Should Not be Considered a Routine Part of CLA-BSI Prevention

The most recent SHEA/IDSA guideline lists several approaches that should not be used to prevent CLA-BSIs including the following.[35] First, antimicrobial prophylaxis for short-term tunneled catheters should not be used either for insertion or while catheters are in use. Second, central venous catheters should not be routinely replaced.

Finally, positive-pressure needleless connectors with mechanical valves should not be routinely used.

Evidence that Implementation of Guidelines Prevents CLA-BSI

The current guidelines emphasize education of persons inserting and maintaining central venous catheters regarding methods to prevent CLA-BSI. The key in preventing infections is adherence to strict aseptic technique in inserting and maintaining the catheters. In 2004, the Institute for Healthcare Improvement (IHI) launched the 100,000 Lives Campaign.[99] This initiative introduced 2 concepts, the first being the use of a "bundle" of interventions for reducing HAIs. For prevention of CLA-BSI the bundle included at insertion hand hygiene, maximal barrier precautions, chlorhexidine skin antisepsis, and optimal catheter site selection (subclavian vein preferred site in adults for nontunneled catheters), as well as daily review of line necessity with prompt removal of unnecessary lines. The second concept was measurement of adherence with these process measures, and frequent feedback of adherence to the staff who insert and maintain catheters.

Increased education of staff with implementation of bundles, checklists, and/or central line carts has been demonstrated to significantly reduce CLA-BSI.[100–103]

DIAGNOSIS
Bloodstream Infections

In evaluating a new fever in an ICU patient, blood cultures should be obtained when clinical evaluation does not strongly suggest a noninfectious source.[104] Blood cultures should also be obtained when bacteremia/fungemia is suspected in non-ICU patients with a fever or other signs of sepsis. Cultures should always be obtained before the initiation of antibiotics.[105] Before obtaining a blood culture from a peripheral vein, skin disinfection should preferentially be performed with 2% chlorhexidine gluconate in 70% isopropyl alcohol.[104] Acceptable alternatives include alcohol or tincture of iodine (1%–2% iodine in alcohol) but not povidone-iodine.[105] The yield of detecting bacteremia/fungemia via a blood culture increases with the amount of blood drawn per culture[105–107] and the number of cultures obtained.[108,109] In adults 20 to 30 mL should be drawn at a single time from a single site. For ICU febrile patients (other than neonates), one should obtain 3 to 4 sets of blood cultures within the first 24 hours of the onset of fever.

For patients with a central venous line, one blood culture should be drawn by venipuncture and at least one culture should be drawn through the catheter,[104] because blood cultures obtained through a catheter are associated with a higher rate of false-positive results than percutaneously obtained cultures.[110,111] Ideally, the distal port of the catheter should be used to obtain the culture. Before obtaining cultures, the catheter hub should be disinfected with alcohol, tincture of iodine, or alcoholic chlorhexidine (>0.5%), allowing adequate drying time to mitigate blood culture contamination.[105] For cultures of an anti-infective catheter tip, specific inhibitors should be used in the culture media.[105]

CLA-BSI

Background
Prospective studies have demonstrated that 25% to 45% of episodes of sepsis in patients with central venous catheters represent true device-related bloodstream infection.[112] Recommendations for diagnosing central venous catheter-associated infections that include detailed diagnostic algorithms have been published.[105,113,114] Central venous catheters are associated with several infective processes. Exit-site

infections are characterized by erythema, induration, and/or tenderness within 2 cm of the catheter exit site; they may also be associated with other signs and symptoms of infection, including fever and purulent discharge from the exit site. Tunnel infections are characterized by tenderness, erythema, and/or induration greater than 2 cm from the catheter exit site, and along the subcutaneous track of a tunneled catheter. Pocket infections are defined as infected fluid in the subcutaneous pocket of a total implanted intravascular device and are often associated with tenderness, erythema, and/or induration over the pocket. Spontaneous rupture and drainage, or necrosis of the overlying skin may occur. All 3 infective processes (ie, exit site, tunnel infection, and pocket infection) may or may not be associated with bacteremia or fungemia. When catheter infection is suspected and there is a catheter exit exudate, the drainage should be collected and sent for Gram strain and culture.[105] Phlebitis, which may result in induration, erythema, warmth, pain, and/or tenderness around the catheter exit site, may mimic infection.

Catheter colonization is defined as significant growth of a microorganism in a quantitative or semiquantitative culture of the catheter tip, subcutaneous catheter segment, or catheter hub. Catheter colonization is a major risk factor for catheter-related bloodstream infection.

Clues to a colonized catheter being the source of bacteremia or fungemia include the following: high-grade bacteremia or fungemia (ie, multiple positive cultures); abrupt onset of fever and symptoms, especially with shock; symptoms/signs of sepsis (eg, hypotension) without obvious source (ie, no identifiable site); evidence of septic thrombophlebitis of the central vein in which the catheter resides; continued bacteremia/fungemia despite appropriate anti-infective therapy; symptoms/signs of sepsis plus catheter malfunction; or bacteremia/fungemia with certain organisms (ie, coagulase-negative staphylococci, *Candida* spp, *Malassizia* spp, *Bacillus* spp, atypical mycobacteria, or *Corynebacterium jeikeium*).

The IDSA Guideline has suggested one of the two following microbiological methods to confirm diagnosis of CLA-BSI.[105] First, simultaneous quantitative blood cultures drawn through the central venous catheter and peripheral vein with at least a 3-fold greater colony count from the blood obtained from the catheter hub than that obtained from the peripheral vein. Second, differential time to positivity with the growth of microbes from a blood sample drawn from a catheter hub at least 2 hours before microbial growth is detected in a blood sample obtained from a peripheral vein. The IDSA states that growth of more than 15 colony-forming units (CFU) from a 5-cm segment of the catheter tip by semiquantitative (roll-plate) culture or growth of greater than 10^2 CFU from a catheter by a quantitative (sonication) broth culture reflects catheter colonization. The isolation of the same organism(s) from a peripheral blood culture and from a culture of the catheter tip provides a definitive diagnosis of CLA-BSI.

Microbiologic methods for the diagnosis of CLA-BSI are summarized in **Table 1** and are discussed below. Cultures of catheters should only be performed when catheter-related bloodstream infection is suspected. No single test is clearly superior for the diagnosis of CLA-BSI with short-term catheters. For the diagnosis of CLA-BSI in patients with long-term catheters, quantitative blood cultures are the most accurate test, but differential time to positivity also has a high degree of accuracy.

Simultaneous quantitative blood culture

Obtaining paired quantitative blood cultures simultaneously from a central venous catheter and via a peripheral venipuncture has been demonstrated to be both sensitive and specific for the diagnosis of CLA-BSI.[115–118] The IDSA recommended using as a cutoff at least a 3-fold greater colony count from the catheter than for blood obtained from a peripheral vein as the predictor for CLA-BSI.

Differential time to positivity of blood cultures drawn via the catheter versus via venipuncture

Differential time to positivity of simultaneous qualitative blood cultures obtained through the catheter and via a peripheral venipuncture is now widely used due to its simplicity and accuracy.[119–125] Current radiometric blood culture systems, in which blood cultures are continuously monitored from growth, make it easy to assess the differential time to positivity. A CLA-BSI should be highly suspected if both sets of blood cultures yield the same organism and the set drawn via the catheter becomes positive 120 minutes or more earlier than the culture drawn peripherally. The interpretation of this diagnostic method could be compromised if antibiotics are given intraluminally at the time of drawing blood through the catheter, in which case colonized catheters may become falsely negative.[113]

Other diagnostic methods that do not require catheter removal

A single quantitative blood culture drawn through a central venous catheter has been shown to be useful in the diagnosis of CLA-BSI.[115,126,127] The best threshold for defining infection appears to be greater than or equal to 100 CFU/mL. Unfortunately, this method cannot distinguish between high-grade bacteremia and CLA-BSI.

Endoluminal brush consists of passing a tapered nylon brush on a steel wire though the catheter hub and lumen, withdrawing the brush, and immediately placing it in a transport container. The container is sonicated and vortexed, and microbes are detected by the pour plate method. As this technique has important risks including arrhythmias, embolization, and inciting bacteremia, it has not been widely used.[113]

Blood drawn via a catheter can be centrifuged and stained with acridine orange. Although the technique has exhibited good sensitivity (improved by acridine orange staining followed by a Gram stain), it has not gained wide acceptance.[113]

Semiquantitative culture of a subcutaneous segment of the catheter (roll-plate)

The semiquantitative roll-plate method for culturing the distal tip of a central venous catheter is a well-described and validated method for detecting catheter colonization.[128–131] The catheter tip (5-cm segment) is rolled at least 4 times against a blood agar plate and then incubated overnight; a colony count of at least 15 CFU suggests catheter colonization. A diagnosis of CLA-BSI is made if the same organism(s) is isolated from a peripheral blood culture and the catheter tip. However, as the method only detects extraluminal contamination, it is less accurate for detecting colonization of long-term (ie, >30 days) catheters in which intraluminal contamination is more common.

Quantitative culture of subcutaneous catheter segments

Several methods have been developed to obtain organisms colonizing both the intraluminal and extraluminal catheter surfaces including sonication,[130,132] vortexing,[133] and centrifugation.[134] Sonication, the most common method, involves placing a 5-cm catheter segment in a 10-mL broth container and then sonicating the container for 1 minute followed by vortexing for 15 seconds; 0.1 mL of the sonicated/vortexed broth and 0.1 mL of a 1:100 dilution of the broth are streaked on blood agar plates and incubated at 35°C.[113] A count of greater than 100 CFU/mL is considered positive.

Table 1
Laboratory methods for diagnosing central line-associated bloodstream infections (CLA-BSI)

Method	Diagnostic Criteria	Advantages	Disadvantages	Sensitivity	Specificity
Simultaneous quantitative blood cultures	Blood culture via catheter yields CFU ≥3× higher than CFU via peripheral vein	Recommended by the IDSA Defines CLA-BSI Does not require catheter removal	Very labor intensive Costly	93%	97%–100%
Differential time to positivity of blood culture via catheter versus peripheral vein	Blood culture via catheter turns positive ≥2 h before simultaneous culture from peripheral vein	Recommended by IDSA Defines CLA-BSI Does not require catheter removal Data currently available with most automated blood culture systems	Use of antibiotics via catheter (or use of lock) may impair interpretation	89%–90%	72%–87%
Quantitative blood culture via catheter	Blood culture via catheter is ≥100 CFU/mL	Does not require catheter removal	Unable to differentiate between CLA-BSI and high-grade bacteremia	81%–86%	85%–96%
Acridine orange leukocyte cytospin	Presence of any organisms	Does not require catheter removal	Limited data of utility	87%	94%
Endoluminal brush	Quantitative culture >100 CFU/mL	Does not require catheter removal	Limited data of utility May precipitate arrhythmia, embolization May cause bacteremia	95%	84%
Semiquantitative culture of catheter tip	≥15 CFU/mL from 5-cm segment of catheter tip (reflects catheter colonization)	Recommended by IDSA Defines catheter colonization (same organism isolated from peripheral vein defines CLA-BSI) Available in most hospital labs	Requires catheter removal Most obtain SQ catheter segment aseptically Does not allow culture of intraluminal organisms	45%–84%	85%

Method	Definition	Advantages	Disadvantages/Comments	Sensitivity	Specificity
Qualitative culture of catheter tip	$\geq 10^2$ CFU from 5 cm segment of catheter tip (reflects catheter colonization)	Recommended by IDSA Defines catheter colonization (same organism isolated from peripheral vein defines CLA-BSI) Excellent sensitivity and specificity	Requires catheter removal Most obtain SQ catheter segment aseptically More labor intensive than semiquantitative method	82%–83%	89%–97%
Qualitative culture of catheter tip	Any growth	Simple for lab to perform	Specifically NOT recommended by IDSA Requires catheter removal Most obtain SQ catheter tip aseptically Less accurate than semiquantitative or quantitative methods	79%–96%	72%–78%
Microscopy of Gram-stained SQ catheter segment	Direct visualization of organisms	Results rapidly available May aid in treatment decisions (ie, may detect gram-positive cocci, gram-negative bacilli)	Requires catheter removal Limited data of utility Only detects extraluminal colonization	84%–100%	97%–100%
Microscopy of acridine orange-stained SQ catheter segment	Direct visualization of organisms	Result rapidly available May aid in treatment decisions (ie, may detect gram-positive cocci, gram-negative bacilli)	Requires catheter removal Limited studies demonstrating utility Only detects extraluminal colonization	84%–100%	97%–100%

Abbreviations: IDSA, Infectious Disease Society of America; SQ, subcutaneous.

Data from Raad I, Hanna H, Maki D. Intravascular catheter-related infections: advances in diagnosis, prevention, and management. Lancet Infect Dis 2007;7: 645–57; Eggimann P. Diagnosis of intravascular catheter infection. Curr Opin Infect Dis 2007;353–9; and Mermel LA, Allon M, Bouza E, et al. Clinical practice guidelines for the diagnosis and management of intravascular catheter-related infection: 2009 update by the Infectious Disease Society of America. Clin Infect Dis 2009;49:1–45.

Other diagnostic methods requiring catheter removal

Microscopy of removed catheters has been done following staining with Gram stain or acridine orange. However, these techniques have not been widely used because they are considered to be labor intensive.

SURVEILLANCE OF CLA-BSI

A consensus guideline recommends that all hospitals measure their CLA-BSI rate using the definitions developed by the NHSN.[35] The numerator consists of the number of CLA-BSIs in each unit assessed. The denominator consists of total number of catheter days in each unit assessed. This ratio (ie, CLA-BSI/number of catheter days) is multiplied by 1000 so that the measure is expressed as number of CLA-BSIs per 1000 catheter days. The CDC recommends that surveillance should be undertaken in the following units: ICUs, special care areas (eg, bone marrow transplant units), neonatal ICUs, and any other inpatient location in the facility where denominator data can be collected. It is recommended that hospitals benchmark their data using the published reports from the NHSN network.[13] The data should be risk adjusted by stratifying by type of patient-care unit.

The NHSN criteria for defining a CLA-BSI are available on the NHSN Web site (http://www.cdc.gov/nhsn/PDFs/pscManual/4PSC_CLABScurrent.pdf). In brief, a central venous catheter is defined as an intravascular catheter that terminates at or close to the heart or in one of the great vessels (eg, aorta, superior or inferior vena cava, internal jugular vein, subclavian vein), which is used for infusion, withdrawal of blood, or hemodynamic monitoring. For patients older than 1 year laboratory-confirmed CLA-BSI must meet one of the following criteria. (1) Patient has a recognized pathogen cultured from one or more blood cultures and the organism cultured from blood is not related to an infection at another site. (2) Patient has at least one of the following signs or symptoms: fever, chills, or hypotension; signs and symptoms and positive laboratory results are not related to an infection at another site; and common skin contaminant (ie, diphtheroids [*Corynebacterium* spp], *Bacillus* [not *B anthracis*] spp, *Propionibacterium* spp, coagulase-negative staphylococci [including *S epidermis*], viridans group streptococci, *Aerococcus* spp, *Micrococcus* spp) is cultured from 2 or more blood cultures drawn at separate locations. Additional details regarding the NHSN surveillance definitions and methods are available on the CDC Web page.

MANAGEMENT OF CLA-BSI
General Recommendations

The management of CLA-BSI has been recently reviewed (**Box 2**).[105,113,135,136] If the patient has severe sepsis or septic shock, additional therapy is warranted.[137] The following recommendations for management are largely based on the most current IDSA guideline.[105] Empiric therapy is often initiated for suspected CLA-BSI. The initial choice of antibiotics depends on the patient's risk factors for infection, underlying diseases, and likely pathogens associated with the specific intravascular device.[105] As gram-positive cocci are the most common pathogen causing CLA-BSI, vancomycin is the drug of choice for empiric therapy. If the health care facility has a preponderance of methicillin-resistant *S aureus* isolates with a minimum inhibitory concentration for vancomycin greater than 2 µg/mL or the patient has a contraindication to vancomycin, the preferred alternative is daptomycin.[138] Initial therapy for gram-negative bacilli should be based on local frequency patterns of different pathogens and local antimicrobial susceptibility data (eg, fourth-generation cephalosporin, carbapenem, or β-lactam/β-lactamase combination with or without an aminoglycoside). Empiric

Box 2
Approach to the management of patients with CLA-BSI

Short-term central venous catheter related bloodstream infection

Uncomplicated: Bloodstream infection and fever resolves within 72 hours in a patient who has no intravascular hardware and no evidence of endocarditis or supportive thrombophlebitis. For infections due to *S aureus* patient is also without malignancy or immunosuppression.

1. Coagulase-negative staphylococci

   Remove catheter and treat with systemic antibiotics for 5–7 days.

   If catheter is retained, treat with a systemic antibiotic and antibiotic lock therapy for 10–14 days.

2. *Staphylococcus aureus*

   Remove catheter and treat with systemic antibiotics for $\geq$14 days.

3. *Enterococcus* spp

   Remove catheter and treat with systemic antibiotics for 7–14 days.

4. Gram-negative bacilli

   Remove catheter and treat with systemic antibiotics for 7–14 days.

5. *Candida* spp

   Remove catheter and treat with antifungal therapy for 14 days after the first negative blood culture.

Complicated

1. Suppurative thrombophlebitis, endocarditis, or osteomyelitis

   Remove catheter and treat with systemic antibiotics for 4–6 weeks; 6–8 weeks for osteomyelitis in adults.

Long-term central venous catheter or port-related bacteremia or fungemia

Uncomplicated infection

1. Coagulase-negative *Staphylococcus*

   May retain catheter/port and use systemic antibiotics for 10–14 days.

   Remove catheter or port if there is clinical deterioration, persisting or relapsing bacteremia; workup for complicated infection and treat accordingly.

2. *Staphylococcus aureus*

   Remove the infected catheter/port and treat with 4–6 weeks of antimicrobial therapy, unless the patient has exceptions listed in Guideline.[a]

3. *Enterococcus* spp

   May retain catheter/port and use systemic antibiotic lock therapy for 7–14 days.

   Remove catheter or port if there is clinical deterioration, persisting or relapsing bacteremia; workup for complicated infection and treat accordingly.

4. Gram-negative bacilli

   Remove catheter/port and treat for 7–14 days.

   For catheter/port salvage, use systemic and antibiotic lock therapy for 10–14 days; if no response, remove catheter/port, rule out endocarditis or suppurative thrombophlebitis, and if not present treat with antibiotics for 10–14 days.

5. *Candida* spp

   Remove catheter/port and treat with antifungal therapy for 14 days after the first negative blood culture.

[a] *Adapted from* Mermel LA, Allon M, Bouza E, et al. Clinical practice guidelines for the diagnosis and management of intravascular catheter-related infection: 2009 update by the Infectious Disease Society of America. Clin Infect Dis 2009;49:1–45.

antibiotics should be chosen that cover *P aeruginosa* in patients who are neutropenic, septic, or known to be colonized with *P aeruginosa*. In critically ill patients with a femoral line, empiric therapy should cover gram-negative bacilli and *Candida* spp. Also, empiric coverage should include agents active against gram-negative bacilli and *Candida* spp in patients with any of the following risk factors: total parenteral nutrition, prolonged use of broad-spectrum antibiotics, hematologic malignancy, stem cell transplantation, solid organ transplantation, femoral catheterization, or multisite colonization with *Candida* spp.

Catheter Removal

For short-term catheters, removal is recommended for CLA-BSI caused by gram-negative bacilli, *S aureus*, *Enterococcus* spp, fungi, and mycobacteria. In the setting of CLA-BSI, antibiotic lock therapy may be attempted to salvage a central venous line colonized with coagulase-negative staphylococci.

Long-term catheters should be removed from patients with CLA-BSI if any of the following conditions are present: severe sepsis; suppurative thrombophlebitis; endocarditis; bloodstream infection that continues despite more than 72 hours of antimicrobial therapy to which the infecting pathogens are susceptible; or infections due to *S aureus*, *P aeruginosa*, fungi, or mycobacteria. In uncomplicated CLA-BSI involving long-term catheters, due to pathogens other than *S aureus*, *P aeruginosa*, *Bacillus* spp, *Micrococcus* spp, propionibacteria, fungi, or mycobacteria, catheter salvage might be attempted in select patients, such as those who have limited vascular access options and who require long-term intravascular access for survival. When treatment is attempted without catheter removal, both systemic and lock therapy should be used. If catheter salvage is attempted, additional blood cultures should be obtained and the catheter removed if blood culture results remain positive following 72 hours or more of appropriate antibiotic therapy.

Antibiotic Lock Therapy

Antibiotic lock therapy has showed great promise in permitting salvage of infected catheters. For CLA-BSI it should only be used in conjunction with systemic antimicrobial therapy, with both regimens administered for 7 to 14 days. Lock therapy may be used to attempt salvage of short-term catheters colonized with coagulase-negative staphylococci. It may be indicated for attempted salvage of long-term catheters without signs/symptoms of exit site or tunnel infections in patients for whom catheter salvage is indicated (see **Box 2**). For patients with negative peripheral blood cultures and multiple positive cultures drawn via the catheter, antibiotic lock therapy may be attempted without systemic therapy for 10 to 14 days for coagulase-negative staphylococci or gram-negative bacilli.

Although ethanol lock therapy has shown promise, the most recent IDSA guideline states that at the present time there are insufficient data to recommend this mode of therapy.

SUMMARY

Central venous access is an important treatment modality in the current management of critically ill patients or those requiring long-term venous access (eg, hemodialysis, chemotherapy). Recent studies suggest that by strict adherence to current guidelines for insertion and maintenance, the incidence of CLA-BSI can be dramatically reduced. Proper diagnosis and treatment of CLA-BSI can in some cases allow potential catheter retention, as well as reduce the morbidity and mortality associated with infection.

REFERENCES

1. Klevens RM, Edwards JR, Richards CL, et al. Estimating health care-associated infections and deaths in U.S. hospitals, 2002. Public Health Rep 2007;122: 160–6.
2. Wenzel RP, Edmond MB. The impact of hospital-acquired bloodstream infections. Emerg Infect Dis 2001;7:174–7.
3. Jarvis WR. Selected aspects of the socioeconomic impact of nosocomial infections: morbidity, mortality, costs, and prevention. Infect Control Hosp Epidemiol 1996;17:552–7.
4. Stone PW, Braccia D, Larson E. Systematic review of economic analyses of health care-associated infections. Am J Infect Control 2005;33:501–9.
5. Anderson DJ, Kirkland KB, Kaye KS, et al. Underresourced hospital infection control and prevention programs: penny wise, pound foolish? Infect Control Hosp Epidemiol 2007;28:767–73.
6. Jarvis WR, Edwards JR, Culver DH, et al. Nosocomial infection rates in adult and pediatric intensive care units in the United States. Am J Med 1991;91(Suppl 3B): 185s–91s.
7. Vincent J-L, Bihari DJ, Suter PM, et al. The prevalence of nosocomial infection in intensive care units in Europe. JAMA 1995;274:639–44.
8. Vincent J-L, Rello J, Marshall J, et al. International study of the prevalence and outcomes of infection in intensive care units. JAMA 2009;302:2323–9.
9. Mermel LA. Prevention of central venous catheter-related infections: what works other than impregnated or coated catheters? J Hosp Infect 2007;65:30–3.
10. Garner JS, Jarvis WR, Emori TB, et al. CDC definitions for nosocomial infections, 1988. Am J Infect Control 1988;16:128–40.
11. Horan TC, Gaynes RP. Surveillance of nosocomial infections. In: Mayhall CG, editor. Hospital epidemiology and infection control. 3rd edition. Baltimore (MD): Lipincott, Williams & Wilkins; 2004. p. 1659–702.
12. Centers for Disease Control and Prevention. National Nosocomial Infection Surveillance (NNIS) system report, data summary from January 1992 through June 2004, issued October 2004. Am J Infect Control 2004;32:470–85.
13. Edwards JR, Peterson KD, Andrus ML, et al. National Healthcare Safety Network (NHSN) report, data summary for 2006 through 2007, issued November 2008. Am J Infect Control 2008;36:609–26.
14. Weber DJ, Sickbert-Bennett EE, Brown V, et al. Comparison of hospitalwide surveillance and targeted intensive care unit surveillance of healthcare-associated infections. Infect Control Hosp Epidemiol 2007;28:1361–6.
15. Scott RD. The direct medical costs of healthcare-associated infections in U.S. hospitals and the benefits of prevention. Available at: http://www.cdc.gov/ncidod/dhqp/pdf/Scott_CostPaper.pdf. Accessed January 2, 2010.
16. Edmond MB, Wallace SE, McClish DK, et al. Nosocomial bloodstream infections in United States hospitals: a three-year analysis. Clin Infect Dis 1999;29:239–44.
17. Biedenbach DJ, Moet GJ, Jones RN. Occurrence and antimicrobial resistance pattern comparisons among bloodstream isolates from the SENTRY antimicrobial surveillance program (1997–2202). Diagn Microbiol Infect Dis 2004;50: 59–69.
18. Diekema DJ, Pfaller MA, Jones RN. Age-related changes in pathogen frequency and antimicrobial susceptibility of bloodstream isolates in North America SENTRY Antimicrobial Surveillance Program, 1997–2000. Int J Antimicrob Agents 2002;20:412–8.

19. Hidron AI, Edwards JR, Patel J, et al. Antimicrobial-resistant pathogens associated with healthcare-associated infections: annual summary of data reported to the National Healthcare Safety Network at the Centers for Disease Control and Prevention, 2006–2007. Infect Control Hosp Epidemiol 2008;29:996–1011.
20. Fridkin SK. Increasing prevalence of antimicrobial resistance in intensive care units. Crit Care Med 2001;29(Suppl 4):N64–9.
21. Maki DG, Cobb L, Garman JK, et al. An attachable silver-impregnated cuff for prevention of infection with central venous catheters: a prospective randomized multicenter trial. Am J Med 1988;85:307–14.
22. Guidet B, Nicola I, Barakett V, et al. Skin versus hub cultures to predict colonization and infections of central venous catheter in intensive care patients. Infection 1994;22:43–8.
23. Salzman MB, Isenberg HD, Shapiro JF, et al. A prospective study of the catheter hub as the portal of entry for microorganisms causing catheter-related sepsis in neonates. J Infect Dis 1993;167:487–90.
24. Salzman MB, Rubin LG. Relevance of the catheter hub as a portal for microorganisms causing catheter-related infections. Nutrition 1997;13(Suppl):15S–7S.
25. Macias AE, Heurtas M, Ponce de Leon S, et al. Contamination of intravenous fluids: a continuing cause of hospital bacteremia. Am J Infect Control 2010; 38(3):217–21.
26. Alonso-Echanove J, Edwards JR, Richards MJ, et al. Effect of nurse staffing and antimicrobial-impregnated central venous catheters on the risk for bloodstream infections in intensive care units. Infect Control Hosp Epidemiol 2003;24: 916–25.
27. Lorente L, Henry C, Martin MM, et al. Central venous catheter-related infection in a prospective and observational study of 2,595 catheters. Crit Care 2005;9: R631–5.
28. Almuneef MA, Memish ZA, Balkhy HH, et al. Rate, risk factors and outcomes of catheter-related bloodstream infection in a paediatric intensive care unit in Saudi Arabia. J Hosp Infect 2006;62:207–13.
29. Hamilton HC, Foxcroft D. Central venous access sites for the prevention of venous thrombosis, stenosis and infection in patients requiring long-term intravenous therapy [review]. Cochrane Database Syst Rev 2007;3:CD004084. DOI:10.1002/14651858.pub2:CD004084.
30. Maki DG, Kluger DM, Crnich CJ. The risk of bloodstream infection in adults with different intravascular devices; a systematic review of 200 published prospective studies. Mayo Clin Proc 2006;81:1159–71.
31. Safdar N, Kluger DM, Maki DG. A review of risk factors for catheter-related bloodstream infection caused by percutaneously inserted, noncuffed central venous catheters. Medicine 2002;81:466–79.
32. O'Grady NP, Alexander M, Dellinger EP, et al. Guideline for the prevention of intravascular catheter-related infections. Clin Infect Dis 2002;35:1281–307.
33. Bishop L, Dougherty L, Bodenham A, et al. Guidelines on the insertion and management of central venous access devices in adults. Int J Lab Hematol 2007;29:261–78.
34. Ramritu P, Halton K, Cook D, et al. Catheter-related bloodstream infections in intensive care units: a systematic review with meta-analysis. J Adv Nurs 2008; 62:3–21.
35. Marschall J, Mermel LA, Classen D, et al. Strategies to prevent central line-associated bloodstream infections in acute care hospitals. Infect Control Hosp Epidemiol 2008;29(Suppl 1):S22–30.

36. Goede MR, Coopersmith CM. Catheter-related bloodstream infection. Surg Clin North Am 2009;89:463–74.
37. Centers for Disease Control and Prevention. Guideline for hand hygiene in health-care settings: recommendations of the Healthcare Infection Control Practices Advisory Committee and the HICPAC/SHEA/APIC/IDSA Hand Hygiene Task Force. MMWR Recomm Rep 2002;51(RR–16):1–45.
38. Rosenthal VD, Guzman S, Safdar N. Reduction in nosocomial infection with improved hand hygiene in intensive care units of a tertiary care hospital in Argentina. Am J Infect Control 2005;33:392–7.
39. Yilmaz G, Koksal I, Aydin K, et al. Risk factors of catheter-related bloodstream infections in parenteral nutrition catheterization. JPEN J Parenter Enteral Nutr 2007;31:284–7.
40. Berenholtz SM, Pronovost PJ, Lipsett PA, et al. Eliminating catheter-related bloodstream infections in the intensive care unit. Crit Care Med 2004;32:2014–20.
41. Mermel LA, McCormick RD, Springman SR, et al. The pathogenesis and epidemiology of catheter-related infection with pulmonary artery Swan-Ganz catheters: a prospective study utilizing molecular subtyping. Am J Med 1991;91(Suppl 3B):197S–205S.
42. Raad II, Hohn DC, Gilbreath BJ, et al. Prevention of central venous catheter-related infections by using maximal sterile barrier precautions during insertion. Infect Control Hosp Epidemiol 1994;15:231–4.
43. Hu KK, Lipsky BA, Veenstra DL, et al. Using maximal sterile barriers to prevent central venous catheter-related infection: a systematic evidence-based review. Am J Infect Control 2004;32:142–6.
44. Young EM, Commiskey ML, Wilson SJ. Translating evidence into practice to prevent central-venous catheter-associated bloodstream infections: a systems-based intervention. Am J Infect Control 2006;34:503–6.
45. Maki DG, Ringer M, Alvarado CJ. Prospective randomized trial of povidone-iodine, alcohol, and chlorhexidine for prevention of infection associated with central venous and arterial catheters. Lancet 1991;338:339–43.
46. Humar A, Ostromecki A, Direnfeld J, et al. Prospective randomized trial of 10% povidone-iodine versus 0.5% tincture of chlorhexidine as cutaneous antisepsis for prevention of central venous catheter infection. Clin Infect Dis 2000;31:1001–7.
47. Chaiyakunapruk N, Veenstra DL, Lipsky BA, et al. Chlorhexidine compared with povidone-iodine solution for vascular catheter-side care: a meta-analysis. Ann Intern Med 2002;136:792–801.
48. Chaiyakunapruk N, Veenstra DL, Lipsky BA, et al. Vascular catheter site care; the clinical and economic benefits of chlorhexidine gluconate compared with povidone iodine. Clin Infect Dis 2003;37:764–71.
49. Valles J, Fernandez I, Alcaraz D, et al. Prospective randomized trial of 3 antiseptic solutions for prevention of catheter colonization in an intensive care unit for adult patients. Infect Control Hosp Epidemiol 2008;29:847–53.
50. Goetz AM, Wagener MM, Muder RR. Risk of infection due to central venous catheters: effect of site of placement and catheter type. Infect Control Hosp Epidemiol 1998;19:842–5.
51. Hind D, Calvert N, McWiliams R, et al. Ultrasonic location devices for central venous cannulation: meta-analysis. BMJ 2003;327:361.
52. Venkataraman ST, Thompson AE. Femoral vascular catheterization in critically ill infants and children. Clin Pediatr (Phila) 1997;36:311–9.

53. Sheridan RL, Weber JM. Mechanical and infectious complications of central venous cannulation in children: lessons learned from a 10-year experience placing more than 1000 catheters. J Burn Care Res 2006;27:713–8.
54. Stenzel JP, Green TP, Fuhrman RP, et al. Percutaneous central venous catheterization in a pediatric intensive care unit: a survival analysis of complications. Crit Care Med 1989;17:984–8.
55. Randolph AG, Cook DJ, Gonzales CA, et al. Tunneling short-term central venous catheters to prevent catheter-related infection: a meta-analysis of randomized, controlled trials. Crit Care Med 1998;26:1452–7.
56. Salzman MB, Isenberg HD, Rubin LG. Use of disinfectants to reduce microbial contamination of hubs of vascular catheters. J Clin Microbiol 1993;31:475–9.
57. Luebke MA, Arduino MJ, Duda DL, et al. Comparison of the microbial barrier properties of a needleless and a conventional needle-based intravenous access system. Am J Infect Control 1998;26:437–41.
58. Casey AL, Worthington T, Lambert PA, et al. A randomized, prospective clinical trial to access the potential infection risk associated with the PosiFlow needleless connector. J Hosp Infect 2003;54:288–93.
59. Lederle FA, Parenti CM, Berskow LC, et al. The idle intravenous catheter. Ann Intern Med 1992;116:737–8.
60. Parenti CM, Lederle FA, Impola CL, et al. Reduction of unnecessary intravenous catheter use. Arch Intern Med 1994;154:1829–32.
61. Gillies D, Walen NM, Morrison AL, et al. Optimal timing for intravenous administration set replacements. Cochrane Database Syst Rev 2005;4: CD003588. DOI:10.1002/14651858.pub2:CD003588.
62. Zakrzewska-Bode A, Muytjens HL, Liem KD, et al. Mupirocin resistance in coagulase-negative staphylococci, after topical prophylaxis for the reduction of colonization of central venous catheters. J Hosp Infect 1995;31:189–93.
63. Flowers RH, Schwenzer KJ, Kopel RF, et al. Efficacy of an attachable subcutaneous cuff for the prevention of intravascular catheter-related infection. A randomized, controlled trial. JAMA 1989;10:878–83.
64. van de Wetering MD, van Woensel JB. Prophylactic antibiotics for preventing early central venous catheter gram positive infections among oncology patients. Cochrane Database Syst Rev 2007;24:CD003295.
65. Niel-Weise BS, Stijnen T, van den Broek PJ. Anti-infective-treated central venous catheters: a systematic review of randomized controlled trials. Intensive Care Med 2007;33:2058–68.
66. Niel-Weise BS, Stijnen T, van den Broek PJ. Anti-infective-treated central venous catheters for total parental nutrition or chemotherapy: a systematic review. J Hosp Infect 2008;69:114–23.
67. Casey AL, Mermel LA, Nightingale P, et al. Antimicrobial central venous catheters in adults: a systematic review and meta-analysis. Lancet Infect Dis 2008;8: 763–77.
68. Ramitu P, Halton K, Collington P, et al. A systematic review comparing the relative effectiveness of antimicrobial-coated catheters in intensive care units. Am J Infect Control 2008;36:104–17.
69. Hockenhull JC, Dwan KM, Smith GW, et al. The clinical effectiveness of central venous catheters treated with anti-infective agents in preventing catheter-related bloodstream infections: a systematic review. Crit Care Med 2009;37:702–12.
70. Weber DJ, Rutala WA. Use of germicides in the home and the healthcare setting: is there a relationship between germicide use and antibiotic resistance? Infect Control Hosp Epidemiol 2006;27:1107–19.

71. Sampath LA, Tambe SM, Modak SM. In vitro and in vivo efficacy of catheters impregnated with antiseptics or antibiotics: evaluation of the risk of bacterial resistance to the antimicrobials in the catheters. Infect Control Hosp Epidemiol 2001;22:640–6.
72. Munson EL, Heard SO, Doern GV. In vitro exposure of bacteria to antimicrobial impregnated-central venous catheters does not directly lead to the emergence of antimicrobial resistance. Chest 2004;126:1628–35.
73. Raad I, Darouiche R, Dupuis J, et al. Central venous catheters coated with minocycline and rifampin for the prevention of catheter-related colonization and bloodstream infections: a randomized, double-blind trial. Ann Intern Med 1997;127:267–74.
74. Darouiche RO, Raad I, Heard SO, et al. A comparison of two antimicrobial-impregnated central venous catheters. N Engl J Med 1999;340:1–8.
75. Chatzinikolaou I, Finkel K, Hanna H, et al. Antibiotic-coated hemodialysis catheters for the prevention of vascular catheter-related infections: a prospective, randomized study. Am J Med 2003;115:352–7.
76. Hanna H, Benjamin R, Chatzinikolaou I, et al. Long-term silicone central venous catheters impregnated with minocycline and rifampin decrease rates of catheter-related bloodstream infection in cancer patients: a prospective randomized clinical trial. J Clin Oncol 2004;22:3163–71.
77. Chelliah A, Heydon KH, Zaoutis TE, et al. Observational trial of antibiotic-coated central venous catheters in critically ill pediatric patients. Pediatr Infect Dis J 2007;26:816–20.
78. Bhutta A, Gilliam C, Honeycutt M, et al. Reduction of bloodstream infections associated with catheters in paediatric intensive care unit: stepwise approach. BMJ 2007;334:362–5.
79. Lim KS, Kam PC. Chlorhexidine—pharmacology and clinical applications. Anaesth Intensive Care 2008;36:502–12.
80. Milstone AM, Passaretti CL, Perl TM. Chlorhexidine: expanding the armamentarium for infection control and prevention. Clin Infect Dis 2008;46:274–81.
81. Munoz-Price LS, Hota B, Stemer A, et al. Prevention of bloodstream infections by use of daily chlorhexidine baths for patients at a long-term acute care hospital. Infect Control Hosp Epidemiol 2009;30:1031–5.
82. Climo MW, Sepkowitz KA, Zuccotti G, et al. The effect of daily bathing with chlorhexidine on the acquisition of methicillin-resistant Staphylococcus aureus, vancomycin-resistant Enterococcus and healthcare-associated bloodstream infections: results of a quasi-experimental multicenter trial. Crit Care Med 2009;37:1858–65.
83. Bleasdale SC, Trick WE, Gonzalez IM, et al. Effectiveness of chlorhexidine bathing to reduce catheter-associated bloodstream infections in medical intensive care unit patients. Arch Intern Med 2007;167:2073–9.
84. Garland JS, Alex CP, Mueller CD, et al. A randomized trial comparing povidone-iodine to a chlorhexidine gluconate-impregnated dressing for prevention of central venous catheter infections in neonates. Pediatrics 2001;107:1431–6.
85. Levy I, Katz J, Solter E, et al. Chlorhexidine-impregnated dressing for prevention of colonization of central venous catheters in infants and children. Pediatr Infect Dis 2005;24:676–9.
86. Timsit J-F, Schwebel C, Bouadma L, et al. Chlorhexidine-impregnated sponges and less frequent dressing changes for prevention of catheter-related infections in critically ill adults. JAMA 2009;301:1231–41.

87. Ho KM, Litton E. Use of chlorhexidine-impregnated dressing to prevent vascular and epidural catheter colonization and infection: a meta-analysis. J Antimicrob Chemother 2006;58:281–7.

88. Kethireddy S, Safdar N. Urokinase lock or flush solution for prevention of bloodstream infections associated with central venous catheters for chemotherapy: a meta-analysis of prospective randomized trials. J Vasc Access 2008;9:51–7.

89. Safdar N, Maki DG. Use of vancomycin-containing lock or flush solutions for prevention of bloodstream infection associated with central venous access devices: a meta-analysis of prospective, randomized trials. Clin Infect Dis 2006;43:474–84.

90. Maiefski M, Rupp ME, Hermsen ED. Ethanol lock technique: review of the literature. Infect Control Hosp Epidemiol 2009;30:1096–108.

91. Jaffer Y, Selby NM, Taal MW, et al. A meta-analysis of hemodialysis catheter lock solutions in the prevention of catheter-related infection. Am J Kidney Dis 2008; 51:233–41.

92. Labriola L, Crott R, Jadoul M. Preventing haemodialysis catheter-related bacteraemia with an antimicrobial lock solution: a meta-analysis of prospective randomized trials. Nephrol Dial Transplant 2008;23:1666–72.

93. James MT, Conley J, Tonelli M, et al. Meta-analysis: antibiotics for prophylaxis against hemodialysis catheter-related infections. Ann Intern Med 2008;148: 596–605.

94. Yahav D, Rozen-Zvi B, Gafter-Gvili A, et al. Antimicrobial lock solutions for the prevention of infections associated with intravascular catheters in patients undergoing hemodialysis: systematic review and meta-analysis of randomized, controlled trials. Clin Infect Dis 2008;47:83–93.

95. Henrickson KJ, Axtell RA, Hoover SM, et al. Prevention of central venous catheter-related infections and thrombotic events in immunocompromised children by the use of vancomycin/ciprofloxacin/heparin flush solution: a randomized, multicenter, double-blind trial. J Clin Oncol 2000;18:1269–78.

96. Barriga FJ, Varas M, Potin M, et al. Efficacy of a vancomycin solution to prevent bacteremia associated with an indwelling central venous catheter in neutropenic and non-neutropenic cancer patients. Med Pediatr Oncol 1997;28:196–200.

97. Carratala J, Niubo J, Fernandez-Sevilla A, et al. Randomized, double-blind, trial of an antibiotic-lock technique for prevention of Gram-positive central venous catheter-related infection in neutropenic patients with cancer. Antimicrob Agents Chemother 1999;43:2200–4.

98. Garland JS, Alex CP, Hendrickson KJ, et al. A vancomycin-heparin lock solution for prevention of nosocomial bloodstream infection in critically ill neonates with peripherally inserted central venous catheters: a prospective, randomized study. Pediatrics 2005;116:e198–205.

99. Berwick DM, Calkins DR, McCannon EJ, et al. The 100,000 live campaign. JAMA 2006;295:324–7.

100. Pronovost P, Needham D, Berenholtz S, et al. An intervention to decrease catheter-related bloodstream infections in the ICU. N Engl J Med 2006;355:2727–32.

101. Zack J. Zeroing in on zero tolerance for central line-associated bacteremia. Am J Infect Control 2008;36:e176–7.

102. Jeffries HE, Mason W, Brewer M, et al. Prevention of central venous catheter-associated bloodstream infections in pediatric intensive care units: a performance improvement collaborative. Infect Control Hosp Epidemiol 2009;30: 645–51.

103. Costello JM, Morrow DF, Graham DA, et al. Systematic intervention to reduce central line-associated bloodstream infection rates in a pediatric cardiac intensive care unit. Pediatrics 2008;121:915–23.
104. O'Grady NP, Barie PS, Bartlett JG, et al. Guidelines for evaluation of new fever in critically ill adult patients: 2008 update from the American College of Critical Care Medicine and the Infectious Disease Society of America. Crit Care Med 2008;36:1330–49.
105. Mermel LA, Allon M, Bouza E, et al. Clinical practice guidelines for the diagnosis and management of intravascular catheter-related infection: 2009 update by the Infectious Disease Society of America. Clin Infect Dis 2009;49:1–45.
106. Mermel LA, Maki DG. Detection of bacteremia in adults: consequence of culturing of inadequate volume blood. Ann Intern Med 1993;119:270–2.
107. Cockrill FR, Wilson JW, Vetter EA, et al. Optimal testing parameters for blood cultures. Clin Infect Dis 2004;38:1724–30.
108. Washington JA. Blood cultures: principles and techniques. Mayo Clin Proc 1975;50:91–8.
109. Lee A, Mirrett S, Reller LB, et al. Detection of bloodstream infections in adults: how many blood cultures are needed? J Clin Microbiol 2007;45:3546–8.
110. Everts RJ, Vinson EN, Adholla PO, et al. Contamination of catheter-drawn blood cultures. J Clin Microbiol 2001;39:3393–4.
111. Falagas ME, Kazantzi MS, Bliziotis IA. Comparison of utility of blood cultures from intravascular catheters and peripheral veins: a systematic review and decision analysis. J Med Microbiol 2008;57:1–8.
112. Tacconelli E, Tumbarello M, Pittiruti M, et al. Central venous catheter-related sepsis in a cohort of 366 hospitalised patients. Eur J Clin Microbiol 1997;16:203–9.
113. Raad I, Hanna H, Maki D. Intravascular catheter-related infections: advances in diagnosis, prevention, and management. Lancet Infect Dis 2007;7:645–57.
114. Eggimann P. Diagnosis of intravascular catheter infection. Curr Opin Infect Dis 2007;20:353–9.
115. Capdevila JA, Planes AM, Palomar M, et al. Value of differential quantitative blood cultures in the diagnosis of catheter-related sepsis. Eur J Clin Microbiol Infect Dis 1992;11:403–7.
116. Douard MC, Arlet G, Longuet P, et al. Diagnosis of venous access port-related infections. Clin Infect Dis 1999;29:1197–202.
117. Chatzinikolaou I, Hanna H, Hachem R, et al. Differential quantitative blood cultures for the diagnosis of catheter-related bloodstream infections associated with short- and long-term catheters: a prospective study. Diagn Microbiol Infect Dis 2004;50:167–72.
118. Catton JA, Dobbins BM, Kite P, et al. In situ diagnosis of intravascular catheter-related bloodstream infection: a comparison of quantitative culture, differential time to positivity, and endoluminal brushing. Crit Care Med 2005;33:787–91.
119. Blot F, Schmidt E, Nitenberg G, et al. Earlier positivity of central-venous- versus peripheral-blood cultures is highly predictive of catheter-related sepsis. J Clin Microbiol 1998;36:105–9.
120. Blot F, Nitenberg G, Chachaty E, et al. Diagnosis of catheter-related bacteraemia: a prospective comparison of the time to positivity of hub-blood versus peripheral-blood cultures. Lancet 1999;354:1071–7.
121. Malgrange VB, Escande MC, Theobald S. Validity of earlier positivity of central venous blood cultures in comparison with peripheral blood cultures for

diagnosing catheter-related bacteremia in cancer patients. J Clin Microbiol 2001;39:274–8.

122. Gaur AH, Flynn PM, Giannini MA, et al. Difference in time to detection: a simple method to differentiate catheter-related from non-catheter-related bloodstream infection in immunocompromised pediatric patients. Clin Infect Dis 2003;37: 469–75.

123. Raad I, Hanna HA, Alakeck B, et al. Differential time to positivity: a useful method for diagnosing catheter-related bloodstream infections. Ann Intern Med 2004;140:18–25.

124. Gaur AH, Flynn PM, Heine DJ, et al. Diagnosis of catheter-related bloodstream infections among pediatric oncology patients lacking a peripheral culture, using differential time to detection. Pediatr Infect Dis J 2005;24:445–9.

125. Bouza E, Alvarado N, Alcala L, et al. A randomized and prospective study of 3 procedures for the diagnosis of catheter-related bloodstream infection without catheter withdrawal. Clin Infect Dis 2007;44:820–6.

126. Wing EJ, Norden CW, Shadduck RK, et al. Use of quantitative bacteriologic techniques to diagnose catheter-related sepsis. Arch Intern Med 1979;139: 482–3.

127. Siegman-Igra Y, Anglim AM, Shapiro DE, et al. Diagnosis of vascular catheter-related bloodstream infection: a meta-analysis. J Clin Microbiol 1997;35:928–36.

128. Maki DG, Weise CE, Sarafin HW. A semiquantitative culture method of identifying intravenous-catheter-related infection. N Engl J Med 1977;296:1305–9.

129. Rello J, Coll P, Prats G. Laboratory diagnosis of catheter-related bacteremia. Scand J Infect Dis 1991;23:583–8.

130. Raad II, Sabbagh MF, Rand RH, et al. Quantitative tip culture methods and diagnosis of central venous catheter-related infections. Diagn Microbiol Infect Dis 1992;15:13–20.

131. Safdar N, Fine JP, Maki DG. Meta-analysis: methods for diagnosing intravascular device-related bloodstream infections. Ann Intern Med 2005;142:451–66.

132. Sherertz RJ, Raad II, Belani A, et al. Three-year experience with sonicated vascular catheter cultures in a clinical microbiology laboratory. J Clin Microbiol 1990;28:76–82.

133. Brun-Buisson C, Abrouk F, Legrand P, et al. Diagnosis of central venous catheter-related sepsis. Critical level of quantitative tip cultures. Arch Intern Med 1987;147:873–7.

134. Bjornson HS, Colley R, Bower RH, et al. Association between microorganism growth at the catheter insertion site and colonization of the catheter in patients receiving total parenteral nutrition. Surgery 1982;92:720–7.

135. Bouza E, Burillo A, Munzo P. Empiric therapy for intravenous central line infections and nosocomially-acquired acute bacterial endocarditis. Crit Care Clin 2008;24:293–312.

136. Sabatier C, Ferrer R, Valles J. Treatment strategies for central venous catheter infections. Expert Opin Pharmacother 2009;10:2231–43.

137. Morrell MR, Micek ST, Kollef MH. The management of severe sepsis and septic shock. Infect Dis Clin North Am 2009;23:485–501.

138. Fowler VG, Boucher HW, Corey GR, et al. Daptomycin versus standard therapy for bacteremia and endocarditis caused by Staphylococcus aureus. N Engl J Med 2006;355:653–65.

Urinary Tract Infections

Carol E. Chenoweth, MD[a,b,*], Sanjay Saint, MD, MPH[c,d]

KEYWORDS

- Prevention • Catheter • Urinary tract infection • Intervention
- Catheter-associated urinary tract infections

Health care-associated urinary tract infections (UTI) account for up to 40% of infections in hospitals and 23% of infections in the intensive care unit (ICU). Most UTIs develop in patients with indwelling urinary catheters. Urinary catheters interfere with normal host immune defenses and allow formation of biofilm, which enables bacterial colonization and affects the specific etiologic organisms found in catheter-associated UTI (CAUTI). These factors have important implications for prevention of UTI in the catheterized patient.

PATHOGENESIS

The normal human urinary tract has innate defense mechanisms that prevent attachment and migration of pathogens into the bladder; these include length of the urethra and micturition.[1,2] In addition, the urinary tract epithelium secretes inhibitors of bacterial adhesion (ie, Tamm-Horsfall proteins and mucopolysaccharides).[2] Urine characteristics, such as osmolality and pH, inhibit growth of microorganisms. Urinary catheterization interferes with all of these normal host defenses.

Most microorganisms causing CAUTI enter the bladder by ascending the urethra from the perineum. First, organisms migrate in the mucous film surrounding the external aspect of the catheter. Organisms entering the bladder from this extraluminal route are primarily endogenous organisms, colonizing the patient's intestinal tract and perineum.[3] In one study of 173 CAUTIs, 115 (66%) were acquired from extraluminal migration of organisms. A smaller proportion of infections (34%) was acquired from intraluminal contamination of the collection system.[3] Organisms acquired

[a] Division of Infectious Diseases, Department of Internal Medicine, University of Michigan Health System, 1500 East Medical Center Drive, 3119 Taubman Center, Ann Arbor, MI 48109-5378, USA
[b] Department of Infection Control and Epidemiology, University of Michigan Health System, Ann Arbor, MI, USA
[c] Division of General Medicine, Department of Internal Medicine, University of Michigan Health System, 300 North Ingalls, Room 7E08, Ann Arbor, MI 48109-0429, USA
[d] Veterans Affairs Ann Arbor Healthcare System, Ann Arbor, MI, USA
* Corresponding author.
E-mail address: cchenow@umich.edu

Infect Dis Clin N Am 25 (2011) 103–115
doi:10.1016/j.idc.2010.11.005
0891-5520/11/$ – see front matter © 2011 Elsevier Inc. All rights reserved.

intraluminally are usually exogenous and result from cross-transmission of organisms from the hands of health care personnel.[2,3] Rarely, organisms such as *Staphylococcus aureus* cause upper UTI from hematogenous spread.

Although most CAUTI are caused by *Enterobacteriaceae* from the patient's own gastrointestinal tract, microorganisms in healthcare-associated UTI may be transmitted from one patient to another by healthcare workers. Approximately 15% of episodes of healthcare-associated bacteriuria occur in clusters from intrahospital transmission.[2,4] Most of these hospital-based outbreaks have been associated with improper hand hygiene by health care personnel.

Biofilms that form on urinary catheters are unique and have important implications for prevention of CAUTIs. Biofilms, composed of clusters of microorganisms and extracellular matrix (primarily polysaccharide materials), form on both the extraluminal and intraluminal surfaces of urinary catheters.[2] Typically, the biofilm is composed of one type of microorganism, although polymicrobial biofilms are possible. Organisms in the biofilm grow slower than organisms growing within the urine itself, and microorganisms within the biofilm may ascend the catheter in 1 to 3 days. Some organisms in the biofilm, especially *Proteus* species, have the ability to hydrolyze urea and increase urine pH. This allows mineral precipitation, which leads to mineral encrustations along the catheter or renal calculi.[2] Biofilm formation is also important, because it provides a protective environment from antimicrobial agents and immune cells. Antimicrobials penetrate poorly into biofilms, and microorganisms grow more slowly in biofilms, rendering many antimicrobials less effective.[2,5]

EPIDEMIOLOGY

CAUTIs account for approximately 40% of all hospital-acquired infections, but make up a smaller proportion of health care-associated infections in the ICU setting. The rate of CAUTI varies by ICU type; rates of CAUTIs reported through the National Healthcare Safety Network (NHSN) in 2006 and 2007 ranged from 7.7 infections per 1000 catheter days in burn ICUs to 3.1 infections per 1000 catheter days in medical/surgical ICUs. Rates of CAUTIs in pediatric ICUs are reported at 5 UTIs per 1000 catheter days, but CAUTIs are infrequently identified in neonatal ICUs.[2,6–9] CAUTIs occur in general care wards at equivalent to or higher rates than in the ICU setting, ranging from 4.7 UTIs per 1000 catheter days in adult step-down units to 16.8 infections per 1000 catheter days in rehabilitation units.[9]

Microbial Etiology

Enterobacteriaceae represent the most common pathogens associated with hospital-wide catheter-related UTI. Other predominant pathogens, especially in the ICU setting, include *Candida* species, enterococci, and *Pseudomonas aeruginosa*.[2,9] While most infections (80%) associated with short-term indwelling urinary catheters are caused by single organisms, infections in long-term catheters are polymicrobial in 77% to 95% of cases, and 10% have more than five species of organisms present.[10] Among data reported from NHSN, between 2006 and 2007, 24.8% of all *E coli* isolates from patients with CAUTIs were resistant to fluoroquinolones.[11] In addition, many *Enterobacteriaceae* produce extended-spectrum beta-lactamases, in some cases, resulting in resistance to all noncarbapenem beta-lactam antimicrobials. In 2006 and 2007, 21.2% of *Klebsiella pneumoniae* and 5.5% of *E coli* isolates from patients with CAUTIs were resistant to ceftriaxone or ceftazidime. Some *Klebsiella* species also produce carbapenemases, allowing resistance to carbapenems. In

2006 and 2007, 10.1% of all *K pneumoniae* isolates from patients with CAUTIs were resistant to carbapenems.[11]

Risk Factors

Duration of catheterization is the most important, consistent risk factor for catheter-associated bacteriuria; approximately 97% of UTIs in the ICU are associated with an indwelling urinary catheter (**Box 1**). Bacteriuria develops quickly at an average daily rate of 3% to 10% per day of catheterization. Bacteriuria will develop in 26% of patients with a catheter in place for 2 to 10 days. All patients catheterized for a month will develop bacteriuria, and long-term catheterization is defined as catheterization for greater than 1 month.[2]

Females have a higher risk of bacteriuria than males (relative risk [RR] 1.7 to 3.7).[10] Heavy bacterial colonization of the perineum also has been associated with increased risk of bacteriuria. Other patient factors identified in one or more studies include

Rapidly fatal underlying illness
Age greater than 50 years
Nonsurgical disease
Hospitalization on an orthopedic or urological service
Catheter insertion after the 6th day of hospitalization
Catheter inserted outside the operating room
Diabetes mellitus
Serum creatinine greater than 2 mg/dl at the time of catheterization.

Nonadherence to catheter care recommendations also has been associated with increased risk of bacteriuria. Systemic antimicrobial agents have a protective effect on bacteriuria (RR 2.0 to 3.9).[10]

Risk factors for UTI-associated bacteremia are less clearly understood than for catheter-associated bacteriuria, because bacteremia occurs in fewer than 4% of CAUTIs.[12,13] Krieger and colleagues[12] followed 1233 patients with hospital-acquired UTI; secondary bloodstream infections developed in 32 patients (2.6%). Risk factors

---

Box 1
Risk factors for CAUTI

Patient-Level Risk Factors

Female sex

Age >50

Severe underlying illness

Nonsurgical disease

Diabetes mellitus

Serum creatinine >2 mg/dL

Modifiable Risk Factors

Duration of catheterization

Nonadherence to appropriate catheter care

Catheter insertion after 6th day of hospitalization

Catheter insertion outside operating room

for bloodstream infections from a urinary source included infections caused by *Serratia marcescens* and male sex. No other factors were found to significantly predispose to bacteremia in patients with UTIs in this study. More recently, Saint and colleagues[14] conducted a case–control study at a Veterans Affairs hospital to determine the risk factors for bacteremia in patients with hospital-acquired bacteriuria. Significant predictors of bacteremia were immunosuppressant therapy within 14 days of bacteriuria (odds ratio [OR] 8.13), history of malignancy (OR 1.94), male sex (OR 1.88), cigarette use in the past 5 years (OR 1.26), and number of hospital days before bacteriuria (OR, 1.03). Corticosteroid use within 7 days of bacteriuria predicted bacteremia in patients younger than 70 years (OR 14.24); similarly, patients younger than 70 years were more likely to develop bacteremia if they had diabetes mellitus (OR 6.19).[14] Clearly identifying predictors for health care-associated urinary tract-related bacteremia may lead to the targeting of appropriate preventive practices at those at highest risk.

DIAGNOSIS AND SURVEILLANCE

Most studies of CAUTI use bacteriuria as the primary outcome, and hence the term bacteriuria is often used interchangeably with UTI in the published literature. The distinction is clinically important, as asymptomatic catheter-associated bacteriuria is rarely associated with adverse outcomes and generally does not require treatment.[13] In general, bacteriuria in a catheterized patient is defined as growth of at least 10^2 colony forming units (CFUs)/mL of a predominant pathogen.[4]

The NHSN surveillance definition for health care-associated UTI allows for standardization and interhospital comparison of infection rates.[15] For adult patients, there are two possible definitions for symptomatic UTI. In the first definition, a patient must have at least one sign or symptom (temperature >38°C, urgency, frequency, dysuria, or suprapubic tenderness) and a positive urine culture ($\geq 10^5$ CFUs/mL with no more than two species of microorganisms). The second definition allows that a patient have at least two signs or symptoms with at least one laboratory finding:

Positive urine dipstick for leukocyte esterase or nitrite
Pyuria with at least three white blood cells per high-power field
Positive urine Gram's stain
Two urine cultures with at least 10^2 CFUs/mL of the same pathogen
One urine culture with $\leq 10^5$ CFUs/mL of a single pathogen in a patient being treated with antimicrobials
Physician diagnosis or treatment of a UTI.

Asymptomatic bacteriuria in a patient who has had a urinary catheter in the previous 7 days is defined as a urine culture growing more than 10^5 CFUs/mL in the absence of signs or symptoms. For a patient who has not had a catheter within the previous 7 days, two positive urine cultures are required.[15]

Clinical diagnosis of CAUTI remains challenging. Pyuria is not a reliable indicator of UTI in the setting of catheterization.[16,17] Musher and colleagues[16] found that most catheterized patients with bacteriuria had pyuria, but 30% of patients with pyuria did not have bacteriuria. Diagnosis of UTI in patients with long-term urinary catheters is particularly difficult, as bacteriuria is invariably present. Systemic symptoms of infection may be the only indications of UTI, especially in patients who have spinal cord injuries.[18] Clinical recognition of UTI remains an important issue, as most antimicrobial use on a general medicine ward in one study was related to a diagnosis of UTI, most often asymptomatic bacteriuria.[19]

Surveillance for CAUTI traditionally has not been a priority for most hospitals, perhaps because of lack of resources required to perform full hospital surveillance and the low priority given to CAUTI compared with other health care-associated infections.[20,21] Since the Centers for Medicare and Medicaid Services has included CAUTI as one of the hospital-acquired complications that will not be reimbursed, hospitals have renewed interest in CAUTI.[22] The symptomatic CAUTI rate per 1000 urinary catheter days is the most widely accepted measure used in surveillance, and is endorsed by the Centers for Disease Control and Prevention (CDC), Infectious Diseases Society of America-The Society for Healthcare Epidemiology of America compendium, and Association for Professionals in Infection Control and Epidemiology.[23–25] Other process or proxy measures include rates of asymptomatic bacteriuria, percentage of patients with indwelling catheters, percentage of catheterization with accepted indications, and duration of catheter use.

PREVENTING CAUTIs

Several recent guidelines exist regarding prevention of CAUTI (**Box 2**).[23–25] General strategies are formulated for prevention of all health care-associated infections, while targeted strategies are focused at risk factors specific for CAUTI.

General Strategies for Prevention

Strict adherence to hand hygiene is recommended for prevention of all health care-associated infections, including UTI.[26] The urinary tract of hospitalized patients and patients in long-term care facilities represents a significant reservoir for multidrug-resistant organisms (MDROs). Indwelling devices, including urinary catheters, increase the risk of colonization with MDROs. Therefore limiting use of invasive devices is an important strategy for prevention of MDROs. Use of contact precautions

---

Box 2
Key strategies for prevention of CAUTI

Avoid use of indwelling urinary catheters

    Placement only for appropriate indications

    Institutional protocols for placement, including in the perioperative setting

Alternatives to indwelling catheterization

    Intermittent catheterization

    Condom catheter

    Portable bladder ultrasound scanner to avoid indwelling catheterization

Early removal of indwelling catheters

    Checklist or daily plan

    Nurse-based interventions

    Electronic reminders

Proper techniques for insertion and maintenance of catheters

    Sterile insertion Closed drainage system

    Avoid routine bladder irrigation

Consider antiseptic or antimicrobial catheters in some settings

with gowns and gloves is recommended as part of a multifaceted strategy for prevention of transmission of MDROs.[27] Repeated antimicrobial treatment for infections related to long-term catheterization is another significant risk for colonization with MDROs, yet some of this use may be inappropriate.[19] Reduction in use of broad-spectrum antimicrobials, as part of an overall antimicrobial stewardship program, is an important strategy to prevent development of antimicrobial resistance associated with urinary catheters.[28] A recent study revealed that a 1-hour educational session reduced the inappropriate use of antibiotic therapy for inpatients with positive urine cultures.[29]

Specific Strategies for Prevention

Several guidelines have been developed or updated recently for the prevention of CAUTI.[23–25] Nevertheless, a recent survey of hospitals nationwide identified that more than half of hospitals did not have a system for monitoring urinary catheters; three-quarters did not monitor duration of catheterization, and nearly one-third did not conduct any surveillance for UTIs.[20] The implementation of a bladder bundle for preventing CAUTI has started in the Michigan Hospital Association Keystone initiative (**Box 3**).[30]

Limitation of Use and Early Removal of Urinary Catheters

Because indwelling urinary catheters are the primary risk factor for health care-associated UTIs, the most effective strategy for CAUTI prevention is limitation or avoidance of catheterization.[31] Studies have shown that urinary catheters are placed for inappropriate indications in 21% to 50% of catheterized patients.[32–34] Physicians are frequently unaware that their patient has a urinary catheter; in one study, 28% of physicians were unaware that their patient had a catheter, with lack of awareness increasing with increased level of training.[35] This unawareness has been correlated with inappropriate catheter use.[35] In addition, physician orders for catheter placement or documentation of presence of catheter occurs in less than 50% of patients with indwelling catheters.[36]

To limit placement of indwelling urinary catheters, catheters should be inserted only for appropriate indications (**Box 4**). Every health care institution should develop written guidelines and criteria for indwelling urinary catheterization based upon these widely accepted indications.[25] Physician orders should be required for insertion of any urinary catheter, and institutions should implement a system for documenting

---

Box 3
The "ABCDE" for preventing CAUTI

Adherence to general infection control principles (eg, hand hygiene, surveillance and feedback, aseptic insertion, proper maintenance, education) is important.

Bladder ultrasound may avoid indwelling catheterization.

Condom catheters or other alternatives to an indwelling catheter such as intermittent catheterization should be considered in appropriate patients.

Do not use the indwelling catheter unless absolutely necessary.

Early removal of the catheter using a reminder or nurse-initiated removal protocol appears to be warranted.

Data from Saint S, Olmsted RN, Fakih MG, et al. Translating health care-associated urinary tract infection prevention research into practice via the bladder bundle. Jt Comm J Qual Patient Saf 2009;35(9):449–55.

Box 4
Appropriate indications for the placement of urinary catheters

Acute anatomic or functional urinary retention or obstruction

Urinary incontinence in the setting of open perineal or sacral wounds

Perioperative use for selected surgical procedures

    Surgical procedures of anticipated long duration

    Urologic procedures

    Intraoperatively for patients with urinary incontinence

    Need for intraoperative urinary monitoring or expected large volume of intravenous infusions

Accurate monitoring of urine output

Improve comfort for end-of-life care or patient preference

Data from Gould CV, Umscheid CA, Agarwal RK, et al. CDC guideline for prevention of catheter-associated urinary tract infections. 2009; Saint S, Lipsky BA. Preventing catheter-related bacteriuria: should we? Can we? How? Arch Intern Med 1999;159(8):800–8.

---

placement of catheters.[25] Insertion of catheters for convenience or for incontinence in the absence of another compelling indication should be avoided. For the most impact, interventions for limiting placement of urinary catheter may be targeted at hospital locations where initial placement often occurs, such as emergency departments and operating rooms.[34] Surveillance for symptomatic CAUTI rate per 1000 urinary catheter days or another outcome measure may help with determining success of targeted interventions.

Nurse-driven interventions have demonstrated effectiveness in reducing duration of catheterization. A nurse-based reminder to physicians to remove unnecessary urinary catheters in a Taiwanese hospital resulted in a reduction in CAUTIs from 11.5 to 8.3 UTIs per 1000 catheter days.[37] Nurse-initiated reminders to physicians of the presence of urinary catheters also decrease the number of catheter days.[38,39] Such interventions are easy to implement and may consist of either a written notice or a verbal contact with the physician regarding the presence of a urinary catheter and alternative options. Electronic reminders, however, may be more cost-effective.[39] Specifically, computerized physician order entry systems may be used more efficiently to reduce both placement of catheters and duration of catheterization. Cornia and colleagues[40] found that a computerized reminder reduced the duration of catheterization by 3 days. In some settings, an infection preventionist may have the capability of working with the information technology department to integrate catheter protocols into electronic physician order entry sets.

Perioperative Management of Urinary Retention

Specific protocols for the management of postoperative urinary retention may be beneficial in reducing duration of urinary catheterization. In one large cohort study, 85% of patients admitted for major surgical procedures had perioperative indwelling catheters; patients with duration of catheterization greater than 2 days were significantly more likely to develop UTIs and were less likely to be discharged to home.[41] Older surgical patients are particularly at risk for prolonged catheterization; 23% of surgical patients older than 65 years of age were discharged to skilled nursing facilities with an indwelling catheter in place and were substantially more likely to have rehospitalization or death within 30 days.[42]

A large prospective trial of patients undergoing orthopedic procedures incorporated a multifaceted protocol for perioperative catheter management consisting of: limiting catheterization to surgeries longer than 5 hours or to total hip and knee replacements; removal of urinary catheters on postoperative day 1 after total knee arthroplasty and postoperative day 2 after total hip arthroplasty. Implementation of this protocol resulted in a two-thirds reduction in the incidence of UTIs.[43]

The question of whether antibiotics given at the time of catheter removal may prevent CAUTI has been addressed in recent studies. In a prospective randomized study of patients undergoing abdominal surgery with urinary catheters in place an average of 7 days, patients who received three doses of trimethoprim-sulfamethoxazole at the time of urinary catheter removal had 16.7% few CAUTIs than patients without prophylaxis.[44] Previous studies in patients with shorter duration of catheterization did not show a benefit of prophylactic antibiotics at the time of catheter removal.[45] Larger studies will be necessary to confirm the benefit of antibiotic prophylaxis at the time of removal of urinary catheters that have been in place for a week or more.

Alternatives to Indwelling Urinary Catheters

Intermittent urinary catheterization may reduce the risk of bacteriuria and UTI compared with indwelling urinary catheterization. Patients with neurogenic bladder and long-term urinary catheters, in particular, may benefit from intermittent catheterization.[24] Several studies of intermittent catheterization in postoperative patients have demonstrated increased risk of urinary retention and bladder distention following surgery.[46–48] A recent meta-analysis demonstrated reduced risk of asymptomatic and symptomatic bacteriuria with use of intermittent catheterization compared with indwelling catheterization (RR of 2.9) in patients following hip or knee surgery.[46] Incorporating use of a portable bladder ultrasound scanner with intermittent catheterization may attenuate this risk and reduce the need for indwelling catheterization.[49,50]

A recent randomized trial demonstrated a decrease in the composite outcome of bacteriuria, symptomatic UTI, or death in patients with condom, or external catheters when compared with those with indwelling catheters; the benefit was primarily in those men without dementia.[51] Condom catheters also may be more comfortable and less painful than indwelling catheters in some men.[51,52] Therefore, condom catheters should be considered as an alternative to indwelling catheters in appropriately selected male patients without urinary retention or bladder outlet obstruction.

Aseptic Techniques for Insertion and Maintenance of Urinary Catheters

If urinary catheterization is necessary, aseptic catheter insertion and maintenance is essential for prevention of CAUTI. Urinary catheters should be inserted by a trained health care professional using aseptic technique.[24,53] Cleaning the meatus before catheter insertion is recommended, but there is currently no consensus regarding the use of sterile water versus an antiseptic preparation.[24,53] A study comparing sterile water with 0.1% chlorhexidine cleaning of the meatal area before insertion demonstrated no difference in the development of bacteriuria.[54] Ongoing daily meatal cleaning using an antiseptic also has not shown clear benefit, and may actually increase rates of bacteriuria compared with routine care with soap and water.[55,56] Sterile lubricant jelly should be used for insertion to reduce urethral trauma, but it does not need to possess antiseptic properties.[24] Routine exchange of urinary catheters is not recommended, except for mechanical reasons, as reduction in bacteriuria associated with exchange of catheters is only transient.[53,57] However, exchange of long-term catheters at the time of treatment of symptomatic UTI may be appropriate.[58]

Closed urinary catheter collection systems reduce the risk of CAUTI and are now the standard of care in the United States. Opening the closed system should be avoided; sampling urine may be performed aseptically from a port or from the drainage bag using sterile technique when large samples are required.[25,53] Instilling antiseptic agents or irrigating the bladder with antimicrobial or antiseptic agents as a prophylactic measure has been shown to increase infection.[59]

Anti-infective Catheters

Antiseptic or antimicrobial impregnated urinary catheters have been studied extensively as an adjunctive measure for preventing CAUTI. Catheters coated with silver oxide are no longer available, as they lacked efficacy when compared with the currently available silver alloy catheters.[60] Antimicrobial catheters are typically coated with nitrofurazone, minocycline, or rifampin, but other agents are being evaluated in newer catheters.[61]

In a large meta-analysis, silver alloy catheters significantly reduced the incidence of asymptomatic bacteriuria (RR 0.54, confidence interval [CI] 0.43 to 0.67) in adult patients catheterized less than 7 days. However, for duration of catheterization greater than 7 days, the reduction in asymptomatic bacteriuria was less pronounced (RR 0.64, 95% CI 0.51 to 0.80). Additionally, antibiotic impregnated catheters were found to decrease the rate of asymptomatic bacteriuria (RR 0.52, 95% CI 0.34 to 0.78) for duration of catheterization less than 7 days but demonstrated no benefit in duration of catheterization greater than 7 days.[62] Another systematic review demonstrated similar results.[63] There are few studies that have evaluated antiseptic and antibiotic-coated catheters in long-term urinary catheterization; thus, no conclusions can be drawn in this setting.[64]

While anti-infective urinary catheters appear to reduce bacteriuria in patients with short-term (less than 7 days) urinary catheters, there is no convincing evidence that use of these catheters prevents CAUTI, UTI-related bacteremia, or mortality. Therefore, there is no consensus for routine use of anti-infective urinary catheters to prevent CAUTI.[24] A recent national qualitative study revealed that hospitals using anti-infective catheters often based their decisions on hospital-specific pilot studies.[20]

Finally, systemic antimicrobial therapy may reduce the risk of CAUTI.[10] However, use of systemic antimicrobial therapy specifically for the purpose of preventing CAUTI is not recommended because of issues of cost, potential adverse effects, and possible selection for multidrug-resistant organisms.[10,25] Methenamine has breakdown products that acidify the urine and have antimicrobial properties. In small studies, this agent has been found to reduce bacteriuria, pyuria, and symptomatic UTI.[10] Use of methenamine for prevention of CAUTI is not currently recommended, but further studies are indicated.

In summary, UTI is the most frequent health care-associated infection and predominantly occurs in patients with indwelling urinary catheters. Usual microorganisms causing catheter-associated UTI include enteric gram-negative bacilli, enterococci, *Candida* species, and *P aeruginosa*. Antimicrobial resistance is of particular concern in urinary pathogens. Duration of catheterization is the most important risk factor for development of UTI. Strategies for preventing CAUTI should primarily be focused on limiting the use and duration of indwelling catheters, use of aseptic technique for catheter insertion, and adherence to proper catheter care. The recently published memory aide "ABCDE" (see **Box 3**) provides a useful way of highlighting the most important preventive methods.[30]

REFERENCES

1. Warren JW. Catheter-associated urinary tract infections. Int J Antimicrob Agents 2001;17(4):299–303.
2. Saint S, Chenoweth CE. Biofilms and catheter-associated urinary tract infections. Infect Dis Clin North Am 2003;17:411–32.
3. Tambyah PA, Halvorson KT, Maki DG. A prospective study of pathogenesis of catheter-associated urinary tract infections. Mayo Clin Proc 1999;74:131–6.
4. Maki DG, Tambyah PA. Engineering out the risk of infection with urinary catheters. Emerg Infect Dis 2001;7(2):1–6.
5. Donlan RM. Biofilms and device-associated infections. Emerg Infect Dis 2001; 7(2):1–4.
6. Gaynes RP, Edwards JR, Jarvis WR, et al. Nosocomial infections among neonates in high-risk nurseries in the United States. Pediatrics 1996;98(3):357–61.
7. Langley JM, Hanakowski M, LeBlanc JC. Unique epidemiology of nosocomial urinary tract infection in children. Am J Infect Control 2001;29:94–8.
8. NNIS System. National Nosocomial Infectious Surveillance (NNIS) system report, data summary from January 1992 through June 2004, issued October 2004. Am J Infect Control 2004;32:470–85.
9. Edwards JR, MStat, Peterson KD, et al. National Healthcare Safety Network (NHSN) report, data summary for 2006 through 2007, issued November 2008. Am J Infect Control 2008;36:609–26.
10. Chenoweth CE, Saint S. Urinary tract infections. In: Jarvis WR, editor. Bennett & Brachman's hospital infections. 5th edition. Philadelphia: Lippincott Williams & Wilkins; 2007. p. 507–16.
11. Hidron AI, Edwards JR, Patel J, et al. NHSN annual update: antimicrobial-resistant pathogens associated with healthcare-associated infections: annual summary of data reported to the National Healthcare Safety Network at the Centers for Disease Control and Prevention, 2006–2007. Infect Control Hosp Epidemiol 2008;29(11):996–1011.
12. Krieger JN, Kaiser DL, Wenzel RP. Urinary tract etiology of bloodstream infections in hospitalized patients. J Infect Dis 1983;148(1):57–62.
13. Tambyah PA, Maki DG. Catheter-associated urinary tract infection is rarely symptomatic: a prospective study of 1497 catheterized patients. Arch Intern Med 2000;160(5):678–82.
14. Saint S, Kaufman SR, Rogers MA, et al. Risk factors for nosocomial urinary tract-related bacteremia: a case–control study. Am J Infect Control 2006;34(7):401–7.
15. Horan TC, Andrus M, Dudeck MA. CDC/NHSN surveillance definition of health care-associated infection and criteria for specific types of infections in the acute care setting. Am J Infect Control 2008;36:309–32.
16. Musher DM, Thorsteinsson SB, Airola VM II. Quantitative urinalysis: diagnosing urinary tract infection in men. JAMA 1976;236:2069–72.
17. Tambyah PA, Maki DG. The relationship between pyuria and infection in patients with indwelling urinary catheters: a prospective study of 761 patients. Arch Intern Med 2000;160(5):673–7.
18. Biering-Sorenson F, Bagi P, Hoiby N. Urinary tract infections in patients with spinal cord lesions: treatment and prevention. Drugs 2001;61(9):1275–87.

19. Gandhi T, Flanders SA, Markovitz E, et al. Importance of urinary tract infection to antibiotic use among hospitalized patients. Infect Control Hosp Epidemiol 2009; 30(2):193–5.
20. Saint S, Kowalski CP, Forman J, et al. A multicenter qualitative study on preventing hospital-acquired urinary tract infection in US hospitals. Infect Control Hosp Epidemiol 2008;29(4):333–41.
21. Saint S, Kowalski CP, Kaufman SR, et al. Preventing hospital-acquired urinary tract infection in the United States: a national study. Clin Infect Dis 2008;46(2): 243–50.
22. Saint S, Meddings JA, Calfee D, et al. Catheter-associated urinary tract infection and the Medicare rule changes. Ann Intern Med 2009;150(12):877–84.
23. Association for Professionals in Infection Control and Epidemiology I. Guide to the elimination of catheter-associated urinary tract infections (CAUTI). 2008.
24. Gould CV, Umscheid CA, Agarwal RK, et al. CDC Guideline for prevention of catheter-associated urinary tract infections 2009. Infect Control Hosp Epidemiol 2010;31(4):319–26.
25. Lo E, Nicolle L, Classen D, et al. Strategies to prevent catheter-associated urinary tract infections in acute care hospitals. Infect Control Hosp Epidemiol 2008; 29(Suppl 1):S41–50.
26. Boyce JM, Pittet D. Guideline for hand hygiene in health-care settings. Recommendations of the Healthcare Infection Control Practices Advisory Committee and the HICPAC/SHEA/APIC/IDSA Hand Hygiene Task Force. Society for Healthcare Epidemiology of America/Association for Professionals in Infection Control/ Infectious Diseases Society of America. MMWR Recomm Rep 2002;51(RR-16): 1–45 [quiz: CE41–4].
27. Siegel JD, Rhinehart E, Jackson M, et al. 2007 Guideline for isolation precautions: preventing transmission of infectious agents in health care settings. Am J Infect Control 2007;35:S65–164.
28. Dellit TH, Owens RC, McGowan JE Jr, et al. Infectious Diseases Society of America and the Society for Healthcare Epidemiology of America guidelines for developing an institutional program to enhance antimicrobial stewardship. Clin Infect Dis 2007;44(2):159–77.
29. Pavese P, Saurel N, Labarere J, et al. Does an educational session with an infectious diseases physician reduce the use of inappropriate antibiotic therapy for inpatients with positive urine culture results? A controlled before-and-after study. Infect Control Hosp Epidemiol 2009;30(6):596–9.
30. Saint S, Olmsted RN, Fakih MG, et al. Translating health care-associated urinary tract infection prevention research into practice via the bladder bundle. Jt Comm J Qual Patient Saf 2009;35(9):449–55.
31. Nicolle LE. The prevention of hospital-acquired urinary tract infection. Clin Infect Dis 2008;46(2):251–3.
32. Gardam MA, Amihod B, Orenstein P, et al. Overutilization of indwelling urinary catheters and the development of nosocomial urinary tract infections. Clin Perform Qual Health Care 1998;6(3):99–102.
33. Jain P, Parada JP, David A, et al. Overuse of the indwelling urinary tract catheter in hospitalized medical patients. Arch Intern Med 1995;155(13):1425–9.
34. Munasinghe RL, Yazdani H, Siddique M, et al. Appropriateness of use of indwelling urinary catheters in patients admitted to the medical service. Infect Control Hosp Epidemiol 2001;22(10):647–9.
35. Saint S, Wiese J, Amory JK, et al. Are physicians aware of which of their patients have indwelling catheters? Am J Med 2000;109:476–80.

36. Conybeare A, Pathak S, Imam I. The quality of hospital records of urethral catheterisation. Ann R Coll Surg Engl 2002;84(2):109–10.
37. Huang WC, Wann SR, Lin SL, et al. Catheter-associated urinary tract infections in intensive care units can be reduced by prompting physicians to remove unnecessary catheters. Infect Control Hosp Epidemiol 2004;25(11):974–8.
38. Fakih MG, Dueweke C, Meisner S, et al. Effect of nurse-led multidisciplinary rounds on reducing the unnecessary use of urinary catheterization in hospitalized patients. Infect Control Hosp Epidemiol 2008;29(9):815–9.
39. Saint S, Kaufman SR, Thompson M, et al. A reminder reduces urinary catheterization in hospitalized patients. Jt Comm J Qual Patient Saf 2005;31(8): 455–62.
40. Cornia PB, Amory JK, Fraser S, et al. Computer-based order entry decreases duration of indwelling urinary catheterization in hospitalized patients. Am J Med 2003;114(5):404–7.
41. Wald HL, Ma A, Bratzler DW, et al. Indwelling urinary catheter use in the postoperative period: analysis of the national surgical infection prevention project data. Arch Surg 2008;143(6):551–7.
42. Wald HL, Epstein AM, Radcliff TA, et al. Extended use of urinary catheters in older surgical patients: a patient safety problem? Infect Control Hosp Epidemiol 2008; 29(2):116–24.
43. Stephan F, Sax H, Wachsmuth M, et al. Reduction of urinary tract infection and antibiotic use after surgery: a controlled, prospective, before-after intervention study. Clin Infect Dis 2006;42(11):1544–51.
44. Pfefferkorn U, Sanlav L, Moldenhauer J, et al. Antibiotic prophylaxis at urinary catheter removal prevents urinary tract infections: a prospective randomized trial. Ann Surg 2009;249(4):573–5.
45. Wazait HD, Patel HR, van der Meulen JH, et al. A pilot randomized double-blind placebo-controlled trial on the use of antibiotics on urinary catheter removal to reduce the rate of urinary tract infection: the pitfalls of ciprofloxacin. BJU Int 2004;94(7):1048–50.
46. Niel-Weise BS, van den Broek PJ. Urinary catheter policies for short-term bladder drainage in adults. Cochrane Database Syst Rev 2005;3:CD004203.
47. Michelson JD, Lotke PA, Steinberg ME. Urinary bladder management after total joint replacement surgery. N Engl J Med 1988;319(6):321–6.
48. Oishi CS, Williams VJ, Hanson PB, et al. Perioperative bladder management after primary total hip arthroplasty. J Arthroplasty 1995;10(6):732–6.
49. Moore DA, Edwards K. Using a portable bladder scan to reduce the incidence of nosocomial urinary tract infections. Medsurg Nurs 1997;6(1):39–43.
50. Stevens E. Bladder ultrasound: avoiding unnecessary catheterizations. Medsurg Nurs 2005;14(4):249–53.
51. Saint S, Kaufman SR, Rogers MA, et al. Condom versus indwelling urinary catheters: a randomized trial. J Am Geriatr Soc 2006;54(7):1055–61.
52. Saint S, Lipsky BA, Baker PD, et al. Urinary catheters: what type do men and their nurses prefer? J Am Geriatr Soc 1999;47(12):1453–7.
53. Pratt RJ, Pellowe C, Loveday HP, et al. Guidelines for preventing infections associated with the insertion and management of short-term indwelling urethral catheters in acute care. J Hosp Infect 2001;47:S39–46.
54. Webster J, Hood RH, Burridge CA, et al. Water or antiseptic for periurethral cleaning before urinary catheterization: a randomized controlled trial. Am J Infect Control 2001;29(6):389–94.

55. Burke JP, Garibaldi RA, Britt MR, et al. Prevention of catheter-associated urinary tract infections. Efficacy of daily meatal care regimens. Am J Med 1981;70(3): 655–8.

56. Saint S, Lipsky BA. Preventing catheter-related bacteriuria: should we? Can we? How? Arch Intern Med 1999;159(8):800–8.

57. Tenney JH, Warren JW. Bacteriuria in women with long-term catheters: paired comparison of indwelling and replacement catheters. J Infect Dis 1988;157(1): 199–202.

58. Raz R, Schiller D, Nicolle LE. Chronic indwelling catheter replacement before antimicrobial therapy for symptomatic urinary tract infection. J Urol 2000; 164(4):1254–8.

59. Warren JW, Platt R, Thomas RJ, et al. Antibiotic irrigation and catheter-associated urinary tract infections. N Engl J Med 1978;299(11):570–3.

60. Saint S, Elmore J, Sullivan S, et al. The efficacy of silver alloy-coated urinary catheters in preventing urinary tract infection: a meta-analysis. Am J Med 1998;105: 236–41.

61. Stensballe J, Tvede M, Looms D, et al. Infection risk with nitrofurazone-impregnated urinary catheters in trauma patients: a randomized trial. Ann Intern Med 2007;147(5):285–93.

62. Schumm K, Lam T. Types of urethral catheters for management of short-term voiding problems in hospitalised adults. Cochrane Database Syst Rev 2008;2: CD004013.

63. Johnson JR, Kuskowski MA, Wilt TJ. Systematic review: antimicrobial urinary catheters to prevent catheter-associated urinary tract infection in hospitalized patients. Ann Intern Med 2006;144(2):116–26.

64. Jahn P, Preuss M, Kernig A, et al. Types of indwelling urinary catheters for long-term bladder drainage in adults. Cochrane Database Syst Rev 2007;3: CD004997.

Prevention of Health Care–Acquired Pneumonia and Transmission of *Mycobacterium tuberculosis* in Health Care Settings

Jerry M. Zuckerman, MD[a,b,]*

KEYWORDS

- Pneumonia • Ventilator associated • Tuberculosis
- Infection control • Review

Health care–acquired pneumonia (HAP) is associated with significant morbidity and mortality. These infections most frequently arise from a patient's indigenous flora, although occasionally they result from exposure to environmental pathogens such as *Legionella* and *Aspergillus*. This article reviews infection prevention strategies to reduce the incidence of HAP. These strategies focus on lowering the risk of aspiration, decreasing the amount of oropharyngeal colonization, shortening the duration of mechanical ventilation, and preventing environmental exposures. Successful implementation of these prevention strategies usually requires a multidisciplinary approach and standardization of protocols. This article also discusses strategies to prevent transmission of *Mycobacterium tuberculosis* within health care settings. Patients with tuberculosis (TB) pose a risk to other patients and health care workers (HCWs) and outbreaks in health care settings occur when appropriate infection control measures are not used. All health care facilities should have an operational TB infection control plan that emphasizes the use of a hierarchy of controls (administrative, environmental, and personal respiratory protection) to prevent the transmission of *M tuberculosis*.

[a] Department of Medicine, Jefferson Medical College, 111 South 11th Street, Philadelphia, PA 19107, USA
[b] Infection Prevention and Control Department, Albert Einstein Medical Center, 5401 Old York Road, Philadelphia, PA 19141, USA
* Division of Infectious Diseases, Department of Medicine, Albert Einstein Medical Center, Klein Building-Suite 331, 5401 Old York Road, Philadelphia, PA 19141.
E-mail address: Zuckermj@einstein.edu

Infect Dis Clin N Am 25 (2011) 117–133
doi:10.1016/j.idc.2010.11.014
0891-5520/11/$ – see front matter © 2011 Elsevier Inc. All rights reserved.

id.theclinics.com

HAP
Epidemiology

In 2002, an estimated 250,000 HAPs were reported in hospitals in the United States, accounting for 15% of all health care–associated infections. HAP was estimated to be the cause of, or associated with, 36,000 hospital deaths.[1] Approximately 50% of these pneumonias occurred in hospital settings outside of the intensive care units (ICUs). In a prospective study, HAP in non-ICU patients occurred at a rate of 3 ± 1.4 cases per 1000 hospital admissions.[2] In the ICU setting, most HAPs are associated with mechanical ventilation. Pneumonias are reported as ventilator associated if the patient was intubated and ventilated at the time of, or within 48 hours before, the onset of infection.[3] Around 10% to 20% of patients receiving mechanical ventilation for more than 48 hours develop ventilator-associated pneumonia (VAP).[4–6] The risk of developing VAP seems to be greatest during the first 5 days of intubation (3% per day). This risk decreases to 2% per day during days 5 to 10 of mechanical ventilation and 1% thereafter.[7]

From 2006–2008, nearly 9000 VAPs were reported to the Centers for Disease Control and Prevention's (CDC's) National Healthcare Safety Network (NHSN) by health care facilities participating in this surveillance system. VAP rates varied according to the characteristics of the unit, including patient population, unit size, and type, and whether or not the unit was located in a major teaching hospital. Burn and trauma units had the highest VAP rates with 10.7 and 8.1 infections per 1000 ventilator days, respectively. Neurologic, neurosurgical, and surgical ICUs had rates of 6.7, 5.3, and 4.9, respectively. VAP rates for medical ICUs or medical/surgical ICUs ranged from 1.9 to 2.9.[8] Ventilator use, defined as the number of ventilator days divided by the number of patient days, in adult ICUs ranged from a mean of 0.27 for medical cardiac units to a mean of 0.57 for trauma ICUs.

The consequences of HAP may be significant. For example, patients who developed HAP after having elective intra-abdominal surgery had a longer length of stay ([LOS] 11.03 days) and a 10-fold greater risk of in-hospital mortality than those patients who did not develop HAP postoperatively. In addition, HAP was independently associated with a 4.13-fold increased risk of being discharged to a skilled nursing facility and a 75% mean increase in total hospital charges.[9] Patients who develop VAP have significantly longer durations of mechanical ventilation, longer lengths of stay (LOSs) in the ICU and hospital, and higher mortality than those patients who do not develop VAP.[4–6,10] A recent economic analysis estimates that the attributable costs of VAP per patient range from $14,806 to $27,520, adjusted to 2007 dollars, and the annual aggregate attributable patient hospital costs range from $0.78 to $1.45 billion dollars in the United States.[11]

Case Definitions

At present, there is no gold standard for establishing the diagnosis of HAP. The diagnosis can be influenced by surveillance strategies, diagnostic techniques, and microbiology and laboratory tests performed. The diagnosis is also subject to significant interobserver variability.[12] Cultures of the respiratory tract are very sensitive but not specific for the diagnosis of pneumonia. Clinical signs and symptoms are also nonspecific and may be associated with other common conditions found in the health care setting. For example, pulmonary embolus, atelectasis, respiratory distress syndrome, pulmonary hemorrhage, and myocardial infarction all may mimic the clinical findings of pneumonia.[13] A detailed discussion on establishing the diagnosis and treatment of VAP is beyond the scope of this review.

For reporting to the NHSN, HAP is identified by using a combination of radiographic, clinical, and laboratory criteria. A physician's diagnosis alone is not sufficient to meet the NHSN's surveillance definition of HAP. Radiographic criteria include 2 or more chest radiographs with at least one of the following findings: new or progressive and persistent infiltrate, consolidation, or cavitation. Clinical criteria include at least one of the following: fever, leukopenia, leukocytosis, or altered mental status for adults 70 years or older. In addition, patients must have at least 2 of the following: new onset of purulent sputum, change in character of sputum, increased respiratory secretions, or increased suctioning requirements; new-onset or worsening cough, dyspnea, or tachypnea; rales or bronchial breath sounds; worsening gas exchange, increased oxygen requirements, or increased ventilator demand. If patients meet these clinical criteria, they are classified as PNU1 according to NHSN algorithms. A PNU2 classification is assigned to those patients who have the aforementioned criteria plus additional specified culture or serologic test results, such as positive blood or pleural fluid culture results, positive quantitative culture results from bronchoalveolar lavage (BAL) or protected specimen brushing, 5% or more BAL-obtained cells containing intracellular bacteria on direct microscopic examination, histopathologic examination showing evidence of pneumonia, detection of viral antigen or antibody from respiratory secretions, or detection of Legionella pneumophila serogroup 1 antigens in urine. Pneumonias that develop in immunocompromised patients and meet certain radiographic, clinical, and laboratory criteria are classified as PNU3. Specific details of the case surveillance definitions and complete radiographic, clinical, and laboratory criteria can be found at http://www.cdc.gov/nhsn/PDFs/pscManual/6pscVAPcurrent.pdf.[3]

Risk Factors

Aspiration of oropharyngeal organisms is the most likely route for bacteria to enter the lower respiratory tract. Using radioisotope tracers, aspiration was found to occur in 45% of 20 healthy adults and 7 of 10 patients with depressed consciousness.[14] In a study of patients on mechanical ventilation, tracheal secretions were assayed for pepsin, a marker for gastric contents. Of nearly 6000 tracheal secretions collected, 31% were pepsin positive and 89% of the 360 study patients had at least 1 aspiration event. Patients who developed pneumonia by day 4 of mechanical ventilation were twice as likely to have pepsin-positive tracheal secretions (42%) compared with those without pneumonia (21%). Risk factors for aspiration included backrest elevation less than 30°, vomiting, gastric feedings, a Glasgow Coma Scale score less than 9, and gastroesophageal reflux disease.[15] Hospital-acquired pneumonia may also develop via inhalation of aerosols containing microorganisms such as Legionella or Aspergillus or less frequently by hematogenous spread.[16]

Risk factors for HAP include increased bacterial colonization of the aerodigestive tract, aspiration into the respiratory tract, or prolonged use of mechanical ventilatory support.[16] Nonmodifiable risk factors are intrinsic to the patient, underlying diagnosis, or procedure. These nonmodifiable risk factors include admission diagnoses of burns, trauma or diseases of the central nervous system, age greater than 70 years, underlying lung disease, thoracoabdominal surgery, depressed level of consciousness, and prior episode of large-volume aspiration.[16] Modifiable risk factors for the development of VAP include gastric acid suppression, frequency of ventilator circuit changes, supine positioning, pooling of subglottic secretions, and antibiotic usage.[17]

Prevention of HAP

Infection prevention efforts to reduce HAP have focused on reducing the risk of aspiration of oropharyngeal secretions, decreasing the duration of mechanical ventilation, and/or preventing oropharyngeal or gastric colonization. Most strategies have focused on the prevention of VAP.

Aspiration of oropharyngeal secretions is a common event, especially in patients on mechanical ventilation. It has been hypothesized that maintaining patients in the semirecumbent position reduces the likelihood of aspiration and subsequent development of pneumonia. Using radiolabeled enteral feeds, mean radioactive counts in endobronchial secretions were significantly higher in samples taken from patients in the supine position compared with those from patients in the semirecumbent position.[18] A randomized trial in mechanically ventilated patients reported a 4-fold reduction in the rate of VAP in patients maintained in the semirecumbent position (45°) versus the supine position (0°).[19] The validity of this study has been questioned because confirmation of the semirecumbent position was monitored only once daily and the supine group was maintained at 0° elevation rather than a standard 10° to 15° elevation.[20]

Although advocated in several guidelines, the feasibility of maintaining patients in a semirecumbent position has been challenged. In a prospective multicenter trial, mechanically ventilated patients were maintained either in a semirecumbent position (target backrest elevation of 45°) or in a supine position (target backrest elevation of 10°). The patients' positions were continuously monitored during the first week of mechanical ventilation. The target backrest elevation of 45° in the semirecumbent group was not achieved during 85% of the study period. The average head of bed elevation achieved was 23° to 28° compared with an average head of bed elevation of 10° to 16° in the supine group.[21] There was no difference in VAP, mortality rates, duration of ventilation, or LOS in the ICU between the 2 groups. The benefit of a comprehensive educational program and standardized orders to maintain mechanically ventilated patients in a semirecumbent position was evaluated in an observational study. Despite the interventions, the target backrest elevation of 45° was achieved in less than 30% of mechanically ventilated patients in the postintervention period.[22] Possible methods to ensure better reliability of keeping the head of the bed elevated include using documentation on nursing flow sheets, enlisting the aid of respiratory therapists, involving families in the process, using visual cues, and providing feedback to the staff on compliance with this measure.[23]

Another approach to decreasing the risk of aspiration is via subglottic suctioning of secretions that may pool above the endotracheal tube cuff. Continuous drainage of subglottic secretions has been associated with a decreased incidence and delayed onset of VAP, reduction in duration of mechanical ventilation, and shorter LOS in the ICU.[24] Suctioning of oral secretions before each positional change has also been shown to reduce the incidence of VAP, the duration of mechanical ventilation, and LOS in the ICU.[25]

Shortening the duration of mechanical ventilation in intubated patients by minimizing sedation and using spontaneous breathing trials may reduce the incidence of pneumonia. The goal of sedation and analgesia in critically ill patients is to optimize patient comfort and minimize distress while avoiding accumulation of drugs and metabolites, which may delay the patient's recovery. The Society of Critical Care Medicine's guidelines for the use of sedatives and analgesics in critically ill patients stress the need to avoid oversedation by setting and titrating medications to a sedation goal using a validated sedation assessment scale.[26] Systematic tapering of the dose or daily interruption of the sedation is also recommended to minimize prolonged sedative effects. Daily sedation interruption in mechanically ventilated patients has been advocated as a way to reduce the duration of ventilatory support and therefore the risk of VAP. In a single-center trial of 128 adults on mechanical ventilation, the group assigned to daily interruption of sedation until the patient was awake (or until they required resumption of sedation because of agitation or discomfort) had a shorter duration of ventilation and shorter median LOS in the ICU than the group that had sedatives managed at the clinician's discretion.[27] A retrospective review of the data showed that the intervention group had a decrease in the number of complications, including the incidence of VAP.[28] Additional clinical trials using sedation protocols in mechanically ventilated patients generally show similar benefits in shortening the duration of mechanical ventilation or reducing ICU LOS and are summarized in a recent review.[29] Similarly, weaning protocols using spontaneous breathing trials for up to 2 hours led to a significant reduction in the duration of mechanical ventilation compared with weaning that was physician driven.[30]

In the multicenter Awakening and Breathing Controlled trial, a protocol pairing daily interruption of sedation with spontaneous breathing trials (intervention group) was compared with usual care with patient-targeted sedation along with a daily spontaneous breathing trial (control group).[31] Patients in the intervention group had significantly more ventilator-free days and decreased LOSs in both the ICU and hospital. More patients in the daily sedation interruption group self-extubated, but the number of patients who required reintubation after self-extubation was similar for the intervention and control groups.

Sedation protocols and daily sedation interruptions are not routinely implemented in many ICUs despite evidence demonstrating its beneficial effect in decreasing the duration of mechanical ventilation. Two studies demonstrated that 30% to 50% of patients in the ICU who were assessed were deeply sedated.[32,33] A 2004 Web-based survey of members of the Society of Critical Care Medicine revealed that 64% reported having a sedation protocol in their units and daily sedation interruption was used by only 40% of the providers. Reasons reported for the absence of a sedation protocol included lack of a physician order, lack of nursing support, and fear of oversedation. Barriers to the use of daily sedation interruption included lack of nursing acceptance, concerns about patient-initiated device removal, and concerns about inducing either respiratory compromise or discomfort in ventilated patients.[34] Even when guidelines and protocols exist, adherence to them is often poor.[35]

To improve adherence to sedation protocols, one institution had a pharmacist evaluate mechanically ventilated patients on continuous sedation on a daily basis to ensure adherence to the institution's previously approved sedation guidelines. The mean duration of mechanical ventilation was significantly reduced from 14 days in the preintervention group to 7.4 days in the postintervention group. The durations of ICU and hospital stays were also significantly decreased.[36] In another study, a nurse-implemented sedation protocol resulted in a decreased incidence of VAP and duration of mechanical ventilation.[37] Concerns about the feasibility and safety of performing a daily sedation interruption protocol outside the context of a research trial have been expressed.[38] Safety screening before initiation of sedation interruption or spontaneous breathing trial, along with close observation, is essential to avoid potential harm to patients.[29] Suggestions for improving the implementation of these processes include having protocols for daily sedation interruption and/or spontaneous breathing trials, using a sedation scale to avoid oversedation, assessing compliance each day on multidisciplinary rounds, and posting compliance with the intervention to encourage change and motivate staff.[23]

Other interventions to prevent VAP have focused on eradicating or preventing oropharyngeal colonization. Oropharyngeal decontamination with a topical antimicrobial paste consisting of gentamicin, colistin, and vancomycin, applied every 6 hours, lowered the incidence of VAP to 10% compared with 23% and 31% in 2 control groups. Duration of mechanical ventilation, length of ICU stay, and mortality were similar in all groups.[39] A meta-analysis of 7 randomized control trials demonstrated that oral application of topical chlorhexidine resulted in a 30% relative reduction in the risk of VAP but no decrease in mortality. The greatest reduction in VAP was seen in patients who had undergone cardiac surgery.[40] The benefit of chlorhexidine may be greater with 2% chlorhexidine solution than with preparations containing a lower concentration.[41–43] A comprehensive oral care program, which included deep suctioning every 6 hours, oral tissue cleansing every 4 hours or as needed, and toothbrushing twice daily, was studied by comparing outcomes in the pre- and postintervention periods. Compliance with the oral care program was 80%. The VAP rate decreased from 12 per 1000 ventilator days to 8 per 1000 ventilator days and was associated with a significant decrease in duration of mechanical ventilation, length of ICU stay, and mortality.[44] Other trials have not demonstrated any benefit of toothbrushing alone or in combination with topical oral chlorhexidine in reducing the incidence of VAP.[45,46]

Selective decontamination of the digestive tract (SDD) and selective oropharyngeal decontamination (SOD) has been studied extensively with most trials demonstrating a decrease in the rates of HAPs. Antimicrobial prophylaxis is used to prevent gastric and oral colonization while keeping the anaerobic intestinal flora intact. SDD consists of topical nonabsorbable antimicrobial agents applied to the oropharynx and stomach combined with the administration of systemic antimicrobials for 3 to 4 days. A recent Cochrane review demonstrated that there was a significant decrease in lower respiratory tract infections (odds ratio [OR], 0.28) and mortality (OR, 0.75) in patients who received a combination of topical and systemic antibiotic prophylaxis.[47] The use of topical prophylaxis alone resulted in a significant decrease in respiratory tract infections but not in mortality. A crossover study in 13 ICUs in the Netherlands compared the efficacy of SDD, SOD, and standard care on mortality. Although crude unadjusted mortality was similar between all treatment arms, there was an absolute reduction in the 28-day mortality of 3.5% in the SDD group and 2.9% in the SOD arm compared with the standard care group after adjustment for covariates.[48] One trial has investigated the impact of SDD on antimicrobial resistance. None of the patients in either the SDD or control group were colonized with methicillin-resistant *Staphylococcus aureus* and 1% were colonized with vancomycin-resistant enterococci. Colonization with gram-negative bacteria resistant to ceftazidime, ciprofloxacin, imipenem, polymyxin E, or tobramycin occurred less frequently in patients in the SDD group (16%) than in those in the control group (26%).[49] This trial was performed in ICUs with a low prevalence of resistant organisms and may not be applicable to other units where resistance is more common. Until additional data are available about the effect of SDD on the emergence of resistant organisms, the routine use of SDD remains an unresolved issue.[16,50]

A silver-coated endotracheal tube has been studied as another approach to prevent bacterial colonization of the oropharynx. In a prospective single-blind randomized trial, use of a silver-coated endotracheal tube resulted in a significant decrease in VAP and delayed time to VAP occurrence. However, there was no difference in duration of intubation, length of ICU or hospital stay, or mortality.[51]

Several interventions, such as frequency of ventilator circuit changes or type of humidification process, do not affect the incidence of VAP. Current recommendations do not recommend changing ventilator circuits on a routine schedule. Circuit changes should be performed when there is visual and/or known contamination of the circuit.[16] Current guidelines also do not recommend preferential use of passive (heat and moisture exchangers) or active humidifiers because comparative trials between the 2 types of humidifiers have not demonstrated any difference in the incidence of VAP.[52,53]

Successful implementation of evidence-based guidelines and conversion of research evidence into clinical practice is often fraught with difficulties. The Society of Healthcare Epidemiology and the Infectious Diseases Society of America have published a compendium of practice recommendations and strategies to prevent VAP.[12] The guidelines recommend direct observation of compliance with VAP-specific process measures (hand hygiene, semirecumbent positioning of eligible patients, daily sedation interruption and assessment of readiness to wean, and regular antiseptic oral care). The incidence of VAP should be determined by performing ongoing surveillance of ventilated patients for clinical, microbiological, and radiographic evidence of pneumonia. Process and outcome measures should be reported regularly to senior hospital leaders, nursing leaders, and clinicians who care for patients at risk for VAP.

The Institute of Healthcare Improvement (IHI) promotes the use of a "ventilator bundle," a collection of care processes to reduce the incidence of VAP and other serious complications associated with mechanical ventilation.[23] IHI's bundle is composed of 4 elements: (1) maintaining head of bed elevation greater than 30°, (2) daily sedation interruption and assessment of readiness to wean, (3) peptic ulcer prophylaxis, and (4) deep vein thrombosis prophylaxis. As part of an IHI-sponsored collaborative project, 35 ICUs submitted data on VAP rates and compliance with the ventilator bundle. On average, the VAP rate decreased by 44.5% in ICUs that demonstrated at least a 20% improvement in adherence to the ventilator bundle. Those units that had a compliance of 95% or more had the greatest reduction (59%) in VAP rates.[54] Successful implementation of the bundle usually required ICUs to change work processes, such as implementing multidisciplinary ICU rounds, establishing daily patient goals, or using weaning protocols by respiratory therapists. A proactive approach involving staff education, process and outcome measurement, and feedback to staff can result in increased compliance with the bundle elements and subsequent reduction in VAP rates.[55] Some investigators have questioned the validity of studies that report success with the ventilator bundle, citing methodological flaws, including publication and selection bias, confounders related to case mix or adjunct measures used, and definitions and diagnostic techniques used to define VAP.[56]

Prevention of Health Care–Acquired Legionella or Aspergillus Pneumonia

Sometimes HAP may arise secondary to environmental pathogens rather than from the patient's indigenous flora. Legionella and Aspergillus are the 2 most common environmental pathogens associated with HAP. The overall incidence of HAP due to Legionella spp is unknown, although institutional outbreaks and sporadic cases have been reported.[16] HAP due to Legionella spp may be underrecognized because diagnostic tests for Legionella are not routinely performed. Legionella spp are found in aquatic environments and have been isolated from cooling towers, evaporative condensers, and heated potable water distribution systems within health care facilities. Growth of Legionella is enhanced by temperatures between 25°C and 42°C, stagnation, and scale and sediment within water systems. Transmission occurs either by inhalation of aerosols of water contaminated with Legionella spp from cooling towers, showers, faucets, and room-air humidifiers or via aspiration of contaminated potable water. The likelihood of developing an infection depends on the intensity of the exposure and the exposed person's health status.

Two approaches have been advocated to prevent legionnaires disease in facilities that have not had any known hospital-acquired cases of Legionella. The first approach is based on periodic routine culturing of a facility's potable water system for Legionella. If any sample is culture positive, clinicians are advised to send diagnostic tests for Legionella from patients who develop HAP. The relationship between the results of environmental surveillance and the risk for legionellosis remains unknown. In a surveillance study, *Legionella* was isolated from 14 of 20 hospital water systems. Of these 14 hospitals, 6 had high-level colonization with more than 30% of the distal outlets being culture positive and 4 of these facilities had cases of hospital-acquired *Legionella* pneumonia. No cases of hospital-acquired *Legionella* pneumonia occurred in hospitals in which environmental samples were culture negative.[57] Decontamination of the potable water system is recommended when 30% or more of the samples are culture positive for *Legionella* species.[58]

An alternative approach to preventing legionnaires disease advocates maintaining a high index of suspicion and ordering appropriate diagnostic tests for patients who develop HAP and are at increased risk for *Legionella* infections. If a definite case or 2 possible cases of health care–acquired legionellosis are identified, then an epidemiologic and environmental investigation should be initiated and appropriate remediation measures instituted. These measures may include increasing the temperature at which heated water is maintained, hyperchlorination, treatment of water with chlorine dioxide, use of a copper-silver ionization system, physical cleaning or replacement of hot water storage tanks, and removal of dead legs in the water distribution system. Culturing of a facility's water system may help to identify the suspected source of infection or to assess the effectiveness of decontamination protocols.[59]

Aspergillus is a ubiquitous fungus that may cause HAP in severely immunocompromised patients. Pulmonary aspergillosis is acquired by inhalation of fungal spores. If host immune defenses are inadequate, then invasive pulmonary disease may occur, resulting in significant morbidity and mortality. Risk factors for invasive pulmonary aspergillosis (IPA) include severe neutropenia, prolonged (>2 weeks) neutropenia, high-dose corticosteroids, hematopoietic stem cell transplantation, and solid organ transplants.[16]

Outbreaks of IPA have been associated with hospital renovation and construction projects, which increase the number of *Aspergillus* spores in the air. An infection control risk assessment by a multidisciplinary team should be performed before the start of any renovation or construction project to determine the need for dust and moisture containment measures and other safeguards to protect susceptible patients.[60] Appropriate barriers should be erected to contain the spread of contaminated dust particles. Shutting off return air vents in the construction area, exhausting air and dust to the outside, using high-efficiency particulate air (HEPA) filters and controlling the direction of air flow are some of the adjustments that can be made to the ventilation system. Other measures to control dust in the air and on surfaces include the use of wet mops and damp wipes to clean the work area and equipment, use of vacuums with HEPA filters, minimizing traffic in the work area, and ensuring proper removal of solid debris. Relocation of high-risk patients to alternative areas may be necessary, and transport of patients should occur via routes that minimize their exposure to construction material or equipment.[59] There is additional discussion of this topic in an article by Geoge Alangaden in the same issue.

TB

The incidence of TB in the United States steadily declined throughout the twentieth century until the mid-1980s when a resurgence of cases occurred. Factors that contributed to this increase in TB included societal issues (homelessness, injecting drug use), decreased public health support, increased immigration of persons from countries with a high incidence of TB, and the emergence of the AIDS epidemic.[61] Interventions, such as greater use of directly observed therapy, increased testing and treatment of latent TB infections in individuals at risk for developing active disease, and strengthening of infection control procedures in hospitals successfully reversed the trend of increasing TB. Since 1992, the rate of TB cases in the United States has decreased by 60% to a record low in 2008 of 4.2 cases per 100,000 populations (12,898 incident cases).[62]

Transmission of TB in Health Care Facilities

Between 1985 and 1992, there were outbreaks of TB, some with multidrug-resistant strains, in health care facilities that resulted in TB transmission to other patients and HCWs. These outbreaks occurred because of the failure to recognize and diagnose TB, resulting in delayed initiation of effective antituberculous therapy and failure to initiate airborne precautions in hospitalized patients or to maintain precautions until patients were no longer infectious to others. They were also associated with lapses in infection control procedures, including failure to maintain proper ventilation in isolation rooms and the inadequate use of proper respiratory protection.[63] These outbreaks and further transmission of TB within health care facilities were successfully curtailed by the widespread implementation of infection control measures recommended by the CDC in 1990 and 1994.[63–67]

Transmission of TB occurs via airborne particles (droplet nuclei) containing *M tuberculosis*. Infectious droplet nuclei, 1 to 5 μm in size, are generated by individuals with pulmonary or laryngeal TB when they cough or talk. Droplet nuclei remain airborne for prolonged periods of time and are small enough when inhaled to evade the mucociliary defenses in airways before being deposited in alveoli. The likelihood of TB being transmitted to another individual depends on the concentration of infectious droplet nuclei in the air and the duration of exposure. Patients with TB are more infectious if they have a cough, cavitation on chest radiograph, a positive acid-fast bacilli (AFB) sputum smear result, and laryngeal involvement or if they undergo a cough-inducing or aerosol-generating procedure. Environmental factors that contribute to increased risk of transmission include exposure to TB in small enclosed spaces, insufficient dilution and removal of infectious droplet nuclei from the air, and recirculation of contaminated air. The transmission, pathogenesis, diagnosis, and treatment of latent and active TB are described extensively elsewhere.[68–70]

Components of a TB Infection Control Program

In 2005, the CDC published revised guidelines for preventing the spread of TB within health care settings.[71] These guidelines recommend that all health care settings have a TB infection control program to ensure prompt detection, isolation, and treatment of persons who have suspected or confirmed TB. The recommended TB control plan relies on a hierarchy of controls, including administrative, environmental, and respiratory protection, and is based on an annual risk assessment performed for the setting. The rest of this article summarizes the salient features of these guidelines. The reader is advised to review the document (available at http://www.cdc.gov/tb/publications/guidelines/infectioncontrol.htm) for a more in-depth discussion.[71]

Administrative measures are the most important level of control to reduce the risk of exposure to persons who have suspected or confirmed TB. These measures include written protocols to ensure the prompt detection and isolation of suspect cases, timeliness of diagnostic tests, education of HCWs regarding TB, and implementation of a screening program for employees who may be exposed to TB. Process measures, such as the time interval to initiation of airborne precautions and/or treatment in suspect or confirmed TB cases, duration of airborne infection isolation (AII) and compliance with discontinuation of airborne precautions criteria should be used to assess the effectiveness of the TB control plan. Infection control investigations are warranted if an HCW is diagnosed with TB disease, person-to-person transmission of *M tuberculosis* is suspected, or there are lapses in TB infection control practices resulting in exposed patients and/or HCWs. Genotyping or restriction fragment length polymorphism analysis of TB isolates can facilitate the identification of TB outbreaks, including those associated with transmission within health care settings.[72]

The primary risk for health care–associated transmission is the unsuspected or undiagnosed patient with infectious TB. A high index of suspicion and prompt triage and initiation of TB airborne precautions is essential to minimize the exposure risk. Failure to appropriately isolate cases can be avoided by carefully reviewing the patient's medical history including questions about (1) a history of TB exposure, infection, or disease; (2) signs or symptoms consistent with TB disease (cough for >3 weeks duration, loss of appetite, unexplained weight loss, night sweats, fever, bloody sputum, hoarseness, fatigue, or chest pain); and (3) presence of comorbidities or use of medications that increase their risk for TB.[73] A decision instrument for predicting which patients with pneumonia do not require admission to a TB isolation room was derived retrospectively and validated prospectively in 11 university-affiliated US emergency departments. According to this study, patients unlikely to have TB are those without a history of TB or previous positive tuberculin skin test result, are not immigrants or homeless, have not been recently incarcerated, do not have any recent weight loss, and do not have apical infiltrates or cavitary lesions on their chest radiographs.[74]

When TB is suspected, patients should remain isolated in an AII room until TB disease is considered unlikely and an alternative diagnosis is established or 3 consecutive negative AFB sputum test results are obtained. Sputum samples should be collected in 8- to 24-hour intervals and at least one should be an early morning specimen. The yield of AFB sputum smears and mycobacterial cultures increased with repeated sputum induction in one study, but another study suggested that a third sputum sample had little additional diagnostic value.[75,76] For hospitalized individuals in whom TB disease is either confirmed or continues to be suspected, airborne precautions should be maintained until patients have demonstrated a clinical response to antituberculous treatment and are determined to be noninfectious. Ideally, patients should be treated in an AII room until they have received at least 2 weeks of standard antituberculous therapy, demonstrated clinical improvement (resolution of fever, decreased cough), and have 3 consecutive negative AFB sputum smear test results. Once patients are medically stable, they can be discharged to home, even if their sputum smear test results have not converted to negative as long as the following criteria are met: (1) follow-up care and directly observed therapy have been arranged, (2) there are no children younger than 4 years or immunocompromised persons in the household, and (3) all immunocompetent household members have previously been exposed to the patient.

Environmental controls are the second line of defense in TB control programs and focus on preventing the spread and reducing the concentration of airborne TB particles. General ventilation systems dilute and remove contaminated air and can be balanced to control airflow patterns in a room or setting. In areas where infectious airborne droplet nuclei might be present (eg, AII rooms), a single-pass ventilation system is preferred with airflow of at least 6 air changes per hour (12 air changes per hour for new construction).[77] External exhaust of contaminated air is preferred but, if necessary, air may be recirculated through HEPA filters. All inpatient rooms are maintained at negative pressure to surrounding areas. A pressure differential greater than or equal to 0.01 in of water is recommended, and monitoring of the negative pressure should be performed daily when the room is occupied by a patient with suspected or confirmed TB. Other areas that should have negative pressure rooms include bronchoscopy and autopsy suites, sputum induction rooms, clinical laboratories, and other selected examination and treatment rooms in areas such as the emergency department or outpatient offices. Routine preventative maintenance should be scheduled and regular quality control checks performed to ensure that environmental controls are functioning properly. Infection control preventionists should be notified of any malfunction of, or scheduled maintenance on, ventilation systems servicing care areas of patients with TB.

Respiratory protective equipment is the last line of defense in a TB control plan and is used at the point of care at which the risk of exposure to infectious droplet nuclei is reduced but not entirely eliminated. Respirators used for TB protection must be certified to have 95% or greater filtration efficiency when challenged with 0.3-μm-sized particles. Minimizing face-seal leakage of a nonpowered air-purifying respirator is essential to optimize the respirator's protective ability. The amount of face-seal leakage is determined by the fit characteristics of the respirator as well as the ability to properly don it. A user-seal check should be performed before each use to ensure that the respirator is positioned correctly and leakage is minimal. The use of respirators for TB in the United States is regulated by the Occupational Safety and Health Administration's general industry standard for respiratory protection. This standard requires health care settings to have a respirator-protection plan to perform fit testing to ensure proper fit and use and to provide annual training for all HCWs who use respirators.[78]

An employee TB screening program is an essential component of the TB control plan. The need for an employee TB screening program and frequency of screening is determined by the likelihood that suspect or confirmed TB cases will be encountered, ie, the setting's risk classification. A setting in which exposure to TB is unlikely is assigned a low-risk classification. In settings in which HCWs may potentially be exposed to patients with TB, the risk classification depends on the size and location of the setting and the number of confirmed TB cases encountered yearly. Inpatient settings with more than 200 beds are classified as medium risk if 6 or more patients with TB were treated in the preceding year and as low risk if fewer than 6 patients with TB were treated. Inpatient settings with fewer than 200 beds are classified as medium risk if 3 or more patients with TB were treated in the preceding year and as low risk if less than 3 patients with TB were treated. Outpatient, outreach, and home-based health care settings are classified as medium risk if 3 or more patients with TB are seen or low risk if fewer than 3 patients with TB are identified in the preceding year.

All HCWs should receive baseline TB screening on hire with either a 2-step tuberculin skin test (TST) or a single interferon gamma release assay (IGRA) for *M tuberculosis*. In a low-risk setting, further TB screening is not necessary unless an exposure occurs. In a medium-risk setting, TB screening should be performed annually. On serial screening, a conversion occurs when there is an increase of 10 mm or more of induration from previous TST readings or IGRA results are reported as positive in an HCW for whom it was previously negative. Screening programs should calculate a conversion rate for the population tested. Conversion rates above baseline or a cluster of conversions should prompt an investigation to determine if TB transmission is occurring within the setting. In situations in which person-to-person transmission may be occurring, screening should be performed every 8 to 10 weeks until there is no evidence of ongoing transmission. Afterwards, the setting should be classified as medium risk for at least 1 year.

Laboratories play an essential role in the diagnosis and management of TB infections by providing accurate results within acceptable turnaround times. In addition, the processing of TB specimens must be performed in a safe manner to minimize exposure risk of laboratory technicians. The Association of Public Health Laboratories has developed a tool for mycobacteriology laboratories to self-assess the quality of their diagnostic TB practices and to identify areas that may be in need of improvement.[79] Laboratories that process TB specimens are classified as medium risk. TB screening should be performed annually or every 8 to 10 weeks if conversions are documented. Personnel should be thoroughly trained in methods that minimize the production of aerosols. All specimens suspected or known to contain *M tuberculosis* must be handled in a class I or II biological safety cabinet (BSC) with appropriate environmental and respiratory protection controls being used. Proper maintenance of the BSC and handling of clinical specimens is essential to minimize the risk of cross-contamination of specimens.

False-positive culture results for *M tuberculosis* have been reported to occur in an estimated 1% to 3% of TB cases and may be secondary to laboratory cross-contamination, contaminated clinical equipment, or clerical errors.[72] Clinicians should consider the possibility of false-positive culture results if their patients' clinical illnesses are not consistent with TB disease. In addition, false-positive results should be considered when there is a single culture-positive specimen out of many obtained from a particular patient, when there is low colony counts on solid media, or when growth is detected in broth-based media after a prolonged incubation period. In addition false-positive results should be considered when specimens from different patients processed in the same laboratory on the same day are reported positive or isolates have unexpected drug resistance.[80,81] Mycobacteriology laboratories should have a plan for identification, review, and notification of possible false-positive culture results.

SUMMARY

HAP is associated with significant morbidity and mortality. These infections most frequently arise from a patient's indigenous flora, although occasionally they result from exposure to environmental pathogens such as *Legionella* and *Aspergillus*. Infection prevention strategies that reduce the incidence of HAP focus on lowering the risk of aspiration, decreasing the amount of oropharyngeal colonization, shortening the duration of mechanical ventilation, and controlling environmental exposures. Successful implementation of these prevention strategies usually requires a multidisciplinary approach and standardization of protocols. Patients with TB pose a risk to other patients and HCWs, and outbreaks in health care settings have occurred when appropriate infection control measures were not used. All health care facilities should have an operational TB infection control plan that emphasizes the use of a hierarchy of controls (administrative, environmental and personal respiratory protection) to prevent the transmission of *M tuberculosis*.

REFERENCES

1. Klevens RM, Edwards JR, Richards CL Jr, et al. Estimating health care-associated infections and deaths in U.S. hospitals, 2002. Public Health Rep 2007; 122(2):160–6.
2. Sopena N, Sabria M, Neunos 2000 Study Group. Multicenter study of hospital-acquired pneumonia in non-ICU patients. Chest 2005;127(1):213–9.

3. Centers for Disease Control and Prevention. Patient safety component protocol: ventilator-associated pneumonia (VAP) event. The National Healthcare Safety Network (NHSN) manual. Available at: http://www.cdc.gov/nhsn/PDFs/pscManual/6pscVAPcurrent.pdf. Accessed November 23, 2009.

4. Rello J, Ollendorf DA, Oster G, et al. Epidemiology and outcomes of ventilator-associated pneumonia in a large US database. Chest 2002;122(6):2115–21.

5. Safdar N, Dezfulian C, Collard HR, et al. Clinical and economic consequences of ventilator-associated pneumonia: a systematic review. Crit Care Med 2005;33: 2184–93.

6. Warren DK, Shukla SJ, Olsen MA, et al. Outcome and attributable cost of ventilator-associated pneumonia among intensive care unit patients in a suburban medical center. Crit Care Med 2003;31(5):1312–7.

7. Cook DJ, Walter SD, Cook RJ, et al. Incidence of and risk factors for ventilator-associated pneumonia in critically ill patients. Ann Intern Med 1998;129(6):433–40.

8. Edwards JR, Peterson KD, Mu Y, et al. National Healthcare Safety Network (NHSN) report: data summary for 2006 through 2008, issued December 2009. Am J Infect Control 2009;37(10):783–805.

9. Thompson DA, Makary MA, Dorman T, et al. Clinical and economic outcomes of hospital acquired pneumonia in intra-abdominal surgery patients. Ann Surg 2006;243(4):547–52.

10. Ibrahim EH, Tracy L, Hill C, et al. The occurrence of ventilator-associated pneumonia in a community hospital: risk factors and clinical outcomes. Chest 2001; 120(2):555–61.

11. Scott RD II. The direct medical costs of healthcare-associated infections in U.S. hospitals and the benefits of prevention. Available at: http://www.cdc.gov/ncidod/dhqp/pdf/Scott_CostPaper.pdf. Accessed December 15, 2009.

12. Coffin SE, Klompas M, Classen D, et al. Strategies to prevent ventilator-associated pneumonia in acute care hospitals. Infect Control Hosp Epidemiol 2008; 29(Suppl 1):S31–40.

13. Klompas M, Kulldorff M, Platt R. Risk of misleading ventilator-associated pneumonia rates with use of standard clinical and microbiological criteria. Clin Infect Dis 2008;46(9):1443–6.

14. Huxley EJ, Viroslav J, Gray WR, et al. Pharyngeal aspiration in normal adults and patients with depressed consciousness. Am J Med 1978;64(4):564–8.

15. Metheny NA, Clouse RE, Chang YH, et al. Tracheobronchial aspiration of gastric contents in critically ill tube-fed patients: frequency, outcomes, and risk factors. Crit Care Med 2006;34(4):1007–15.

16. Tablan OC, Anderson LJ, Besser R, et al. Guidelines for preventing health-care–associated pneumonia, 2003: recommendations of CDC and the Healthcare Infection Control Practices Advisory Committee. MMWR Recomm Rep 2004; 53(RR-3):1–36.

17. Bonten MJ, Kollef MH, Hall JB. Risk factors for ventilator-associated pneumonia: from epidemiology to patient management. Clin Infect Dis 2004;38(8):1141–9.

18. Torres A, Serra-Batlles J, Ros E, et al. Pulmonary aspiration of gastric contents in patients receiving mechanical ventilation: the effect of body position. Ann Intern Med 1992;116(7):540–3.

19. Drakulovic MB, Torres A, Bauer TT, et al. Supine body position as a risk factor for nosocomial pneumonia in mechanically ventilated patients: a randomised trial. Lancet 1999;354(9193):1851–8.

20. Combes A. Backrest elevation for the prevention of ventilator-associated pneumonia: back to the real world? Crit Care Med 2006;34(2):559–61.

21. van Nieuwenhoven CA, Vandenbroucke-Grauls C, van Tiel FH, et al. Feasibility and effects of the semirecumbent position to prevent ventilator-associated pneumonia: a randomized study. Crit Care Med 2006;34(2):396–402.

22. Helman DL Jr, Sherner JH 3rd, Fitzpatrick TM, et al. Effect of standardized orders and provider education on head-of-bed positioning in mechanically ventilated patients. Crit Care Med 2003;31(9):2285–90.

23. 5 Million Lives Campaign. Getting started kit: prevent ventilator-associated pneumonia how-to guide. Cambridge (MA): Institute for Healthcare Improvement; 2008.

24. Dezfulian C, Shojania K, Collard HR, et al. Subglottic secretion drainage for preventing ventilator-associated pneumonia: a meta-analysis. Am J Med 2005; 118(1):11–8.

25. Chao YF, Chen YY, Wang KW, et al. Removal of oral secretion prior to position change can reduce the incidence of ventilator-associated pneumonia for adult ICU patients: a clinical controlled trial study. J Clin Nurs 2009;18(1):22–8.

26. Jacobi J, Fraser GL, Coursin DB, et al. Clinical practice guidelines for the sustained use of sedatives and analgesics in the critically ill adult. Crit Care Med 2002;30(1):119–41.

27. Kress JP, Pohlman AS, O'Connor MF, et al. Daily interruption of sedative infusions in critically ill patients undergoing mechanical ventilation. N Engl J Med 2000; 342(20):1471–7.

28. Schweickert WD, Gehlbach BK, Pohlman AS, et al. Daily interruption of sedative infusions and complications of critical illness in mechanically ventilated patients. Crit Care Med 2004;32(6):1272–6.

29. Sessler CN, Pedram S. Protocolized and target-based sedation and analgesia in the ICU. Crit Care Clin 2009;25(3):489–513, viii.

30. Ely EW, Baker AM, Dunagan DP, et al. Effect on the duration of mechanical ventilation of identifying patients capable of breathing spontaneously. N Engl J Med 1996;335(25):1864–9.

31. Girard TD, Kress JP, Fuchs BD, et al. Efficacy and safety of a paired sedation and ventilator weaning protocol for mechanically ventilated patients in intensive care (Awakening and Breathing Controlled trial): a randomised controlled trial. Lancet 2008;371(9607):126–34.

32. Weinert CR, Calvin AD. Epidemiology of sedation and sedation adequacy for mechanically ventilated patients in a medical and surgical intensive care unit. Crit Care Med 2007;35(2):393–401.

33. Payen JF, Chanques G, Mantz J, et al. Current practices in sedation and analgesia for mechanically ventilated critically ill patients: a prospective multicenter patient-based study. Anesthesiology 2007;106(4):687–95 [quiz: 891–2].

34. Tanios MA, de Wit M, Epstein SK, et al. Perceived barriers to the use of sedation protocols and daily sedation interruption: a multidisciplinary survey. J Crit Care 2009;24(1):66–73.

35. Bair N, Bobek MB, Hoffman-Hogg L, et al. Introduction of sedative, analgesic, and neuromuscular blocking agent guidelines in a medical intensive care unit: physician and nurse adherence. Crit Care Med 2000;28(3):707–13.

36. Marshall J, Finn CA, Theodore AC. Impact of a clinical pharmacist-enforced intensive care unit sedation protocol on duration of mechanical ventilation and hospital stay. Crit Care Med 2008;36(2):427–33.

37. Quenot JP, Ladoire S, Devoucoux F, et al. Effect of a nurse-implemented sedation protocol on the incidence of ventilator-associated pneumonia. Crit Care Med 2007;35(9):2031–6.

38. Brochard L. Sedation in the intensive-care unit: good and bad? Lancet 2008; 371(9607):95–7.
39. Bergmans DC, Bonten MJ, Gaillard CA, et al. Prevention of ventilator-associated pneumonia by oral decontamination: a prospective, randomized, double-blind, placebo-controlled study. Am J Respir Crit Care Med 2001;164(3):382–8.
40. Chlebicki MP, Safdar N. Topical chlorhexidine for prevention of ventilator-associated pneumonia: a meta-analysis. Crit Care Med 2007;35(2):595–602.
41. Bellissimo-Rodrigues F, Bellissimo-Rodrigues WT, Viana JM, et al. Effectiveness of oral rinse with chlorhexidine in preventing nosocomial respiratory tract infections among intensive care unit patients. Infect Control Hosp Epidemiol 2009; 30(10):952–8.
42. Tantipong H, Morkchareonpong C, Jaiyindee S, et al. Randomized controlled trial and meta-analysis of oral decontamination with 2% chlorhexidine solution for the prevention of ventilator-associated pneumonia. Infect Control Hosp Epidemiol 2008;29(2):131–6.
43. Koeman M, van der Ven AJ, Hak E, et al. Oral decontamination with chlorhexidine reduces the incidence of ventilator-associated pneumonia. Am J Respir Crit Care Med 2006;173(12):1348–55.
44. Garcia R, Jendresky L, Colbert L, et al. Reducing ventilator-associated pneumonia through advanced oral-dental care: a 48-month study. Am J Crit Care 2009;18(6):523–32.
45. Munro CL, Grap MJ, Jones DJ, et al. Chlorhexidine, toothbrushing, and preventing ventilator-associated pneumonia in critically ill adults. Am J Crit Care 2009; 18(5):428–37 [quiz: 438].
46. Pobo A, Lisboa T, Rodriguez A, et al. A randomized trial of dental brushing for preventing ventilator-associated pneumonia. Chest 2009;136(2):433–9.
47. Liberati A, D'Amico R, Pifferi S, et al. Antibiotic prophylaxis to reduce respiratory tract infections and mortality in adults receiving intensive care. Cochrane Database Syst Rev 2009;4:CD000022.
48. de Smet AMGA, Kluytmans JAJW, Cooper BS, et al. Decontamination of the digestive tract and oropharynx in ICU Patients. N Engl J Med 2009;360(1): 20–31.
49. de Jonge E, Schultz MJ, Spanjaard L, et al. Effects of selective decontamination of digestive tract on mortality and acquisition of resistant bacteria in intensive care: a randomised controlled trial. Lancet 2003;362(9389):1011–6.
50. Dodek P, Keenan S, Cook D, et al. Evidence-based clinical practice guideline for the prevention of ventilator-associated pneumonia. Ann Intern Med 2004;141(4): 305–13.
51. Kollef MH, Afessa B, Anzueto A, et al. Silver-coated endotracheal tubes and incidence of ventilator-associated pneumonia: the NASCENT randomized trial. JAMA 2008;300(7):805–13.
52. Siempos II, Vardakas KZ, Kopterides P, et al. Impact of passive humidification on clinical outcomes of mechanically ventilated patients: a meta-analysis of randomized controlled trials. Crit Care Med 2007;35(12):2843–51.
53. Niel-Weise BS, Wille JC, van den Broek PJ. Humidification policies for mechanically ventilated intensive care patients and prevention of ventilator-associated pneumonia: a systematic review of randomized controlled trials. J Hosp Infect 2007;65(4):285–91.
54. Resar R, Pronovost P, Haraden C, et al. Using a bundle approach to improve ventilator care processes and reduce ventilator-associated pneumonia. Jt Comm J Qual Patient Saf 2005;31(5):243–8.

55. Hawe CS, Ellis KS, Cairns CJ, et al. Reduction of ventilator-associated pneumonia: active versus passive guideline implementation. Intensive Care Med 2009;35(7):1180–6.
56. Zilberberg MD, Shorr AF, Kollef MH. Implementing quality improvements in the intensive care unit: ventilator bundle as an example. Crit Care Med 2009;37(1):305–9.
57. Stout JE, Muder RR, Mietzner S, et al. Role of environmental surveillance in determining the risk of hospital-acquired legionellosis: a national surveillance study with clinical correlations. Infect Control Hosp Epidemiol 2007;28(7):818–24.
58. Squier CL, Stout JE, Krsytofiak S, et al. A proactive approach to prevention of health care-acquired Legionnaires' disease: the Allegheny County (Pittsburgh) experience. Am J Infect Control 2005;33(6):360–7.
59. Centers for Disease Control and Prevention. Guidelines for environmental infection control in health-care facilities: recommendations of CDC and the Healthcare Infection Control Practices Advisory Committee (HICPAC). Available at: http://www.cdc. gov/ncidod/dhqp/pdf/guidelines/Enviro_guide_03.pdf. Accessed December 24, 2009.
60. Bartley JM. APIC state-of-the-art report: the role of infection control during construction in health care facilities. Am J Infect Control 2000;28(2):156–69.
61. Burzynski J, Schluger NW. The epidemiology of tuberculosis in the United States. Semin Respir Crit Care Med 2008;29(5):492–8.
62. Centers for Disease Control and Prevention (CDC). Trends in tuberculosis—United States, 2008. MMWR Morb Mortal Wkly Rep 2009;58(10):249–53.
63. Guidelines for preventing the transmission of *Mycobacterium tuberculosis* in health-care facilities, 1994. Centers for Disease Control and Prevention. MMWR Recomm Rep 1994;43(RR–13):1–132.
64. Manangan LP, Bennett CL, Tablan N, et al. Nosocomial tuberculosis prevention measures among two groups of US hospitals, 1992 to 1996. Chest 2000; 117(2):380–4.
65. Wenger PN, Otten J, Breeden A, et al. Control of nosocomial transmission of multidrug-resistant *Mycobacterium tuberculosis* among healthcare workers and HIV-infected patients. Lancet 1995;345(8944):235–40.
66. Dooley SW Jr, Castro KG, Hutton MD, et al. Guidelines for preventing the transmission of tuberculosis in health-care settings, with special focus on HIV-related issues. MMWR Recomm Rep 1990;39(RR–17):1–29.
67. Fuss EP, Israel E, Baruch N, et al. Improved tuberculosis infection control practices in Maryland acute care hospitals. Am J Infect Control 2000;28(2):133–7.
68. Centers for Disease Control and Prevention. Targeted tuberculin testing and treatment of latent tuberculosis infection. American Thoracic Society. MMWR Recomm Rep 2000;49(RR–6):1–51.
69. Diagnostic standards and classification of tuberculosis in adults and children. This official statement of the American Thoracic Society and the Centers for Disease Control and Prevention was adopted by the ATS Board of Directors, July 1999. This statement was endorsed by the Council of the Infectious Disease Society of America, September 1999. Am J Respir Crit Care Med 2000;161 (4 Pt 1):1376–95.
70. Centers for Disease Control and Prevention. Treatment of Tuberculosis, American Thoracic Society, CDC, and Infectious Diseases Society of America. MMWR 2003;52(RR–11):1–77.
71. Jensen PA, Lambert LA, Iademarco MF, et al. Guidelines for preventing the transmission of *Mycobacterium tuberculosis* in health-care settings, 2005. MMWR Recomm Rep 2005;54(RR–17):1–141.

72. National TB Controllers Association/CDC Advisory Group on Tuberculosis Genotyping. Guide to the application of genotyping to tuberculosis prevention and control. Available at: http://www.cdc.gov/tb/programs/genotyping/manual.htm. Accessed December 26, 2009.

73. Iwata K, Smith BA, Santos E, et al. Failure to implement respiratory isolation: why does it happen? Infect Control Hosp Epidemiol 2002;23(10):595–9.

74. Moran GJ, Barrett TW, Mower WR, et al. Decision instrument for the isolation of pneumonia patients with suspected pulmonary tuberculosis admitted through US Emergency Departments. Ann Emerg Med 2009;53(5):625–32.

75. Al Zahrani K, Al Jahdali H, Poirier L, et al. Yield of smear, culture and amplification tests from repeated sputum induction for the diagnosis of pulmonary tuberculosis. Int J Tuberc Lung Dis 2001;5(9):855–60.

76. Leonard MK, Osterholt D, Kourbatova EV, et al. How many sputum specimens are necessary to diagnose pulmonary tuberculosis? Am J Infect Control 2005;33(1): 58–61.

77. Siegel JD, Rhinehart E, Jackson M, et al. 2007 Guideline for isolation precautions: preventing transmission of infectious agents in health care settings. Am J Infect Control 2007;35(10 Suppl 2):S65–164.

78. Occupational Safety and Health Administration. Respiratory Protection. - 1910.134. Available at: http://www.osha.gov/pls/oshaweb/owadisp.show_document?p_ table=STANDARDS&p_id=12716. Accessed December 24, 2009.

79. Association of Public Health Laboratories. *Mycobacterium tuberculosis*: assessing your laboratory. Available at: http://www.aphl.org/aphlprograms/infectious/ tuberculosis/Documents/Mycobacteria_TuberculosisAssessingYourLaboratory. pdf. Accessed December 24, 2009.

80. Burman WJ, Reves RR. Review of false-positive cultures for *Mycobacterium tuberculosis* and recommendations for avoiding unnecessary treatment. Clin Infect Dis 2000;31(6):1390–5.

81. Fitzpatrick L, Braden C, Cronin W, et al. Investigation of laboratory cross-contamination of *Mycobacterium tuberculosis* cultures. Clin Infect Dis 2004;38(6):e52–4.

Surgical Site Infections

Deverick J. Anderson, MD, MPH

KEYWORDS

- Surgical site infection • Health care–acquired infection
- Outcome

Attempts at reducing the rate of surgical site infections (SSIs) date to the early nineteenth century with the study of the epidemiology and prevention of surgical fever by James Young Hamilton.[1] Thereafter, Joseph Lister pioneered his use of antiseptics for the prevention of orthopedic SSIs in 1865. Fortunately, many other advances have been made in surgery and infection control over the past 150 years. However, as medicine has advanced, new types of infection risks have developed. For example, over the past 50 years, the frequency of surgical procedures has increased, procedures have become more invasive, a greater proportion of operative procedures include insertion of foreign objects, and procedures are performed on an increasingly morbid patient population. As a result, SSIs remain a leading cause of morbidity and mortality in modern health care.

EPIDEMIOLOGY AND OUTCOMES
Epidemiology

SSIs are a devastating and common complication of hospitalization, occurring in 2% to 5% of patients undergoing surgery in the United States.[2] As many as 15 million procedures are annually performed in the United States; thus, approximately 300,000 to 500,000 SSIs occur each year.[3] SSI is the second most common type of health care–associated infection (HAI).[4] *Staphylococcus aureus* is the most common cause of SSI, occurring in 20% of SSIs among hospitals that report to the Centers for Disease Control and Prevention (CDC) (**Table 1**)[5] and causes as many as 37% of SSIs that occur in community hospitals.[6] In fact, methicillin-resistant *S aureus* (MRSA) is not only a common pathogen in tertiary care and academic institutions but is also the single most common SSI pathogen in community hospitals.[6]

Outcomes

SSIs lead to increased duration of hospitalization, cost, and risk of death. Each SSI leads to more than 1 week of additional postoperative hospital days.[3,7] The costs

Division of Infectious Diseases, Duke University Medical Center, DUMC Box 102359, Durham, NC 27710, USA
E-mail address: deverick.anderson@duke.edu

Infect Dis Clin N Am 25 (2011) 135–153
doi:10.1016/j.idc.2010.11.004
0891-5520/11/$ – see front matter © 2011 Elsevier Inc. All rights reserved.

Table 1	
The 10 most common pathogens causing SSIs in hospitals that report to the CDC	
Pathogen	Percentage of Infections (%)
S aureus	20
Coagulase-negative staphylococci	14
Enterococci	12
Pseudomonas aeruginosa	8
Escherichia coli	8
Enterobacter species	7
Proteus mirabilis	3
Streptococci	3
Klebsiella pneumoniae	3
Candida albicans	2

Data from National Nosocomial Infections Surveillance (NNIS) report, data summary from October 1986-April 1996, issued May 1996. A report from the National Nosocomial Infections Surveillance (NNIS) System. Am J Infect Control 1996;24(5):380–8; and Mangram AJ, Horan TC, Pearson ML, et al. Guideline for prevention of surgical site infection, 1999. Hospital Infection Control Practices Advisory Committee. Infect Control Hosp Epidemiol 1999;20(4)250–78 [quiz: 279–80].

attributable to SSI range from $3000 to $29,000 per patient per SSI, depending on the type of procedure.[8] In total, SSIs cost the US health care system approximately $10 billion annually.[9] SSI increases mortality risk by 2 to 11 fold.[10] Moreover, 77% of deaths in patients with SSI are attributed directly to the SSIs.[11] SSIs caused by resistant organisms, such as MRSA, lead to even worse outcomes.[12,13]

DIAGNOSIS

Most SSIs that do not involve implants are diagnosed within 3 weeks of surgery.[14] The CDC's National Healthcare Surveillance Network (NHSN) has developed standardized criteria for defining an SSI (**Box 1**).[15] SSIs are classified as either incisional or organ/space (**Fig. 1**). Incisional SSIs are further classified into superficial (involving only skin or subcutaneous tissue of the incision) or deep (involving fascia and/or muscular layers). Organ/space SSIs include infections in a tissue deep to the fascia that was opened or manipulated during surgery. For all classifications, infection can occur within 30 days after the operation if no implant was placed or within 1 year if an implant was placed and the infection is related to the incision. The NHSN defines implant as a nonhuman-derived implantable foreign body (eg, prosthetic heart valve, nonhuman vascular graft, mechanical heart, or joint prosthesis) that is permanently placed in a patient.

Serum laboratory tests can be suggestive but none are specific for SSI. For example, basic hematologic abnormalities, including increasing white blood cell count and neutrophil concentration, are suggestive of infection. For example, leukocytosis of more than 15,000/mm^3 in the setting of hyponatremia (sodium<135 mEq/L) is predictive of necrotizing soft tissue infection.[16] However, many SSIs occur without any hematologic or serologic laboratory abnormalities. Culturing samples of all suspected cases of deep and organ/space infections should be done to guide therapy and determine the susceptibility of the infecting organism. Ideally, culture samples are obtained in the operative setting, and external wound swabs are avoided. Radiographic studies may be adjunctive for the diagnosis of SSI. Computed tomography is more reliable

---

Box 1
Criteria for defining an SSI[a]

Incisional SSI

Superficial: Infection involves skin or subcutaneous tissue of the incision and at least one of the following:

1. Purulent drainage, with or without laboratory confirmation, from the superficial incision

2. Organisms isolated from an aseptically obtained culture from the superficial incision

3. At least one of the following signs or symptoms, pain, localized swelling, erythema, or heat, and superficial incision is deliberately opened by the surgeon (not applicable if culture-negative infection)

4. Diagnosis of superficial incisional SSI by the surgeon

Deep: Infection involves deep soft tissues (eg, fascial and muscle layers) of the incision and at least one of the following:

1. Purulent drainage from the deep incision, excluding organ/space[b]

2. A deep incision that spontaneously dehisces or is deliberately opened by a surgeon when a patient has one or more of the following signs/symptoms, fever (>38°C), localized pain, unless site is culture negative

3. An abscess or other evidence of infection is found on direct examination, during repeat surgery, or by histopathologic or radiological examination[c]

4. Diagnosis of a deep incisional SSI by the surgeon

Organ/space SSI:

Infection involves any part of the anatomy (eg, organs or organ spaces), which was opened or manipulated during an operation and at least one of the following:

1. Purulent drainage from a drain that is placed through the stab wound into the organ/space

2. Organisms isolated from an aseptically obtained culture from the organ/space

3. An abscess or other evidence of infection involving organ/space, which is found on examination (physical, histopathologic, or radiological) or during repeat surgery

4. Diagnosis of an organ/space SSI by the surgeon

[a] For all classifications, infection is defined as occurring within 30 days after the operation if no implant is placed or within 1 year if an implant is in place and the infection is related to the incision.
[b] Report infection that involves both superficial and deep incision sites as a deep incisional SSI.
[c] Report an organ/space SSI that drains through the incision as a deep incisional SSI.
Adapted from Horan TC, Gaynes RP, Martone WJ, et al. CDC definitions of nosocomial surgical site infections, 1992: a modification of CDC definitions of surgical wound infections. Infect Control Hosp Epidemiol 1992;13(10):606–8.

---

than plain radiographs for the detection of free air in soft tissue and the presence of deep abscess.

Diagnosis of SSIs in the setting of an implant or prosthetic joint can be even more difficult. For example, radiographs are often difficult to interpret with the presence of prosthetic material or metal. Cultures directly from explanted material, however, may aid the diagnosis.[17] A recent trial comparing conventional tissue culture with culture of specimens after sonication of explanted joints demonstrated that sonicated specimens had a higher sensitivity for the diagnosis of prosthetic joint infection (PJI)

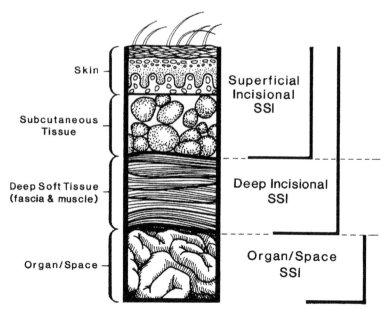

Fig. 1. CDC classification of surgical site infection (public domain). (*From* Horan TC, Gaynes RP, Martone WJ, et al. CDC definitions of nosocomial surgical site infections, 1992: a modification of CDC definitions of surgical wound infections. Infect Control Hosp Epidemiol 1992;13(10):606–8.)

than periprosthetic tissue culture (79% vs 61%, with an even wider difference in the subgroup of patients who had received antibiotics before explant) and similar specificity.[18] However, few microbiology labs have the capability to perform these cultures, and transport of specimens while avoiding contamination may be difficult.

PATHOGENESIS OF INFECTION

The likelihood that an SSI will occur is a complex relationship among (1) microbial characteristics (eg, degree of contamination, virulence of pathogen), (2) patient characteristics (eg, immune status, diabetes), and (3) surgical characteristics (eg, introduction of foreign material, amount of damage to tissues). Similar to taxes and death, microbial contamination of surgical sites is universal, despite the use of cutting-edge technology and expert technique. The pathogens that lead to SSI are acquired from the patient's endogenous flora or, less frequently, exogenously from the operating room (OR) environment.

Endogenous Contamination

The period of greatest risk for infection occurs while the surgical wound is open, that is, from the time of incision to the time of wound closure.[19] Twenty percent of bacterial skin flora resides in skin appendages, such as sebaceous glands, hair follicles, and sweat glands.[20] Thus, modern methods of pre- and perioperative antisepsis can reduce but not eliminate contamination of the surgical site by endogenous skin flora of the surgical patient. As a result, gram-positive cocci from patients' endogenous flora at or near the site of surgery remain the leading cause of SSI.[21]

Inoculation of the surgical site by endogenous flora from remote sites of the patient may also occur infrequently. Experiments using albumin microspheres as tracer particles revealed that 100% of surgical wounds are contaminated with particles (skin squames) from sites from the surgical patient (eg, head, groin), which are distant in location to the surgical wound.[22] Postsurgical inoculation of the surgical site secondary to a remote focus of infection (such as *S aureus* pneumonia) is an even less-frequent cause of SSI.[23]

Exogenous Contamination

Exogenous sources of contamination are occasionally implicated in the pathogenesis of SSI, including colonized or infected surgical personnel, the OR environment, and surgical instruments. Infections due to exogenous sources most commonly occur sporadically, but several exogenous point source outbreaks have been reported.[24–28] Surgical personnel colonized with *S aureus* are occasionally identified as sources of *S aureus* causing SSI.[29] Carriage of group A streptococci by OR personnel has been implicated as a cause of several SSI outbreaks.[24,30–33] It is important to remember, however, that most SSIs are not contracted from exogenous sources.

Unusual environmental pathogens are occasionally implicated in SSIs from sources in the OR. For example, *Rhodococcus bronchialis* was implicated in an outbreak of SSI after coronary artery bypass surgery because of colonization of an OR nurse by her dog.[25] Other unusual pathogens causing SSI include *Legionella pneumophila* after contamination of a prosthetic valve by tap water,[26,34,35] *Mycobacterium chelonae* and *Mycobacterium fortuitum* after breast augmentation,[27,36] *Rhizopus rhizopodiformis* after contamination of adhesive dressings,[28] *Clostridium perfringens* contamination of elastic bandages,[37] and *Pseudomonas multivorans* contamination of a disinfectant solution.[38]

Burden of Inoculation

Although many other factors contribute to the risk of SSI, the burden of pathogens inoculated into a surgical wound intraoperatively remains one of the most accepted risk factors. In fact, the greater the degree of surgical wound contamination, the higher the risk for infection. In the setting of appropriate antimicrobial prophylaxis, wound contamination with greater than 10^5 microorganisms is required to cause SSI.[39,40] However, the bacterial inoculum required to cause SSI may be much lower when foreign bodies are present.[41] For example, the presence of surgical sutures decreases the required inoculum for *S aureus* SSI by two-thirds (from 10^6 to 10^2 organisms).[42] Other models have demonstrated that the minimum inoculum for SSI due to virulent pathogens such as *S aureus* is as few as 10 colony-forming unit (CFU) in the presence of polytetrafluoroethylene vascular grafts[43] and 1 CFU in the proximity of dextran beads.[44]

Pathogen Virulence

Many potential SSI pathogens have intrinsic virulence factors or characteristics that contribute to their ability to cause infection. Several gram-positive organisms, including *S aureus*, coagulase-negative staphylococcus, and *Enterococcus faecalis*, possess microbial surface components recognizing adhesive matrix molecules that allow better adhesion to collagen, fibrin, fibronectin, and other extracellular matrix proteins.[44–47] Most of these same organisms also have the ability to produce a glycocalyx-rich biofilm, which shields the organisms from both the immune system and most antimicrobial agents.[48–50] In addition, once in the wound, some Staphylococci and Streptococci produce exotoxins that lead to host tissue damage,[51] interfere with phagocytosis,[52] and alter cellular metabolism.[53] Many gram-negative pathogens produce endotoxins that stimulate cytokine production and, often, systemic inflammatory response syndrome.[54] Several bacteria possess polysaccharide capsules or other surface components that additionally inhibit opsonization and phagocytosis.[55]

RISK FACTORS

Risk factors for SSI are typically separated into patient-related (preoperative), procedure-related (perioperative), and postoperative categories (**Table 2**). In general, patient-related risk factors for the development of SSI can be categorized as either unmodifiable or modifiable. The most prominent unmodifiable risk factor is age. In a cohort study of more than 144,000 patients, increasing age independently predicted an increased risk of SSI until age 65 years, but at ages 65 years or more, increasing age independently predicted a decreased risk of SSI.[56] Modifiable patient-related risk factors include poorly controlled diabetes mellitus,[57] obesity,[58] tobacco use,[59,60] use of immunosuppressive medications,[61] and length of preoperative hospitalization.[19]

Procedure-related perioperative risk factors include wound class,[62] length of surgery,[63] shaving of hair,[64,65] hypoxia,[66,67] and hypothermia.[68] Of note, the act of surgery itself leads to increased risk of infection. The microbicidal activity of neutrophils harvested after surgery is 25% less than neutrophils harvested before surgery[69]; surgery leads to decreased levels of circulating HLA-DR antigens[70] and a decrease in T-cell proliferation and response[71]; neutrophils exhibit reduced chemotaxis and diminished superoxide production in the setting of perioperative hypothermia.[72] Specific recommendations are available regarding traffic in the OR and OR parameters, such as ventilation, to reduce the risk of exogenous seeding of the surgical wound as a result of personnel in the OR.[11,73] As a rule of thumb, the degree of microbial contamination of the OR air is directly proportional to the number of people in the room[74]; thus, traffic in and out of the room should be limited as much as possible.

Several risk factors that occur during the perioperative period, including hyperglycemia and diabetes mellitus,[57,75] remain important during the immediate postoperative period. Two additional risk variables that are present exclusively in the postoperative period are wound care and postoperative blood transfusions. Postoperative wound care is determined by the technique used for closure of the surgical site. Most wounds are closed primarily (ie, skin edges are approximated with sutures or staples) and these wounds should be kept clean by covering with a sterile dressing for 24 to 48 hours after surgery.[76] A meta-analysis of 20 studies of the associated risk of SSI after receipt of blood products demonstrated that patients who received even a single unit of blood in the immediate postoperative period were at increased risk for SSI (odds ratio, 3.5).[77]

PREVENTION

Methods to prevent SSI were recently summarized in the Society for Healthcare Epidemiology of America/Infectious Disease Society of America Compendium of Strategies to Prevent HAI in Acute Care Hospitals.[78] In particular, emphasis was placed on the importance of perioperative antimicrobial prophylaxis, avoiding shaving, glucose control for cardiac surgery, and measurement and feedback of rates of SSI to surgeons. If feasible, modifiable risk factors for SSI should be addressed. **Table 2** summarizes important risk factors and current guidelines for addressing each risk factor to decrease the risk of SSI.

Table 2
Risk factors for SSI and current recommendations to decrease the risk of SSI

Risk Factors	Recommendations
Intrinsic, patient-related (Preoperative)	
Age	No formal recommendation, relationship to increased risk of SSI may be secondary to comorbidities or immunosenescence[56,63,132]
Glucose control, diabetes mellitus	Control serum blood glucose levels[133]
Obesity	Increase dosing of perioperative antimicrobial agent for morbidly obese patients[134]
Smoking cessation	Encourage smoking cessation within 30 d of procedure[133]
Immunosuppressive medications	No formal recommendation[133]; in general, avoid immunosuppressive medications in the perioperative period if possible
Nutrition	Do not delay surgery to enhance nutritional support[133]
Remote sites of infection	Identify and treat all remote infections before elective procedures[133]
Preoperative hospitalization	Keep preoperative stay as short as possible[133]
Extrinsic, procedure-related (Perioperative)	
Preparation of the patient	
Hair Removal	Do not remove unless presence of hair interferes with the operation[133]; if hair removal is necessary, remove by clipping and do not shave immediately before surgery
Skin preparation	Wash and clean skin around incision site, using approved surgical preparations[133]
Chlorhexidine nasal and oropharyngeal rinse	No formal recommendation in most recent guidelines[133]; Recent RCT of cardiac surgeries showed decreased incidence of postoperative nosocomial infections[116]
Surgical scrub (surgeon's hands and forearms)	Use appropriate antiseptic agent to perform 2–5 min preoperative surgical scrub[133]
Incision site	Use appropriate antiseptic agent[133]
Antimicrobial prophylaxis	Administer only when indicated[133]
Timing	Administer within 1 h of incision to maximize tissue concentration[133]
Choice	Select appropriate agents based on surgical procedure, most common pathogens causing SSI for a specific procedure, and published recommendations[133]
Duration of therapy	Stop agent within 24 h after the procedure[133,135]
Surgeon skill/technique	Handle tissue carefully and eradicate dead space[133]
Incision time	No formal recommendation in most recent guidelines[133]; minimize as much as possible[136]
Maintain oxygenation with supplemental O_2	No formal recommendation in most recent guidelines,[133] RCTs have reported conflicting results in colorectal procedures[66,67,125]

(continued on next page)

Table 2 (continued)	
Risk Factors	**Recommendations**
Maintain normothermia	Avoid hypothermia in surgical patients whenever possible by actively warming the patient to >36°C, particularly in colorectal surgery[137]
OR characteristics	
Ventilation	Follow the American Institute of Architects' recommendations[73,133]
Traffic	Minimize OR traffic[133]
Environmental surfaces	Use an EPA-approved hospital disinfectant to clean visibly soiled or contaminated surfaces and equipment[133]

Abbreviations: EPA, Environmental Protection Agency; O_2, oxygen; RCT, randomized controlled trial.

Perioperative Antimicrobial Prophylaxis

The appropriate use of perioperative antimicrobial prophylaxis is a well-proven intervention to reduce the risk of SSI in elective procedures.[11,40,79] The goal of surgical antimicrobial prophylaxis is to reduce the concentration of potential pathogens at or in close proximity to the surgical incision. Four main principles dictate prophylactic antimicrobial use: (1) use antimicrobial prophylaxis for all elective operations that require entry into a hollow viscus, operations that involve insertion of an intravascular prosthetic device or prosthetic joint, or operations in which an SSI would pose catastrophic risk[80–83]; (2) use antimicrobial agents that are safe, cost-effective, and bactericidal against expected pathogens for specific surgical procedures[11]; (3) time the infusion so that a bactericidal concentration of the agent is present in tissue and serum at the time of incision[79] and; (4) maintain therapeutic levels of the agent in tissue and serum throughout the entire operation (ie, until wound closure).[81,84,85] Thus, the 2 major components of appropriate perioperative antimicrobial prophylaxis are using the appropriate agent at the appropriate dose and giving the agent at the appropriate time.

Administering antimicrobial prophylaxis shortly before incision reduces the rate of SSI.[79] The chosen agent should be given at a time that allows for maximum tissue concentration at the time of incision. The optimal administration time typically occurs within 2 hours before surgery.[86] In one retrospective study of approximately 3000 patients undergoing various elective inpatient procedures, the lowest rates of SSI occurred in the group of patients who received antimicrobial prophylaxis within 1 hour before incision.[79]

Current regulatory process measures state that starting infusion of antimicrobial prophylaxis within 1 hour before incision maximizes benefit (and for vancomycin and fluoroquinolones, within 2 hours before incision).[87] Thus, prophylaxis may be started as soon as 1 minute before incision and the OR team still "gets credit" from a regulatory perspective. Although this practice may follow the letter of the law, it certainly does not follow the spirit. For most agents, antimicrobial prophylaxis is most effective if infusion is started between 60 and 30 minutes before surgery. For example, in one prospective observational study of 3836 surgical patients, antimicrobial prophylaxis given 0 to 29 minutes before surgery was less effective than comparable therapy administered between 30 to 59 minutes before surgery, even after statistical adjustment for other confounding risk factors such as the American Society of Anesthesiologists score, duration of surgery, and wound class.[88] In another study involving 2048 patients undergoing cardiac bypass surgery, patients who received vancomycin 0 to 15 minutes before the beginning of surgery had higher rates of post-operative infection than those who received vancomycin 16 to 60 minutes preoperatively.[89]

If a procedure is expected to last several hours, prophylactic agents should be redosed intraoperatively.[11] For example, cefazolin should be reinfused if a procedure lasts longer than 3 to 4 hours. One retrospective study of 1548 patients undergoing prolonged cardiac procedures (>400 minutes) demonstrated that patients who received intraoperative redosing of cefazolin had significantly fewer SSIs than those who did not receive redosing, even after adjusting for baseline risk (7.7% vs 16.0%; adjusted odds ratio, 0.44; 95% confidence interval [CI], 0.23–0.86).[90]

Although not directly related to the prevention of SSI, an additional measure related to perioperative surgical prophylaxis is the number of doses administered. Single-dose antimicrobial prophylaxis is equivalent to multiple perioperative doses for the prevention of SSI. A meta-analysis of more than 40 studies comparing single doses of parenteral antimicrobials with placebo or multiple doses in hysterectomies; cesarean sections; colorectal procedures; gastric, biliary, transurethral operations; and cardiothoracic procedures demonstrated that administering multiple doses of antibiotics provided no benefit for SSI prevention over a single dose.[91] Similarly, a more recent systematic review of 28 prospective randomized studies comparing single versus multiple doses of perioperative antimicrobials also concluded that there was no additional benefit of more than a single prophylactic dose.[84] Thus, current recommendations state that prophylactic antibiotics should not be given for longer than 24 hours after surgery or longer than 48 hours after cardiothoracic surgery.

Hospitals that improve compliance with the different components of appropriate antimicrobial prophylaxis decrease the rates of SSI. For example, the Center for Medi-care and Medicaid Service created the Surgical Infection Prevention Project and per-formed a large study on the impact of improved antimicrobial prophylaxis process measures. The study, which included 34,133 procedures performed at 56 hospitals, led to an improvement of 27% in antibiotic timing, an improvement of 6% in antibiotic choice, an improvement of 27% in stopping prophylaxis within 24 hours of incision, and, most importantly, a reduction of 27% in the average rate of SSI.[92] A recent study included these 3 antimicrobial prophylaxis process measures as part of a global checklist to improve outcomes after surgical procedures.[93] This prospective quasi-experimental study of approximately 8000 operative patients demonstrated that implementation of a 19-item checklist in 8 institutions throughout the world led to lower rates of postoperative complications and death. Furthermore, the rate of appro-priately administered antimicrobial prophylaxis improved by 60% and the rate of SSI decreased by half.

Avoid Shaving

Preoperative shaving leads to increased rates of SSI by causing microscopic abra-sions of the skin, which become foci for bacterial growth.[7,64,65] Some studies, however, suggest that any form of hair removal, shaving, depilatory, or clipping, leads to increased rates of SSI and should thus be avoided when possible.[64,94,95] Thus, current recommendations state that hair should not be removed from the surgical site unless the hair interferes with the procedure.[11] If hair removal is necessary, the hair should be removed with electric clippers immediately before surgery.[96,97]

Glucose Control

As described earlier, diabetes mellitus is clearly associated with an increased risk of SSI.[57,75] Elevated serum glucose levels in both the pre- and postoperative periods have been associated with an increased risk of SSI.[57,98] For example, in one study of 8910 patients undergoing cardiac surgery, rates of SSI decreased substantially after implementing an intravenous insulin regimen to maintain postoperative glucose levels lesser than 200 mg/dL for the first 48 hours after surgery.[57] In contrast, strict glucose level control in the intraoperative period has not been shown to decrease the risk of SSI and may actually lead to harm.[99] Thus, current recommendations state that (1) every effort should be made to improve control of diabetes mellitus before surgery and (2) postoperative serum glucose concentration should be maintained lesser than 200 mg/dL for the first 48 hours after surgery.

Surveillance and Feedback to Surgeons

Surveillance and reporting of infection rates to surgeons reduce the rate of SSI for all procedure classes.[7,100–102] Two main methods can be used to perform surveillance for SSIs, the direct method and the indirect method. The direct method with daily observation of the surgical site by the surgeon, a trained nurse, or infection control professional is the most accurate method of surveillance.[7,101,103,104] The indirect method of SSI surveillance consists of a combination of the following: review of microbiology reports, surgeon and/or patient surveys, and screening for readmission of surgical patients. The indirect method of SSI surveillance is less time consuming, can be readily performed by infection control personnel during surveillance rounds, and is both reliable (sensitivity, 84%–89%) and specific (specificity, 99.8%) compared with the gold standard of direct surveillance.[105,106] Automated data systems that use hospital databases with administrative claims data, antibiotic days, readmission to the hospital, and return to the OR and/or implementation of a system that imports automated microbiological culture data, surgical procedure data, and general demographic information can broaden indirect SSI surveillance and may obviate direct surveillance.[107–109]

The landmark study on the efficacy of nosocomial infection control study by Haley and colleagues[100] showed that establishing an infection control program that includes the feedback of SSI rates to surgeons can lower the overall rate of SSI by as much as 35% and remains one of the studies on which modern infection control programs are based. No studies have yet revealed the exact mechanism by which feedback to surgeons reduces the rate of SSI. Possible explanations for this reduction from feedback include (1) increased awareness of the problem of SSIs, (2) anxiety created by awareness that patient outcomes are being monitored, or (3) introspection concerning possible systematic, procedural, or technical errors.[19]

Simple rates of SSI provide minimal information for surgeons. Instead, rates of SSI should first be risk stratified using the National Nosocomial Infections Surveillance risk index. Then, rates of SSI for a surgeon and a specific procedure should be benchmarked against internal and external standards. That is, risk-stratified rates of SSI for a specific procedure can be compared with the surgeon's previous rates, rates of other surgeons at the institution, and national rates published by the CDC.

Unresolved issues in the prevention of SSI

Preoperative bathing Showering or bathing with an antiseptic agent, such as chlorhexidine gluconate, povidone-iodine, or triclocarban-medicated soap, decreases the amount of endogenous microbial flora on the skin.[110,111] However, this intervention has not yet been clearly demonstrated to lower rates of SSI in clinical trials.[112–114] In fact, a prospective, randomized, controlled, double-blind trial comparing preoperative showers with soap containing chlorhexidine gluconate with preoperative showers with nonmedicated soap in 1400 patients found no significant difference in infection rates between the 2 groups.[112] Most likely, the lack of benefit is related to the method of application of the antiseptic; for example, chlorhexidine gluconate typically requires several applications for maximum microbial-reducing benefit.[115]

Decolonization of *S aureus* carriage Studies examining the utility of preoperative *S aureus* nasal decolonization with antimicrobial agents have produced inconsistent results. A randomized controlled trial examined the utility of oral and nasal rinses with chlorhexidine gluconate (0.12%) before cardiothoracic surgery for the prevention of postoperative nosocomial infections.[116] Although the overall number of SSIs was not different in the 2 groups, the number of deep SSIs was significantly decreased in the group that received chlorhexidine (1.9% vs 5.2%, $P = .002$). Given the proven benefit, low toxicity, and lack of emerging resistance in long-term clinical studies of chlorhexidine,[117] preoperative treatment with chlorhexidine represents a promising intervention for the prevention of SSIs.

Studies examining the efficacy of decolonization of *S aureus* with mupirocin have generally shown that mupirocin is effective at decolonization, but the impact on SSI remains unclear. One study with historical controls reported that the preoperative application of mupirocin to the nares of operative patients led to a decrease of 67% in the rate of SSI after cardiothoracic surgery (from 7.3% to 2.8%), regardless of *S aureus* carrier status.[118] In addition, a separate nonrandomized analysis of almost 1900 consecutive cardiothoracic procedures showed that the overall rate of SSI was lower in patients who received decolonization with mupirocin (2.7% vs 0.9%, $P = .005$).[117] These findings, however, were not corroborated in a double-blind randomized controlled trial in which 1933 surgical patients randomized to receive preoperative mupirocin were compared with 1931 patients randomized to placebo.[119] Treatment with mupirocin led to lower rates of *S aureus* colonization and lower rates of overall postoperative hospital-acquired infections caused by *S aureus* (3.8% of patients who received mupirocin vs 7.6% of patients who received placebo, $P = .02$). The intervention, however, did not lead to a significant decrease in the rate of SSI caused by *S aureus* (3.6% of patients who received mupirocin vs 5.8% of patients who received placebo; odds ratio, 2.9; 95% CI, 0.8–3.4).[119]

However, *S aureus* resistance to mupirocin has rapidly emerged in some institutions.[120] For example, extensive use of mupirocin correlated with an increase in resistance to mupirocin among *S aureus* strains from 3% to 65% over a 4-year period in one European institution.[121] The emergence of mupirocin resistance is concerning and clearly negates the efficacy of preoperative decolonization. Thus, many experts recommend that decolonization be limited to specific high-risk populations and not administered universally.

Perioperative oxygen supplementation Six randomized controlled trials have evaluated the utility of high inspired oxygen fraction in the perioperative setting.[66,67,122–125] Four studies demonstrated a reduction in the rate of SSI after administration of 80% FiO_2 during and after surgery,[66,67,122,124] one study demonstrated no difference,[123] and one study actually concluded that administration of 80% FiO_2 led to higher rates of SSI.[125] The investigators of a recent meta-analysis that included 5 of the earlier-mentioned trials (including the negative study) concluded that high inspired oxygen decreased the risk of SSI, although significant methodological differences were noted among the studies.[126] No increased risk of harm was noted in the randomized controlled trial that rigorously evaluated adverse outcomes.[123] Thus, supplemental oxygen seems to reduce the risk for SSI in certain surgeries such as colorectal and abdominal surgeries.

TREATMENT

Surgical opening of the incision with removal of necrotic tissue is the primary and most important aspect of therapy for many SSIs.[127] Antimicrobial therapy is an important adjunct to surgical debridement. The type of debridement and duration of the postoperative antimicrobial therapy depend on the anatomic site of infection and invasiveness of the SSI, although deep incisional and organ/space infections almost universally require operative drainage of accumulated pus. A key consideration for both the need for surgical debridement and duration of antimicrobial therapy is whether prosthetic material is present and infected.

Superficial incisional SSI can usually be treated without debridement, with oral antibiotics. Postoperative patients with suspected deep or organ/space SSI, fever (temperature>38.5°C), or tachycardia (heart rate, 110 beats/min) generally require antibiotics in addition to opening of the suture line.[127] Few published data exist to support the use of specific antimicrobial agents or specific therapeutic durations for the treatment of SSI. Decisions regarding the antimicrobial agent and length of therapy for SSI are influenced by the location of the infection (eg, mediastinum, abdominal cavity, joint), depth of infection, adequacy or completeness of surgical debridement, and resistance patterns of the pathogen. As a rule of thumb, effective systemic antimicrobial therapy should be started as soon as a deep incisional or organ/space SSI is suspected. For example, in one study, patients with mediastinitis who received antimicrobial therapy active against the infecting pathogen within 7 days of debridement had a reduction of 60% in mortality rates compared with patients who did not receive effective antimicrobial therapy.[128]

PJI is a unique problem that usually requires surgical debridement and prolonged antimicrobial therapy. Surgical treatment of PJI includes the following different strategies: debridement with retention of the prosthesis, 1- or 2-stage exchange with reimplantation, resection arthroplasty, and amputation.[129] Removal of foreign materials, such as wires, bone wax, and devitalized tissues, greatly improves the likelihood of cure.[130] Traditionally, a 2-stage exchange has been the standard treatment modality used to cure an infected prosthesis. The 2-stage exchange involves debridement and removal of the infected prosthesis followed by prolonged antimicrobial therapy (often up to 6–8 weeks) and subsequent reimplantation of a new prosthesis. The 1-stage exchange involves debridement, removal of the prosthetic joint, and immediate reimplantation of a new prosthesis. In some cases of SSI, the infected prosthesis can be salvaged through early surgical debridement in combination with effective antimicrobial therapy.[131] The likelihood of successful salvage of an infected prosthesis is improved if the following conditions are met: signs and symptoms of PJI are detected within 3 weeks of implantation, the implant remains stable and functional, the surrounding soft tissue remains in good condition, and the patient is treated with appropriate systemic antimicrobials.[129] Most patients with PJI should receive 6 to 8 weeks of intravenous antimicrobial therapy.[129]

SUMMARY

SSIs lead to an excess of health care resource expenditure, patient suffering, and death. Improved adherence to evidence-based preventative measures, particularly those related to appropriate antimicrobial prophylaxis, can decrease the rate of SSI. Diagnosis is difficult, particularly in the setting of a procedure that involved prosthetic material. In general, aggressive surgical debridement in combination with effective antimicrobial therapy are needed to optimize the treatment of SSIs.

REFERENCES

1. Selwyn S. Hospital infection: the first 2500 years. J Hosp Infect 1991;18(Suppl A): 5–64.
2. Graves EJ. National hospital discharge survey: annual summary 1987. National Center for Health Statistics 1989;13 :11.
3. Cruse P. Wound infection surveillance. Rev Infect Dis 1981;3(4):734–7.
4. Wenzel RP. Health care-associated infections: major issues in the early years of the 21st century. Clin Infect Dis 2007;45(Suppl 1):S85–8.
5. National Nosocomial Infections Surveillance (NNIS) report, data summary from October 1986-April 1996, issued May 1996. A report from the National Nosocomial Infections Surveillance (NNIS) System. Am J Infect Control 1998;24(5): 380–8.
6. Anderson DJ, Sexton DJ, Kanafani ZA, et al. Severe surgical site infection in community hospitals: epidemiology, key procedures, and the changing prevalence of methicillin-resistant *Staphylococcus aureus*. Infect Control Hosp Epidemiol 2007;28(9):1047–53.
7. Cruse PJ, Foord R. The epidemiology of wound infection. A 10-year prospective study of 62,939 wounds. Surg Clin North Am 1980;60(1):27–40.
8. Anderson DJ, Kirkland KB, Kaye KS, et al. Underresourced hospital infection control and prevention programs: penny wise, pound foolish? Infect Control Hosp Epidemiol 2007;28(7):767–73.
9. Scott RD. The direct medical costs of healthcare-associated infections in U.S. hospitals and the benefits of prevention. Atlanta (GA): Division of Healthcare Quality Promotion National Center for Preparedness, Detection, and Control of Infectious Diseases Coordinating Center for Infectious Diseases Centers for Disease Control and Prevention; 2009.
10. Kirkland KB, Briggs JP, Trivette SL, et al. The impact of surgical-site infections in the 1990s: attributable mortality, excess length of hospitalization, and extra costs. Infect Control Hosp Epidemiol 1999;20(11):725–30.
11. Mangram AJ, Horan TC, Pearson ML, et al. Guideline for prevention of surgical site infection, 1999. Hospital infection control practices advisory committee. Infect Control Hosp Epidemiol 1999;20(4):250–78 [quiz: 279–80].
12. Cosgrove SE, Qi Y, Kaye KS, et al. The impact of methicillin resistance in *Staphylococcus aureus* bacteremia on patient outcomes: mortality, length of stay, and hospital charges. Infect Control Hosp Epidemiol 2005;26(2):166–74.
13. Cosgrove SE, Sakoulas G, Perencevich EN, et al. Comparison of mortality associated with methicillin-resistant and methicillin-susceptible *Staphylococcus aureus* bacteremia: a meta-analysis. Clin Infect Dis 2003;36(1):53–9.
14. Sands K, Vineyard G, Platt R. Surgical site infections occurring after hospital discharge. J Infect Dis 1996;173(4):963–70.
15. Horan TC, Gaynes RP, Martone WJ, et al. CDC definitions of nosocomial surgical site infections, 1992: a modification of CDC definitions of surgical wound infections. Infect Control Hosp Epidemiol 1992;13(10):606–8.
16. Wall DB, Klein SR, Black S, et al. A simple model to help distinguish necrotizing fasciitis from nonnecrotizing soft tissue infection. J Am Coll Surg 2000;191(3): 227–31.
17. Donlan RM. New approaches for the characterization of prosthetic joint biofilms. Clin Orthop Relat Res 2005;437:12–9.
18. Trampuz A, Piper KE, Jacobson MJ, et al. Sonication of removed hip and knee prostheses for diagnosis of infection. N Engl J Med 2007;357(7):654–63.

19. Wong ES. Surgical site infections. 3rd edition. Baltimore (MD): Lippincott, Williams, and Wilkins; 2004.
20. Tuazon CU. Skin and skin structure infections in the patient at risk: carrier state of Staphylococcus aureus. Am J Med 1984;76(5A):166–71.
21. Altemeier WA, Culbertson WR, Hummel RP. Surgical considerations of endogenous infections—sources, types, and methods of control. Surg Clin North Am 1968;48(1):227–40.
22. Wiley AM, Ha'eri GB. Routes of infection. A study of using "tracer particles" in the orthopedic operating room. Clin Orthop Relat Res 1979;139:150–5.
23. Edwards LD. The epidemiology of 2056 remote site infections and 1966 surgical wound infections occurring in 1865 patients: a four year study of 40,923 operations at Rush-Presbyterian-St Luke's Hospital, Chicago. Ann Surg 1976;184(6):758–66.
24. Berkelman RL, Martin D, Graham DR, et al. Streptococcal wound infections caused by a vaginal carrier. JAMA 1982;247(19):2680–2.
25. Richet HM, Craven PC, Brown JM, et al. A cluster of Rhodococcus (Gordona) bronchialis sternal-wound infections after coronary-artery bypass surgery. N Engl J Med 1991;324(2):104–9.
26. Lowry PW, Blankenship RJ, Gridley W, et al. A cluster of Legionella sternal-wound infections due to postoperative topical exposure to contaminated tap water. N Engl J Med 1991;324(2):109–13.
27. Clegg HW, Foster MT, Sanders WE Jr, et al. Infection due to organisms of the Mycobacterium fortuitum complex after augmentation mammaplasty: clinical and epidemiologic features. J Infect Dis 1983;147(3):427–33.
28. Gartenberg G, Bottone EJ, Keusch GT, et al. Hospital-acquired mucormycosis (Rhizopus rhizopodiformis) of skin and subcutaneous tissue: epidemiology, mycology and treatment. N Engl J Med 1978;299(20):1115–8.
29. Weber S, Herwaldt LA, McNutt LA, et al. An outbreak of Staphylococcus aureus in a pediatric cardiothoracic surgery unit. Infect Control Hosp Epidemiol 2002; 23(2):77–81.
30. McIntyre DM. An epidemic of Streptococcus pyogenes puerperal and postoperative sepsis with an unusual carrier site—the anus. Am J Obstet Gynecol 1968;101(3):308–14.
31. Stamm WE, Feeley JC, Facklam RR. Wound infections due to group A streptococcus traced to a vaginal carrier. J Infect Dis 1978;138(3):287–92.
32. Schaffner W, Lefkowitz LB Jr, Goodman JS, et al. Hospital outbreak of infections with group a streptococci traced to an asymptomatic anal carrier. N Engl J Med 1969;280(22):1224–5.
33. Gyrska P. Postoperative streptococcal wound infection. The anatomy of an epidemic. JAMA 1970;213:1189–91.
34. Tompkins LS, Roessler BJ, Redd SC, et al. Legionella prosthetic-valve endocarditis. N Engl J Med 1988;318(9):530–5.
35. Brabender W, Hinthorn DR, Asher M, et al. Legionella pneumophila wound infection. JAMA 1983;250(22):3091–2.
36. Safranek TJ, Jarvis WR, Carson LA, et al. Mycobacterium chelonae wound infections after plastic surgery employing contaminated gentian violet skin-marking solution. N Engl J Med 1987;317(4):197–201.
37. Pearson RD, Valenti WM, Steigbigel RT. Clostridium perfringens wound infection associated with elastic bandages. JAMA 1980;244(10):1128–30.
38. Bassett DC, Stokes KJ, Thomas WR. Wound infection with Pseudomonas multivorans. A water-borne contaminant of disinfectant solutions. Lancet 1970; 1(7658):1188–91.

39. Krizek TJ, Robson MC. Evolution of quantitative bacteriology in wound management. Am J Surg 1975;130(5):579–84.
40. Houang ET, Ahmet Z. Intraoperative wound contamination during abdominal hysterectomy. J Hosp Infect 1991;19(3):181–9.
41. James RC, Macleod CJ. Induction of staphylococcal infections in mice with small inocula introduced on sutures. Br J Exp Pathol 1961;42:266–77.
42. Elek SD, Conen PE. The virulence of *Staphylococcus pyogenes* for man; a study of the problems of wound infection. Br J Exp Pathol 1957;38(6):573–86.
43. Arbeit RD, Dunn RM. Expression of capsular polysaccharide during experimental focal infection with *Staphylococcus aureus*. J Infect Dis 1987;156(6):947–52.
44. Froman G, Switalski LM, Speziale P, et al. Isolation and characterization of a fibronectin receptor from *Staphylococcus aureus*. J Biol Chem 1987; 262(14):6564–71.
45. Rich RL, Kreikemeyer B, Owens RT, et al. Ace is a collagen-binding MSCRAMM from *Enterococcus faecalis*. J Biol Chem 1999;274(38):26939–45.
46. Switalski LM, Patti JM, Butcher W, et al. A collagen receptor on *Staphylococcus aureus* strains isolated from patients with septic arthritis mediates adhesion to cartilage. Mol Microbiol 1993;7(1):99–107.
47. Liu Y, Ames B, Gorovits E, et al. SdrX, a serine-aspartate repeat protein expressed by *Staphylococcus capitis* with collagen VI binding activity. Infect Immun 2004;72(11):6237–44.
48. Christensen GD, Baddour LM, Simpson WA. Phenotypic variation of *Staphylococcus epidermidis* slime production in vitro and in vivo. Infect Immun 1987; 55(12):2870–7.
49. Mayberry-Carson KJ, Tober-Meyer B, Smith JK, et al. Bacterial adherence and glycocalyx formation in osteomyelitis experimentally induced with *Staphylococcus aureus*. Infect Immun 1984;43(3):825–33.
50. Mills J, Pulliam L, Dall L, et al. Exopolysaccharide production by viridans streptococci in experimental endocarditis. Infect Immun 1984;43(1):359–67.
51. Rogolsky M. Nonenteric toxins of *Staphylococcus aureus*. Microbiol Rev 1979; 43(3):320–60.
52. Dossett JH, Kronvall G, Williams RC Jr, et al. Antiphagocytic effects of staphylococfcal protein A. J Immunol 1969;103(6):1405–10.
53. Dellinger EP. Surgical infections and choice of antibiotics. 15th edition. Philadelphia: W.B. Saunders Co; 1997.
54. Morrison DC, Ryan JL. Endotoxins and disease mechanisms. Annu Rev Med 1987;38:417–32.
55. Kasper DL. Bacterial capsule—old dogmas and new tricks. J Infect Dis 1986; 153(3):407–15.
56. Kaye KS, Schmit K, Pieper C, et al. The effect of increasing age on the risk of surgical site infection. J Infect Dis 2005;191(7):1056–62.
57. Zerr KJ, Furnary AP, Grunkemeier GL, et al. Glucose control lowers the risk of wound infection in diabetics after open heart operations. Ann Thorac Surg 1997;63(2):356–61.
58. Lilienfeld DE, Vlahov D, Tenney JH, et al. Obesity and diabetes as risk factors for postoperative wound infections after cardiac surgery. Am J Infect Control 1988; 16(1):3–6.
59. Nagachinta T, Stephens M, Reitz B, et al. Risk factors for surgical-wound infection following cardiac surgery. J Infect Dis 1987;156(6):967–73.
60. Sorensen LT, Horby J, Friis E, et al. Smoking as a risk factor for wound healing and infection in breast cancer surgery. Eur J Surg Oncol 2002;28(8):815–20.

61. Post S, Betzler M, von Ditfurth B, et al. Risks of intestinal anastomoses in Crohn's disease. Ann Surg 1991;213(1):37–42.

62. Berard F, Gandon J. Postoperative wound infections: the influence of ultraviolet irradiation of the operating room and of various other factors. Ann Surg 1964; 160(Suppl 1):1–192.

63. Pessaux P, Msika S, Atalla D, et al. Risk factors for postoperative infectious complications in noncolorectal abdominal surgery: a multivariate analysis based on a prospective multicenter study of 4718 patients. Arch Surg 2003;138(3):314–24.

64. Mishriki SF, Law DJ, Jeffery PJ. Factors affecting the incidence of postoperative wound infection. J Hosp Infect 1990;16(3):223–30.

65. Seropian R, Reynolds BM. Wound infections after preoperative depilatory versus razor preparation. Am J Surg 1971;121(3):251–4.

66. Belda FJ, Aguilera L, Garcia de la Asuncion J, et al. Supplemental perioperative oxygen and the risk of surgical wound infection: a randomized controlled trial. JAMA 2005;294(16):2035–42.

67. Greif R, Akca O, Horn EP, et al. Supplemental perioperative oxygen to reduce the incidence of surgical-wound infection. Outcomes Research Group. N Engl J Med 2000;342(3):161–7.

68. Melling AC, Ali B, Scott EM, et al. Effects of preoperative warming on the incidence of wound infection after clean surgery: a randomised controlled trial. Lancet 2001;358(9285):876–80.

69. El-Maallem H, Fletcher J. Effects of surgery on neutrophil granulocyte function. Infect Immun 1981;32(1):38–41.

70. Cheadle WG, Hershman MJ, Wellhausen SR, et al. HLA-DR antigen expression on peripheral blood monocytes correlates with surgical infection. Am J Surg 1991;161(6):639–45.

71. Hensler T, Hecker H, Heeg K, et al. Distinct mechanisms of immunosuppression as a consequence of major surgery. Infect Immun 1997;65(6):2283–91.

72. Clardy CW, Edwards KM, Gay JC. Increased susceptibility to infection in hypothermic children: possible role of acquired neutrophil dysfunction. Pediatr Infect Dis 1985;4(4):379–82.

73. Architects AIo. Guidelines for design and construction of hospital and health care facilities. Washington, DC: American Institute of Architects Press; 1996.

74. Ayliffe GA. Role of the environment of the operating suite in surgical wound infection. Rev Infect Dis 1991;13(Suppl 10):S800–4.

75. Latham R, Lancaster AD, Covington JF, et al. The association of diabetes and glucose control with surgical-site infections among cardiothoracic surgery patients. Infect Control Hosp Epidemiol 2001;22(10):607–12.

76. Morain WD, Colen LB. Wound healing in diabetes mellitus. Clin Plast Surg 1990; 17(3):493–501.

77. Hill GE, Frawley WH, Griffith KE, et al. Allogeneic blood transfusion increases the risk of postoperative bacterial infection: a meta-analysis. J Trauma 2003; 54(5):908–14.

78. Anderson DJ, Kaye KS, Classen D, et al. Strategies to prevent surgical site infections in acute care hospitals. Infect Control Hosp Epidemiol 2008;29(Suppl 1): S51–61.

79. Classen DC, Evans RS, Pestotnik SL, et al. The timing of prophylactic administration of antibiotics and the risk of surgical-wound infection. N Engl J Med 1992; 326(5):281–6.

80. Kernodle DS, Kaiser AB. Surgical and trauma related infections, vol. 2. 5th edition. New York: Churchill Livingstone; 2000.

81. Antimicrobial prophylaxis in surgery. Med Lett Drugs Ther 1997;39(1012):97–101.
82. Ehrenkranz NJ. Antimicrobial prophylaxis in surgery: mechanisms, misconceptions, and mischief. Infect Control Hosp Epidemiol 1993;14(2):99–106.
83. Nichols RL. Surgical antibiotic prophylaxis. Med Clin North Am 1995;79(3): 509–22.
84. McDonald M, Grabsch E, Marshall C, et al. Single- versus multiple-dose antimicrobial prophylaxis for major surgery: a systematic review. Aust N Z J Surg 1998;68(6):388–96.
85. Nichols RL. Antibiotic prophylaxis in surgery. J Chemother 1989;1(3):170–8.
86. Page CP, Bohnen JM, Fletcher JR, et al. Antimicrobial prophylaxis for surgical wounds. Guidelines for clinical care. Arch Surg 1993;128(1):79–88.
87. Bratzler DW, Hunt DR. The surgical infection prevention and surgical care improvement projects: national initiatives to improve outcomes for patients having surgery. Clin Infect Dis 2006;43(3):322–30.
88. Weber WP, Marti WR, Zwahlen M, et al. The timing of surgical antimicrobial prophylaxis. Ann Surg 2008;247(6):918–26.
89. Garey KW, Dao T, Chen H, et al. Timing of vancomycin prophylaxis for cardiac surgery patients and the risk of surgical site infections. J Antimicrob Chemother 2006;58(3):645–50.
90. Zanetti G, Giardina R, Platt R. Intraoperative redosing of cefazolin and risk for surgical site infection in cardiac surgery. Emerg Infect Dis 2001;7(5):828–31.
91. DiPiro JT, Cheung RP, Bowden TA Jr, et al. Single dose systemic antibiotic prophylaxis of surgical wound infections. Am J Surg 1986;152(5):552–9.
92. Dellinger EP, Hausmann SM, Bratzler DW, et al. Hospitals collaborate to decrease surgical site infections. Am J Surg 2005;190(1):9–15.
93. Haynes AB, Weiser TG, Berry WR, et al. A surgical safety checklist to reduce morbidity and mortality in a global population. N Engl J Med 2009;360(5):491–9.
94. Moro ML, Carrieri MP, Tozzi AE, et al. Risk factors for surgical wound infections in clean surgery: a multicenter study. Italian PRINOS Study Group. Ann Ital Chir 1996;67(1):13–9.
95. Winston KR. Hair and neurosurgery. Neurosurgery 1992;31(2):320–9.
96. Alexander JW, Fischer JE, Boyajian M, et al. The influence of hair-removal methods on wound infections. Arch Surg 1983;118(3):347–52.
97. Masterson TM, Rodeheaver GT, Morgan RF, et al. Bacteriologic evaluation of electric clippers for surgical hair removal. Am J Surg 1984;148(3):301–2.
98. Wilson SJ, Sexton DJ. Elevated preoperative fasting serum glucose levels increase the risk of postoperative mediastinitis in patients undergoing open heart surgery. Infect Control Hosp Epidemiol 2003;24(10):776–8.
99. Gandhi GY, Nuttall GA, Abel MD, et al. Intensive intraoperative insulin therapy versus conventional glucose management during cardiac surgery: a randomized trial. Ann Intern Med 2007;146(4):233–43.
100. Haley RW, Culver DH, White JW, et al. The efficacy of infection surveillance and control programs in preventing nosocomial infections in US hospitals. Am J Epidemiol 1985;121(2):182–205.
101. Condon RE, Schulte WJ, Malangoni MA, et al. Effectiveness of a surgical wound surveillance program. Arch Surg 1983;118(3):303–7.
102. Olson M, O'Connor M, Schwartz ML. Surgical wound infections. A 5-year prospective study of 20,193 wounds at the Minneapolis VA Medical Center. Ann Surg 1984;199(3):253–9.
103. Kerstein M, Flower M, Harkavy LM, et al. Surveillance for postoperative wound infections: practical aspects. Am Surg 1978;44(4):210–4.

104. Mead PB, Pories SE, Hall P, et al. Decreasing the incidence of surgical wound infections. Validation of a surveillance-notification program. Arch Surg 1986; 121(4):458–61.

105. Baker C, Luce J, Chenoweth C, et al. Comparison of case-finding methodologies for endometritis after cesarean section. Am J Infect Control 1995;23(1): 27–33.

106. Cardo DM, Falk PS, Mayhall CG. Validation of surgical wound surveillance. Infect Control Hosp Epidemiol 1993;14(4):211–5.

107. Chalfine A, Cauet D, Lin WC, et al. Highly sensitive and efficient computer-assisted system for routine surveillance for surgical site infection. Infect Control Hosp Epidemiol 2006;27(8):794–801.

108. Miner AL, Sands KE, Yokoe DS, et al. Enhanced identification of postoperative infections among outpatients. Emerg Infect Dis 2004;10(11):1931–7.

109. Yokoe DS, Noskin GA, Cunnigham SM, et al. Enhanced identification of postoperative infections among inpatients. Emerg Infect Dis 2004;10(11):1924–30.

110. Garibaldi RA. Prevention of intraoperative wound contamination with chlorhexidine shower and scrub. J Hosp Infect 1988;11(Suppl B):5–9.

111. Hayek LJ, Emerson JM, Gardner AM. A placebo-controlled trial of the effect of two preoperative baths or showers with chlorhexidine detergent on postoperative wound infection rates. J Hosp Infect 1987;10(2):165–72.

112. Rotter ML, Larsen SO, Cooke EM, et al. A comparison of the effects of preoperative whole-body bathing with detergent alone and with detergent containing chlorhexidine gluconate on the frequency of wound infections after clean surgery. The European Working Party on Control of Hospital Infections. J Hosp Infect 1988;11(4):310–20.

113. Leigh DA, Stronge JL, Marriner J, et al. Total body bathing with 'Hibiscrub' (chlorhexidine) in surgical patients: a controlled trial. J Hosp Infect 1983;4(3):229–35.

114. Lynch W, Davey PG, Malek M, et al. Cost-effectiveness analysis of the use of chlorhexidine detergent in preoperative whole-body disinfection in wound infection prophylaxis. J Hosp Infect 1992;21(3):179–91.

115. Kaiser AB, Kernodle DS, Barg NL, et al. Influence of preoperative showers on staphylococcal skin colonization: a comparative trial of antiseptic skin cleansers. Ann Thorac Surg 1988;45(1):35–8.

116. Segers P, Speekenbrink RG, Ubbink DT, et al. Prevention of nosocomial infection in cardiac surgery by decontamination of the nasopharynx and oropharynx with chlorhexidine gluconate: a randomized controlled trial. JAMA 2006;296(20): 2460–6.

117. Cimochowski GE, Harostock MD, Brown R, et al. Intranasal mupirocin reduces sternal wound infection after open heart surgery in diabetics and nondiabetics. Ann Thorac Surg 2001;71(5):1572–8 [discussion: 1578–79].

118. Kluytmans JA, Mouton JW, VandenBergh MF, et al. Reduction of surgical-site infections in cardiothoracic surgery by elimination of nasal carriage of *Staphylococcus aureus*. Infect Control Hosp Epidemiol 1996;17(12):780–5.

119. Perl TM, Cullen JJ, Wenzel RP, et al. Intranasal mupirocin to prevent postoperative *Staphylococcus aureus* infections. N Engl J Med 2002;346(24):1871–7.

120. Perl TM. Prevention of *Staphylococcus aureus* infections among surgical patients: beyond traditional perioperative prophylaxis. Surgery 2003;134 (Suppl 5):S10–7.

121. Miller MA, Dascal A, Portnoy J, et al. Development of mupirocin resistance among methicillin-resistant *Staphylococcus aureus* after widespread use of nasal mupirocin ointment. Infect Control Hosp Epidemiol 1996;17(12):811–3.

122. Mayzler O, Weksler N, Domchik S, et al. Does supplemental perioperative oxygen administration reduce the incidence of wound infection in elective colorectal surgery? Minerva Anestesiol 2005;71(1–2):21–5.
123. Meyhoff CS, Wetterslev J, Jorgensen LN, et al. Effect of high perioperative oxygen fraction on surgical site infection and pulmonary complications after abdominal surgery: the PROXI randomized clinical trial. JAMA 2009;302(14): 1543–50.
124. Myles PS, Leslie K, Chan MT, et al. Avoidance of nitrous oxide for patients undergoing major surgery: a randomized controlled trial. Anesthesiology 2007;107(2):221–31.
125. Pryor KO, Fahey TJ 3rd, Lien CA, et al. Surgical site infection and the routine use of perioperative hyperoxia in a general surgical population: a randomized controlled trial. JAMA 2004;291(1):79–87.
126. Qadan M, Akca O, Mahid SS, et al. Perioperative supplemental oxygen therapy and surgical site infection: a meta-analysis of randomized controlled trials. Arch Surg 2009;144(4):359–66 [discussion: 366–7].
127. Stevens DL, Bisno AL, Chambers HF, et al. Practice guidelines for the diagnosis and management of skin and soft-tissue infections. Clin Infect Dis 2005;41(10): 1373–406.
128. Karra R, McDermott L, Connelly S, et al. Risk factors for 1-year mortality after postoperative mediastinitis. J Thorac Cardiovasc Surg 2006;132(3):537–43.
129. Zimmerli W, Trampuz A, Ochsner PE. Prosthetic-joint infections. N Engl J Med 2004;351(16):1645–54.
130. El Oakley RM, Wright JE. Postoperative mediastinitis: classification and management. Ann Thorac Surg 1996;61(3):1030–6.
131. Brandt CM, Sistrunk WW, Duffy MC, et al. Staphylococcus aureus prosthetic joint infection treated with debridement and prosthesis retention. Clin Infect Dis 1997;24(5):914–9.
132. Raymond DP, Pelletier SJ, Crabtree TD, et al. Surgical infection and the aging population. Am Surg 2001;67(9):827–32 [discussion: 832–3].
133. Mangram AJ, Horan TC, Pearson ML, et al. Guideline for prevention of surgical site infection, 1999. Centers for Disease Control and Prevention (CDC) Hospital Infection Control Practices Advisory Committee. Am J Infect Control 1999;27(2): 97–132 [quiz 133–4; discussion: 196].
134. Forse RA, Karam B, MacLean LD, et al. Antibiotic prophylaxis for surgery in morbidly obese patients. Surgery 1989;106(4):750–6 [discussion: 756–7].
135. Bratzler DW, Houck PM. Antimicrobial prophylaxis for surgery: an advisory statement from the National Surgical Infection Prevention Project. Clin Infect Dis 2004;38(12):1706–15.
136. Haley RW, Culver DH, Morgan WM, et al. Identifying patients at high risk of surgical wound infection. A simple multivariate index of patient susceptibility and wound contamination. Am J Epidemiol 1985;121(2):206–15.
137. Kurz A, Sessler DI, Lenhardt R. Perioperative normothermia to reduce the incidence of surgical-wound infection and shorten hospitalization. Study of Wound Infection and Temperature Group. N Engl J Med 1996;334(19):1209–15.

Control of Methicillin-resistant *Staphylococcus aureus*

Andie S. Lee, MD, Benedikt Huttner, MD,
Stephan Harbarth, MD, MS*

KEYWORDS

- MRSA • Epidemiology • Infection prevention
- Active surveillance • Screening • Decolonization

Methicillin-resistant *Staphylococcus aureus* (MRSA) was first described in 1961 and in the following decades it quickly became an important cause of health care-associated infections (HAIs) worldwide. National surveillance data show that MRSA is recovered in about 53% of *S aureus* isolates in the United States[1] and reaches similar levels in parts of Southern Europe.[2] MRSA is an important nosocomial pathogen because of its virulence and survival fitness.[3] In health care facilities there is selective advantage for MRSA survival as a result of antibiotic use.

Strategies to control MRSA have targeted the reservoir of carriers, routes of transmission, and antibiotic pressure (**Fig. 1**). In practice, multiple interventions are often employed to attempt to effectively control MRSA. However, the utility of control measures is debated because of the emergence of community-associated MRSA, an increasing reservoir of health care-associated MRSA, the inability to eradicate endemic MRSA, and the disruption in patient care and costs associated with these strategies.[4]

This article describes approaches to MRSA control in health care settings where MRSA is already endemic. Current controversies surrounding various control measures are discussed. This article does not focus on the control of community-associated MRSA or the search-and-destroy strategy used in some regions with low MRSA prevalence (refer to the national policy document of the Dutch Working Party on Infection Prevention).[5]

Funding support: Work by the authors was supported by the European Commission under the Life Science Health Priority of the 6th Framework Program (MOSAR network contract LSHP-CT-2007-037941 and CHAMP network contract SP5A-CT-2007-044317).
Infection Control Program, University of Geneva Hospitals and Medical School, 4, Rue Gabrielle-Perret-Gentil, CH-1211 Geneva 14, Switzerland
* Corresponding author.
E-mail address: stephan.harbarth@hcuge.ch

Infect Dis Clin N Am 25 (2011) 155–179
doi:10.1016/j.idc.2010.11.002
0891-5520/11/$ – see front matter © 2011 Elsevier Inc. All rights reserved.

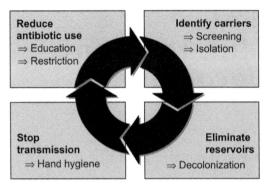

| Reduce antibiotic use ⇒ Education ⇒ Restriction | Identify carriers ⇒ Screening ⇒ Isolation |
| Stop transmission ⇒ Hand hygiene | Eliminate reservoirs ⇒ Decolonization |

Fig. 1. Approaches to the control of endemic methicillin-resistant *Staphylococcus aureus*. (*From* Harbarth S. Control of endemic methicillin-resistant *Staphylococcus aureus*–recent advances and future challenges. Clin Microbiol Infect 2006;12(12):1155; with permission from Wiley-Blackwell publishing.)

EPIDEMIOLOGY

Not all countries and regions are equally affected by MRSA. Some countries, such as the Netherlands or Scandinavian countries, have succeeded in maintaining low levels of MRSA; whereas, in Southern Europe more than 25% of *Staphylococcus aureus* isolates are methicillin resistant.[2] The marked variation in Europe in the proportion of *S aureus* isolates that are methicillin resistant is shown in **Fig. 2**. These differences are at least partly explained by varying antibiotic use and infection control practices.[6]

In recent years, MRSA has emerged in some countries as an important cause of skin and soft-tissue infections in otherwise healthy adults without prior health care

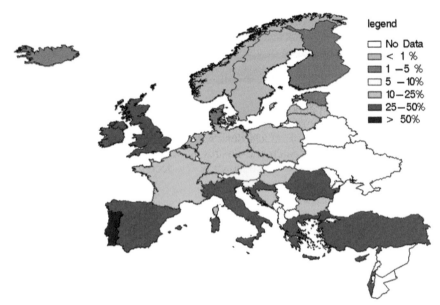

legend
☐ No Data
▨ < 1 %
▨ 1 −5 %
☐ 5 −10%
▨ 10−25%
■ 25−50%
■ > 50%

Fig. 2. Proportion of MRSA among *S aureus* isolates in countries participating in the European Antimicrobial Resistance Surveillance System (EARSS) in 2008. (*Data from* EARSS data. Available at: http://www.ecdc.europa.eu/en/activities/surveillance/EARS-Net/Pages/index.aspx. Accessed December 10, 2010.)

contact.[7,8] These infections are caused by specific strains that differ from hospital-associated strains and are commonly referred to as *community-associated MRSA* (CA-MRSA). They often carry virulence factors, such as the exotoxin Panton-Valentine leukocidin (PVL), that may play a role in fulminant infections, such as severe necrotizing community-onset pneumonia or necrotizing fasciitis.[9,10]

In the United States there is evidence that CA-MRSA strains might replace traditional hospital-associated strains, an assumption also supported by mathematical models.[11–14] A retrospective study from Chicago analyzed hospital-onset MRSA bacteremias between 2000 and 2006 and found that CA-MRSA strains caused an increasing proportion of bacteremias (from 24% to 49%); whereas, total hospital-onset MRSA bloodstream infection (BSI) rates were stable.[13] This phenomenon may not be limited to the United States as demonstrated by a study from Greece that reported PVL-positive MRSA strains as a cause of a quarter of all health care-associated MRSA infections in 2 university hospitals in 2004 to 2005.[15] In addition, livestock-related MRSA, particularly transmission from pigs to humans, is a recently recognized problem and may increasingly be imported into the hospital.[16,17]

The past epidemic waves of *S aureus* have demonstrated that the epidemiology of this pathogen is complex and unpredictable.[18,19] Only time will reveal the extent to which CA-MRSA or livestock-related MRSA will replace the traditional hospital strains and what the clinical consequences of this replacement will be.

CURRENT MRSA INFECTION CONTROL PRACTICES

Recommendations and guidelines for MRSA control have been issued by several professional organizations and national institutions. These documents, among other things, discuss the role of surveillance for MRSA, which may be broadly classified into 2 strategies: routine, clinical culture-based surveillance and active surveillance. Active surveillance uses microbiological cultures or molecular techniques on patient samples to identify patients with asymptomatic MRSA colonization. Samples are usually collected from the anterior nares and other sites, including the perineum and wounds. Active surveillance for MRSA is discussed in detail in a later section of this article. In recent years, several national surveys of MRSA control practices have been conducted both in Europe and in the United States. These surveys demonstrate varying ways in which guidelines have been applied in the real world. Four such surveys are summarized in **Table 1**.

Two studies were conducted exclusively in intensive care units (ICUs). A survey performed in England in 2000 included almost all (96%) ICUs in the country.[20] Overall, there was marked variation in patient and staff screening and infection control procedures. Of note, 35% of ICUs screened staff members and 24% of ICUs did not have an isolation policy for patients with MRSA. In Germany, ICUs participating in the German Nosocomial Infection Surveillance System (KISS) were sent a questionnaire in 2001.[21] There were screening policies for at-risk patients on admission in 58% of ICUs and isolation of MRSA carriers was practiced in 66% of ICUs.

Two surveys that also included non-ICU patient care areas have been conducted in the United States. MRSA control opinions and practices among infectious disease consultants were surveyed in 2002.[22] A total of 71% of respondents favored use of contact precautions. In terms of active surveillance cultures, such as those obtained from the nares, 18% of those surveyed favored their use in general wards and 35% in the ICU ($P<.001$). However, surveillance cultures were only being used in 13% of general wards and 18% of ICUs in which the respondents practiced. Most infectious disease consultants endorsed contact precautions and worked in hospitals that have

Table 1
Surveys of MRSA infection control practices in England, Germany, and the United States

Study	Country Year	Surveillance System/Network	Survey Type	Number of Respondents (%)	Wards Included	Routine Screening	Contact Precautions and Isolation	Decolonization
Hails et al,[20] 2003	England 2000	—	Questionnaire with telephone follow-up	217 (96)	ICUs	97% any routine screening: 75% on admission 11% on discharge 86% patients transferred 53% weekly 35% screen staff	Gloves and aprons: 92% any patient 8% only patients on contact precautions Isolation: 90% isolation cubicles present but made up <25% of total beds in half ICUs 24% no isolation policy	—
Gastmeier et al,[21] 2004	Germany 2001	German Nosocomial Infection Surveillance System (KISS)	Questionnaire	164 (77)	ICUs	58% at-risk patients on admission 82% roommates of patients with MRSA	66% isolate	86% mupirocin 73% antiseptic baths

Sunenshine et al,[22] 2005	United States 2002	Infectious Diseases Society of America (IDSA) Emerging Infections Network (EIN)	Questionnaire to infectious disease consultants	477 (51)	ICUs, transplant, general	Favored screening in the following: 35% ICUs 46% transplant wards 18% general wards Actually screening in the following: 18% ICUs 17% transplant wards 13% general wards	71% favor contact precautions	—
Jarvis et al,[23] 2007	United States 2006	Association for Professionals in Infection Control and Epidemiology, Inc (APIC)	Questionnaire to APIC members	1237	Hospital wide	29% any routine screening 42% from long-term care facilities 33% from other health care facilities 20% repeat admissions	>72% use contact isolation	—

implemented them. In contrast, they were divided about the role of active MRSA surveillance and few infectious disease consultants worked in hospitals that use surveillance cultures on a routine basis. Another study conducted in the United States in 2006 was a large national prevalence survey of MRSA in health care facilities.[23] There were 1237 respondents and all states were represented. Active surveillance testing was used in 29% of hospitals in which the respondents worked.

The situation in surveyed health systems in different countries demonstrates that despite recommendations about screening and isolation of patients with MRSA, there is wide variation in approaches both between and within countries. This variation may reflect the controversies that still exist in many aspects of MRSA control and practical difficulties in implementation of control strategies.

OUTCOMES OF MRSA INFECTION CONTROL PRACTICES

Not only have MRSA control measures between countries varied but so have the outcomes of such strategies. Varying baseline prevalence of MRSA is likely one important factor when assessing the success of different approaches. Another important factor when assessing outcomes of infection control strategies is the type and extent of surveillance systems that are in place. Many countries or regions have implemented prospective surveillance networks that enable early detection of increases in or outbreaks of MRSA. Data available from these surveillance systems may facilitate implementation of early interventions, increasing the likelihood of success. These data are also valuable for feedback to institutions as well as benchmarking and monitoring the success of control strategies. A summary of several national or regional surveillance networks is presented in **Table 2**.

In France, where MRSA rates in the 1990s were high, there is now a favorable trend in MRSA prevalence (**Fig. 3**). This trend is thought to be at least in part attributable to a stringent national MRSA control program that was gradually introduced between 1993 and 2004. The program included strengthening of infection control activities, developing surveillance networks, and mandatory notification of outbreaks to interregional coordination centers and the National Institute for Public Health Surveillance. During 2005 to 2008, 5 quality indicators with public reporting were implemented: infection control structures and activities; use of alcohol-based hand rubs; surveillance of surgical site infection; antibiotic use policy; and incidence of MRSA infection. These measures were associated with a decrease in MRSA bacteremia rates in France during 2001 to 2007.[24]

In the United Kingdom, MRSA bacteremia rates rose during the 1990s, peaking in 2003. Since then, there has been a yearly reduction in rates (**Fig. 4**). Like the French experience, these favorable trends followed the implementation of a national strategy organized through the Department of Health.[25] Mandatory reporting of certain HAIs began in 2001. After MRSA bacteremia rates peaked in 2003, a target was set of 50% reduction in the national total to be achieved by 2008. A hand hygiene campaign ("cleanyourhands")[26] was launched nationally in 2004.[27] In 2005, the Department of Health implemented care bundles, including guidelines on catheter care, MRSA screening, and a care bundle for ventilated patients. Although the hand hygiene promotion campaign is considered a major contributor to subsequent favorable trends in MRSA rates at a national level,[28] it is likely that the multifaceted approach, together with a clear target and support from the Department of Health, has resulted in this marked improvement.

In addition to France and the United Kingdom, there is now a diverse group of European countries with varying baseline MRSA prevalence that have been able to inverse previous worrisome trends of increasing MRSA rates. In contrast, national data from the United States are not yet encouraging. The incidence rate of hospital-onset invasive MRSA infections was 1.02 per 10,000 population in 2005 and decreased 9.4% per year (95% confidence interval [CI], 14.7% to 3.8%; $P = .005$), and the incidence of health care-associated community-onset infections was 2.20 per 10,000 population in 2005 and decreased 5.7% per year (95% CI, 9.7% to 1.6%; $P = .01$).[29] The Surveillance Network–USA, which reports resistance trends from 300 clinical laboratories across the United States, shows that MRSA rates have been steadily increasing since 1998, reaching 53% in 2005 (**Fig. 5**).[1] However, recent data regarding the incidence of MRSA central line-associated BSIs in US ICUs reported favorable trends.[30] Although the proportion of S aureus central line-associated BSIs caused by MRSA increased by 26% ($P = .02$) from 1997 to 2007, overall MRSA central line-associated BSI incidence decreased by 50% ($P<.001$) over this period. The reduction in infections was likely caused by several interventions that were implemented during the study period, including improved hand hygiene practices, standardized line insertion and care practices, improved catheter technology, and shorter periods of catheter use in patients.[31] There was an overall reduction in central line-associated BSI incidence caused by all organisms, including methicillin-sensitive Staphylococcus aureus (MSSA), which suggests that the decline was not caused by MRSA-specific control strategies, such as active surveillance for MRSA.[31]

It is important to compare international figures with caution because of differing definitions, study populations, and duration of follow-up used in reports. It is often difficult to identify the precise determinants of success or failure. Many factors, such as local compliance with programs, resources, facilities, bed occupancy, length of stay, case-mix, staffing, and administrative support, are important in the successful implementation of a program. In addition, the priority given to infection control interventions by senior management and national authorities may explain some of the differences seen.[32]

APPROACHES TO AND CONTROVERSIES IN MRSA CONTROL

When reviewing MRSA control research, there are some important issues to consider before applying results to clinical practice. The literature often reports the results of multiple interventions on outcome measures and it may be difficult to assign the relative contribution of each intervention. It is also important to note that studies reporting outcomes of strategies do so in the context of varying baseline prevalence of MRSA. Thus, the external validity of such results can be an issue. In addition, many studies have suboptimal design and analysis. Reporting bias, where negative studies are less likely to be published, must also be considered.

Research concerning MRSA control interventions has resulted in ongoing debate with regard to the utility of active surveillance cultures, isolation, decolonization, and environmental cleaning. The importance of hand hygiene and informed antibiotic stewardship are less controversial. The potential advantages and disadvantages of these control strategies are summarized in **Table 3** and discussed in the following sections.

Hand Hygiene

Hand hygiene is an integral part of standard infection control measures. The effectiveness of hand hygiene promotion has been demonstrated in reductions in MRSA transmission and rates of HAI.[28,33–35] It is particularly important to perform hand hygiene at the appropriate times with the correct technique. Despite its importance and simplicity, compliance with hand hygiene remains low among health care workers

Table 2
Examples of national and regional surveillance networks of MRSA

Country/Region	Surveillance System/Network Web site	Year Established	Number of Participants	Voluntary/Mandatory Participation	Surveillance Data Collected
United States	National Healthcare Safety Network (NHSN) (previously National Nosocomial Infection Surveillance system, NNIS) http://www.cdc.gov/nhsn	NNIS 1997 NHSN 2005	3000 hospitals	Voluntary (mandatory in some states from 2007)	All health care-associated infections (absolute numbers and rates per patient-days or device-days)
Australia/ New Zealand	Australian Group for Antimicrobial Resistance (AGAR) http://antimicrobial-resistance.com	1985	31 laboratories	Voluntary	Antimicrobial resistance of Staphylococcus aureus (proportion of isolates resistant) Similar data for gram-negatives, Streptococcus pneumoniae, Enterococcus spp, and Haemophilus influenzae Annual data collection (for S aureus)
Europe	European Antimicrobial Resistance Surveillance System (EARSS) http://www.ecdc.europa.eu/en/activities/surveillance/EARS-Net/Page	1999	31 countries (900 public-health laboratories serving more than 1400 hospitals)	Voluntary	Oxacillin resistance of invasive S aureus (proportion of isolates resistant by country) Similar data for S pneumoniae, Enterococcus spp, E coli, K pneumoniae, and P aeruginosa Quarterly data collection

Country	Program	Year	Coverage	Status	Data collected
France	French national nosocomial infection control program (RAISIN) http://www.invs.sante.fr/raisin	2002	755 health care facilities	Mandatory and publicly reported since 2009	MRSA clinical cultures (incidence per 1000 patient-days for patients hospitalized for at least 24 hours). Similar data for extended-spectrum beta-lactamase producers Annual data collection
United Kingdom	*Staphylococcus aureus* bacteremia surveillance scheme (Health Protection Agency) http://www.hpa.org.uk/web/HPAweb&Page&HPAweb AutoListName/Page/1191942169773	2001	All hospitals	Voluntary (before 2004), mandatory (from 2004)	MRSA bacteremia (absolute number and rate per 10,000 bed days)
Germany	Krankenhaus-Infektions-Surveillance-System (KISS) http://www.nrz-hygiene.de/en/nrz/welcome	1997	184 hospitals (MRSA data)	Voluntary	MRSA colonization and infection (cases per 1000 patient-days) Differentiation between health care-associated and community-associated cases Annual data collection

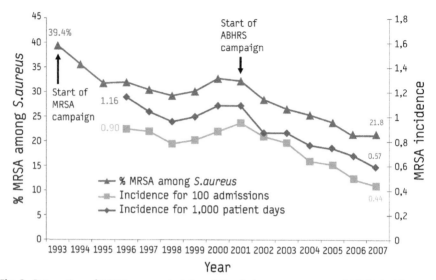

Fig. 3. Proportion of MRSA among isolates of *Staphylococcus aureus* and MRSA incidence in 39 teaching hospitals in the Paris area, 1993 to 2007. ABHRS, alcohol-based hand rub solutions; MRSA, methicillin-resistant *S aureus*. (*From* Azanowsky JM, Brun-Buisson C, Carbonne A, et al. Recent trends in antimicrobial resistance among *Streptococcus pneumoniae* and *Staphylococcus aureus* isolates: the French experience. Euro Surveill 2008;13(46):pii 19035. Available at: http://www.eurosurveillance.org/ViewArticle.aspx?ArticleId=19035. Accessed December 10, 2010; with permission.)

(HCWs).[36] Controversy exists regarding the utility of attempts to further increase hand hygiene compliance in settings where baseline compliance rates are already high (>50%). In this situation, computer modeling suggests that this intervention alone may not result in further significant reduction in MRSA transmission.[37]

Active Surveillance Cultures

The majority of MRSA carriage is asymptomatic and therefore not identified using routine clinical cultures. The latter alone may only identify 18% of actual MRSA

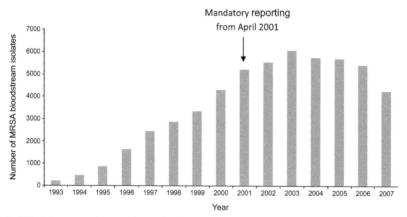

Fig. 4. MRSA bacteremia cases in England, 1994 to 2007. (*From* Liebowitz LD. MRSA burden and interventions. Int J Antimicrob Agents 2009;34(Suppl 3):S12; with permission.)

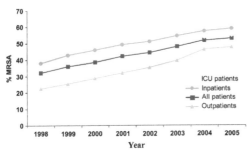

Fig. 5. MRSA trends in the United States (1998 to March 2005), The Surveillance Network–USA. (*From* Styers D, Sheehan DJ, Hogan P, et al. Laboratory-based surveillance of current antimicrobial resistance patterns and trends among *Staphylococcus aureus*: 2005 status in the United States. Ann Clin Microbiol Antimicrob 2006;5:2; with permission.)

patient-days.[38] A significant number of colonized patients will subsequently develop infection, up to 25% in ICUs.[39] Active MRSA surveillance identifies this large reservoir of transmission and infection risk through screening cultures, often of the nares. These colonized patients may then be placed on contact precautions and treatment (usually in the form of topical antibiotics and antiseptics) may be instituted in an attempt to eradicate carriage. Active surveillance may be universal, where all patients admitted to hospital are screened, or targeted, where screening is limited to patient groups at increased risk of colonization, such as those with prior antibiotic use, prolonged hospitalization, ICU admission, hemodialysis, or contact with a known MRSA carrier. Risk factors for MRSA colonization may vary in different regions. HCWs who are MRSA colonized can act as reservoirs for outbreaks and ongoing transmission. HCW screening in settings with endemic MRSA is beyond the scope of this review but is discussed elsewhere.[40]

The use of active surveillance remains controversial due to questions about its effectiveness and costs, especially active surveillance using molecular assays. Active surveillance is considered most useful in patients at high risk of MRSA infection, such as in the ICU or outbreak settings.[41,42] In ICU patients, this intervention has resulted in decreased incidence of MRSA bacteremia, not only in the ICU but hospital wide.[43,44]

Several recent studies have evaluated the effectiveness of universal active MRSA surveillance with conflicting results (**Table 4**). An observational study of universal MRSA screening with polymerase chain reaction (PCR) showed reduction in MRSA disease.[38] In contrast, a prospective crossover study in surgical wards, also using PCR screening, did not find a reduction in infections or acquisition.[45] Other studies have compared molecular and culture-based screening, also with varying results. Two crossover studies conducted in the United Kingdom came to opposite conclusions.[46,47] The first study included medical and surgical units and found no difference in MRSA acquisition rates.[46] Although the number of inappropriate preemptive isolation days was reduced, the investigators concluded that the increased cost of rapid tests was not justified. In contrast, the second study, conducted in surgical units, found a significant reduction in acquisition rates with molecular versus culture-based screening.[47]

Two recent systematic reviews have observed that the quality of published evidence regarding MRSA active surveillance is variable.[48,49] McGinigle and colleagues[48] reviewed studies in adult ICUs and did not identify any randomized controlled trials. They concluded that existing evidence favored use of active surveillance, but the evidence is of poor quality and definitive recommendations cannot be made. This

Table 3
Advantages and disadvantages of various MRSA control strategies

Infection Control Measure	Mode of Action	Potential Advantages	Potential Disadvantages/Barriers to Implementation
Hand hygiene	Reduces cross transmission	Simple Inexpensive Not organism specific	Difficult to sustain high hand hygiene compliance rates
MRSA screening of patients	Early identification of carriers	Identifies reservoir Reduces infection risk for individual patients (eg, by appropriate perioperative antibiotic prophylaxis)	Costs Resources MRSA specific Needs to be linked with other measures (isolation, decolonization) Optimal population and method controversial
Screening and decolonization of health care workers	Reduces reservoir	Complete assessment of reservoir Interruption of MRSA transmission to patients Reduction of infection risk for the individual health care worker Decreased transmission risk to close contacts/community reservoir	Disruption of patient care False reassurance of noncolonized or nonidentified health care workers Ethical considerations (stigmatization) Costs
Isolation	Increased barrier to cross transmission	Interruption of MRSA transmission Decreased risk for noncolonized patients Better compliance with infection control measures	Costs Potential negative psychological effects Possible decrease in quality of care of patients
Decolonization	Reduces reservoir	Interruption of MRSA transmission to other patients Reduces infection risk for individual patients	Not feasible for all patients Side effects of decolonization treatment Risk of mupirocin and chlorhexidine resistance
Routine chlorhexidine body washing	Reduces reservoir	Reduces infection risk for individual patients Not organism specific	Risk of chlorhexidine resistance
Antibiotic stewardship	Reduces selection pressure	Not organism specific (includes *Clostridium difficile*), improved patient care in general	Opposition from physicians and pharmaceutical industry Most effective interventions unclear Long-term effects unclear
Enhanced environmental cleaning	Reduces environmental contamination	Not organism specific Reduction in hand contamination	Strong evidence for efficacy lacking Best strategy unclear

review prompted criticism for omitting some important studies and emphasizing the randomized controlled study design.[50] Poorly conducted randomized trials may be less reliable than other study types, such as well conducted interrupted time series and controlled before-and-after studies, performed over extended periods of time. Importantly, critics emphasize the consistency of positive findings in ICUs.[51] Tacconelli and colleagues[49] conducted a systematic review of studies using molecular screening. Compared with culture-based screening, use of rapid molecular tests was not associated with decreased MRSA acquisition rates. However, when molecular screening was compared with no active surveillance for MRSA, there was a significant decrease in MRSA BSIs and a nonsignificant trend to reduction in surgical-site infections. Both systematic reviews noted that available evidence is heterogeneous in terms of study design and outcome measures.

The costs and adverse effects of universal active MRSA surveillance have also prompted much discussion, particularly with regard to laboratory resources, decolonization, and isolation policies. Ethical issues concerning patient screening without considering the role of colonized staff[52] as well as balancing patient autonomy and protection of the population have also been discussed, particularly for low-risk patients.[53] In addition, practical issues, such as choice of anatomic screening sites and tests, need to be considered. It must also be emphasized that screening alone is not effective. Surveillance results should be followed by appropriate interventions to reduce the risk of transmission.[52]

Some argue that resources are better used to target all HAIs rather than MRSA alone. One hospital used non–MRSA-specific infection control interventions and was able to reduce MRSA infection rates by 70% in their ICUs.[54] Wenzel and colleagues[55] modeled MRSA active surveillance compared with a broader infection-control approach on attributable mortality from BSIs. Based on their findings, they concluded that an MRSA-focused approach alone is inherently flawed. This argument against active surveillance for MRSA has been criticized for the following reasons: its premise that hospitals use active surveillance without implementing other measures, the lack of importance placed on higher mortality caused by MRSA compared with other nosocomial pathogens, underestimation of the impact of MRSA screening on infection rates, and overestimation of screening costs.[56,57]

To add to the debate, guidelines provided by governmental, public health, and professional societies, particularly the Society of Healthcare Epidemiology of America (SHEA) and Centers for Disease Control and Prevention (CDC), differ in their recommendations, mainly concerning routine use of active surveillance for MRSA. The previous SHEA guideline recommended active surveillance for all high-risk patients[58]; whereas, the CDC guideline has a staged approach, recommending it only if other interventions fail.[59] This issue has sparked much debate by supporters of each strategy.[60–63] A subsequent SHEA/Infectious Diseases Society of America (IDSA) practice recommendation issued in 2008 states that a specific recommendation cannot be made because of conflicting research results and differences among institutions. Active surveillance cultures may be useful when other measures fail and, if implemented, should be part of a multifaceted approach.[64]

Screening policies are not only influenced by scientific and economic evidence but also by increasing public and subsequent political pressure. In the United Kingdom and several states in the United States, new laws have made MRSA screening of hospitalized patients mandatory in some locales, prompting much debate.[65–67] Opponents argue that these laws lack the flexibility of allowing health care professionals to respond to changes in local epidemiology and scientific evidence.[65] There are several important considerations when implementing active surveillance programs (**Fig. 6**).

Table 4
Selected studies of universal MRSA screening

Study; Country	Setting	Design	Control Group	Total Duration	Rapid Screening	Decolonization	Admission MRSA Prevalence (%)	Baseline MRSA Infection Rate (per 1000 Patient-Days)	Comments about Additional Interventions	Findings	Primary Outcome
Harbarth et al,[45] 2008; Switzerland	Surgery	Crossover	Yes	24 m	Molecular (in house)	Yes	5.1	0.91	Modified perioperative prophylaxis	No reduction in MRSA infections	Negative
Robicsek et al,[38] 2008; USA	Hospital wide	Before-after	No	45 m	Molecular (commercial modified in house)	Yes (at physician discretion)	6.3	0.89	Staged ICU screening, then universal screening and decolonization	Reduction in MRSA disease	Positive
Keshtgar et al,[114] 2008; UK	Surgery	Before-after	No	12 m	Molecular (commercial)	Yes (plus povidone iodine or silver sulfadiazine for wounds)	4.5	0.39 bacteremia; 1.74 wound infection	Modified perioperative prophylaxis	Reduction in MRSA bacteremia	Positive
Jeyaratnam et al,[46] 2008; UK	Geriatrics, oncology, surgery	Crossover	Yes	14 m	Molecular (commercial) versus selective broth/chromogenic agar	Yes	6.7	1.09	Preemptive isolation if high-risk patients; discharge screening	No reduction in MRSA transmission	Negative

Study	Setting	Design		Duration	Detection method	Decolonization			Intervention	Reduction	Outcome
Chaberny et al,[44] 2008; Germany	Surgery, ICU	Before-after	No	60 m	Chromogenic agar	Elective surgery patients (plus antiseptic shampoo and gargle)	Not stated	0.2–0.4; nosocomial only 0.11–0.23	Biannual feedback of MRSA rates to wards	Reduction in MRSA infections (hospital wide)	Positive
Aldeyab et al,[115] 2009; UK	Surgery, medical/cardiac	Crossover	Yes	8 m	Molecular (commercial) versus chromogenic agar	Not stated	6.8–7.3	Not stated	Discharge screening	No reduction in MRSA transmission	Negative
Hardy et al,[47] 2010; UK	Surgery	Crossover	Yes	16 m	Molecular (commercial) versus chromogenic agar	Yes (with naseptin if high-level mupirocin resistance)	3.6	Not stated	Rescreening every 4 days; Decolonization in 71% molecular versus 41% culture arms	Reduction in MRSA transmission	Positive

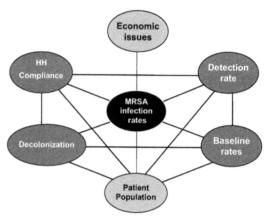

Fig. 6. Important issues to consider when introducing an active surveillance program for MRSA. HH, hand hygiene.

Therefore a tailored approach is necessary and a uniform mandate may not allow a tailored approach to occur. Mandates also remove the autonomy and authority of practitioners to act in their local interests based on local epidemiology.[66] It is clear that the controversies surrounding this issue of government mandates for active surveillance will not be easily resolved. The authors think a reasonable approach is to use targeted rather than universal screening (predominantly with chromogenic agar) based on local MRSA prevalence, risk factors for colonization, and vulnerability of the patient population. This strategy is likely cost-effective if linked to prompt institution of control measures.

Contact Precautions and Isolation

Placing patients who are colonized or infected with MRSA on contact precautions using gowns and gloves may delay colonization of other, noncolonized patients by 5 days and reduce the rate of HAIs by 2.2 times.[68] However, one recent study found no effect of gown use on transmission of MRSA.[69] Masks may reduce the risk of colonization of HCWs with MRSA and may be appropriate in the care of patients with MRSA pulmonary colonization or infection.[58] It is recommended that patients who are MRSA-colonized and -infected are isolated in single rooms or cohorted depending on the availability of single rooms.[59,64,70] Where facilities are limited, patients should be isolated based on a risk assessment of the likelihood of transmission and possible impact of MRSA spread to vulnerable patients.[70]

Observational studies have shown that isolation reduces MRSA acquisition and infections among hospitalized patients.[21,71] However, one prospective study of isolation in the ICU did not show a difference in MRSA transmission.[72] The ICUs in the 2 hospitals in this study used on-admission and weekly active surveillance cultures to determine the incidence of MRSA colonization. No evidence of increased transmission was found after comparison of time periods when patients colonized with MRSA were moved or not moved into single rooms and cohorted bays. This finding may be explained by low screening compliance, delays in notification of results, and poor compliance with general infection control measures. The debate about the utility of contact isolation is also influenced by concerns about the adverse effects of social isolation, feelings of depression, patient satisfaction, and the level of care provided by HCWs to patients in isolation.[73,74] The ethical considerations of such an intervention, which balances patient autonomy with protection of the population, have also been discussed in detail in other publications.[75]

Decolonization

Decolonization of carriers is commonly used for MRSA control in Northwestern Europe and Western Australia but less so in the United States. This intervention aims to suppress or eradicate MRSA carriage to reduce transmission within an institution and subsequent infection risk in individual patients who are colonized.[76] Decolonization is performed with topical nasal antibiotics (eg, mupirocin) and antibacterial body washes (eg, chlorhexidine). Short-term nasal mupirocin is the most effective treatment for eradicating MRSA carriage, with a success rate of approximately 90% 1 week after treatment and up to 60% after longer follow-up.[77] Some health care professionals also use concurrent systemic antibiotics for 7 to 14 days in selected cases.[78]

Recent reviews conclude that there is insufficient evidence to support routine decolonization of all MRSA carriers.[79,80] Decolonization is often used during MRSA outbreaks, particularly if linked to transmission by HCWs. Data looking specifically at ICUs show that the incidence of MRSA colonization and infections was reduced after initiation of decolonization.[81,82] Other reports have also demonstrated that decolonization of S aureus carriers with mupirocin reduces infection rates, particularly in patients undergoing surgery and dialysis.[83] However, decolonization of MRSA carriers did not reduce infection rates in a study of subjects who were predominantly cared for by medical services.[84] It must be noted, however, that eradication of MRSA as opposed to MSSA can be challenging because of the presence of chronic wounds, medical devices, and comorbidities. The success of decolonization may also be influenced by compliance with the decolonization protocols. For example, decolonization is often more effective when it occurs under direct supervision of an HCW rather than when patients are provided instructions to perform decolonization on their own.[85]

The use of decolonization therapy has also raised some concerns. Resistance may emerge with uncontrolled use of mupirocin.[86–88] Previous studies have shown that 1% of subjects on mupirocin and 9% of subjects receiving oral antibiotics developed resistance to the antibiotics used for decolonization.[77] Treatment failure has been associated with colonization with mupirocin-resistant strains at baseline or recovery of resistant strains after treatment with mupirocin when baseline strains were sensitive.[89] Some experts have also questioned the utility of this intervention because of significant rates of recolonization in patients.[90]

Routine Bathing with Chlorhexidine

Studies have evaluated routine bathing with chlorhexidine in subjects in ICUs.[91–93] By reducing the bacterial load on patients' skin, this method may reduce MRSA transmission and infection. A study in 6 ICUs showed that acquisition of MRSA decreased by 32% following the introduction of daily chlorhexidine bathing.[93] With the low number of MRSA BSIs observed, they were unable to document a significant reduction in BSIs caused by MRSA after the intervention. However, recent evidence suggests that chlorhexidine resistance may result in failure of chlorhexidine bathing protocols.[94] Thus caution must be exercised with widespread use of chlorhexidine bathing in ICUs and it may be prudent to monitor for the emergence of resistance to chlorhexidine.

Antibiotic Stewardship

Not surprisingly, selective pressure resulting from prior antibiotic use is a risk factor for MRSA acquisition and transmission.[95,96] A recent meta-analysis of 76 studies showed a 1.8-fold (95% confidence interval [CI] 1.7–1.9) increase in the overall risk of acquiring

MRSA in subjects with recent antibiotic use, particularly fluoroquinolones (risk ratio 3, 95% CI 2.5–3.5).[97] Two studies using robust statistical methods have also shown an association between antibiotic use and MRSA incidence on a hospital level.[98,99] Some studies suggest that reduction in antibiotic use can result in reduction in the incidence of MRSA infections.[100,101] A quasi-experimental study in France showed that a restriction policy that decreased fluoroquinolone use in 1 hospital was associated with a decrease in MRSA isolation rate compared with 3 control hospitals.[102] Because antibiotic use is also linked to the incidence of other nosocomial pathogens, the promotion of appropriate antibiotic use should be a priority for hospitals worldwide.[103,104] Antibiotic stewardship is discussed by Tamma and Cosgrove in detail elsewhere in this issue.

Environmental Cleaning

MRSA is frequently found in the environment close to patients who are colonized.[105,106] Environmental isolates are often closely related to those colonizing patients.[105–107] Numerous inanimate surfaces, such as keyboards, tourniquets, or patient files, can become contaminated with MRSA.[107] This contamination is partly caused by the ability of MRSA to survive on dry surfaces for up to several months.[108] MRSA can be transferred from these surfaces, particularly hand-touch sites, to the hands or gloves of HCWs and then ultimately to patients if hand hygiene is inadequate.[109]

Some observational studies suggest that environmental contamination plays a role in MRSA transmission. In one study, subjects admitted to rooms previously occupied by patients who were colonized had an increased risk of acquiring MRSA.[110] However, environmental contamination was thought to be a minor contributor to overall transmission in this study. MRSA is sensitive to commonly used hospital disinfectants, thus enhanced environmental cleaning has been suggested to reduce environmental contamination and ultimately MRSA acquisition.[107] Cleaning intervention studies are hampered by lack of consensus on how to assess the efficacy of cleaning. Some small-scale studies show that enhanced cleaning can reduce environmental contamination with MRSA.[111,112] However, strong evidence that correlates environmental MRSA contamination and infection rates is lacking.[113]

SUMMARY

Progress in medical therapies has been significant over the last few decades but brings with it difficult challenges, including an increased risk of acquisition and infection with multiresistant pathogens, in particular MRSA. The control of MRSA is paramount in the health care setting and an important public health issue that has become a subject of increasing public and political interest. Successful strategies for MRSA control require a multifaceted approach as well as leadership and administrative support to facilitate implementation of evidence-based interventions. There must also be flexibility to adapt and institute these measures in the context of local epidemiology and available resources.

REFERENCES

1. Styers D, Sheehan DJ, Hogan P, et al. Laboratory-based surveillance of current antimicrobial resistance patterns and trends among Staphylococcus aureus: 2005 status in the United States. Ann Clin Microbiol Antimicrob 2006;5:2.
2. EARSS data. Available at: http://www.ecdc.europa.eu/en/activities/surveillance/EARS-Net/Pages/index.aspx. Accessed December 10, 2010.

3. Cosgrove SE, Qi Y, Kaye KS, et al. The impact of methicillin resistance in Staphylococcus aureus bacteremia on patient outcomes: mortality, length of stay, and hospital charges. Infect Control Hosp Epidemiol 2005;26(2):166–74.

4. Marshall C, Wesselingh S, McDonald M, et al. Control of endemic MRSA-what is the evidence? A personal view. J Hosp Infect 2004;56(4):253–68.

5. Dutch Working Party on Infection Prevention (WIP). Policy for methicillin-resistant Staphylococcus aureus. 2007. Available at: http://www.wip.nl/UK. Accessed November 3, 2010.

6. MacKenzie FM, Bruce J, Struelens MJ, et al. Antimicrobial drug use and infection control practices associated with the prevalence of methicillin-resistant Staphylococcus aureus in European hospitals. Clin Microbiol Infect 2007; 13(3):269–76.

7. Moran GJ, Krishnadasan A, Gorwitz RJ, et al. Methicillin-resistant S. aureus infections among patients in the emergency department. N Engl J Med 2006; 355(7):666–74.

8. Vourli S, Vagiakou H, Ganteris G, et al. High rates of community-acquired, Panton-Valentine leukocidin (PVL)- positive methicillin-resistant S. aureus (MRSA) infections in adult outpatients in Greece. Euro Surveill 2009;14(2):19089 pii.

9. van Belkum A, Melles DC, Nouwen J, et al. Co-evolutionary aspects of human colonisation and infection by Staphylococcus aureus. Infect Genet Evol 2009; 9(1):32–47.

10. Hidron AI, Low CE, Honig EG, et al. Emergence of community-acquired meticillin-resistant Staphylococcus aureus strain USA300 as a cause of necrotising community-onset pneumonia. Lancet Infect Dis 2009;9(6):384–92.

11. Seybold U, Kourbatova EV, Johnson JG, et al. Emergence of community-associated methicillin-resistant Staphylococcus aureus USA 300 genotype as a major cause of health care-associated blood stream infections. Clin Infect Dis 2006; 42(5):647–56.

12. Patel M, Waites KB, Hoesley CJ, et al. Emergence of USA300 MRSA in a tertiary medical centre: implications for epidemiological studies. J Hosp Infect 2008; 68(3):208–13.

13. Popovich KJ, Weinstein RA, Hota B. Are community-associated methicillin-resistant Staphylococcus aureus (MRSA) strains replacing traditional nosocomial MRSA strains? Clin Infect Dis 2008;46(6):787–94.

14. D'Agata EM, Webb GF, Horn MA, et al. Modeling the invasion of community-acquired methicillin-resistant Staphylococcus aureus into hospitals. Clin Infect Dis 2009;48(3):274–84.

15. Chini V, Petinaki E, Meugnier H, et al. Emergence of a new clone carrying Panton-Valentine leukocidin genes and staphylococcal cassette chromosome mec type V among methicillin-resistant Staphylococcus aureus in Greece. Scand J Infect Dis 2008;40(5):368–72.

16. Voss A, Loeffen F, Bakker J, et al. Methicillin-resistant Staphylococcus aureus in pig farming. Emerg Infect Dis 2005;11(12):1965–6.

17. Kock R, Harlizius J, Bressan N, et al. Prevalence and molecular characteristics of methicillin-resistant Staphylococcus aureus (MRSA) among pigs on German farms and import of livestock-related MRSA into hospitals. Eur J Clin Microbiol Infect Dis 2009;28(11):1375–82.

18. Shinefield HR, Ruff NL. Staphylococcal infections: a historical perspective. Infect Dis Clin North Am 2009;23(1):1–15.

19. Chambers HF, Deleo FR. Waves of resistance: Staphylococcus aureus in the antibiotic era. Nat Rev Microbiol 2009;7(9):629–41.

20. Hails J, Kwaku F, Wilson AP, et al. Large variation in MRSA policies, procedures and prevalence in English intensive care units: a questionnaire analysis. Intensive Care Med 2003;29(3):481–3.
21. Gastmeier P, Schwab F, Geffers C, et al. To isolate or not to isolate? Analysis of data from the German nosocomial infection surveillance system regarding the placement of patients with methicillin-resistant Staphylococcus aureus in private rooms in intensive care units. Infect Control Hosp Epidemiol 2004;25(2):109–13.
22. Sunenshine RH, Liedtke LA, Fridkin SK, et al. Management of inpatients colonized or infected with antimicrobial-resistant bacteria in hospitals in the United States. Infect Control Hosp Epidemiol 2005;26(2):138–43.
23. Jarvis WR, Schlosser J, Chinn RY, et al. National prevalence of methicillin-resistant Staphylococcus aureus in inpatients at US health care facilities, 2006. Am J Infect Control 2007;35(10):631–7.
24. Carlet J, Astagneau P, Brun-Buisson C, et al. French national program for prevention of healthcare-associated infections and antimicrobial resistance, 1992–2008: positive trends, but perseverance needed. Infect Control Hosp Epidemiol 2009;30(8):737–45.
25. Liebowitz LD. MRSA burden and interventions. Int J Antimicrob Agents 2009; 34(Suppl 3):S11–3.
26. Available at: http://www.npsa.nhs.uk/cleanyourhands/. Accessed November 3, 2010.
27. National Health Service. Clean, safe care: reducing MRSA and other healthcare associated infections. Available at: http://www.clean-safe-care.nhs.uk. Accessed November 3, 2010.
28. Stone S, Fuller C, Slade R, et al. The success and effectiveness of the world's first national clean your hands campaign in England and Wales 2004–2008: a prospective observational interrupted time-series [abstract O140]. Paper presented at the 19th European Congress of Clinical Microbiology and Infectious Diseases. Helsinki (Finland), May 16, 2009.
29. Kallen AJ, Mu Y, Bulens S, Reingold A, et al. Health care-associated invasive MRSA infections, 2005–2008. JAMA 2010;304(6):641–8.
30. Burton DC, Edwards JR, Horan TC, et al. Methicillin-resistant Staphylococcus aureus central line-associated bloodstream infections in US intensive care units, 1997–2007. JAMA 2009;301(7):727–36.
31. Climo MW. Decreasing MRSA infections: an end met by unclear means. JAMA 2009;301(7):772–3.
32. Humphreys H. Implementing guidelines for the control and prevention of methicillin-resistant Staphylococcus aureus and vancomycin-resistant enterococci: how valid are international comparisons of success? J Hosp Infect 2006; 62(2):133–5.
33. Pittet D, Hugonnet S, Harbarth S, et al. Effectiveness of a hospital-wide programme to improve compliance with hand hygiene. Infection Control Programme. Lancet 2000;356(9238):1307–12.
34. Johnson PD, Martin R, Burrell LJ, et al. Efficacy of an alcohol/chlorhexidine hand hygiene program in a hospital with high rates of nosocomial methicillin-resistant Staphylococcus aureus (MRSA) infection. Med J Aust 2005; 183(10):509–14.
35. Grayson ML, Jarvie LJ, Martin R, et al. Significant reductions in methicillin-resistant Staphylococcus aureus bacteraemia and clinical isolates associated with a multisite, hand hygiene culture-change program and subsequent successful statewide roll-out. Med J Aust 2008;188(11):633–40.

36. World Health Organization (WHO). WHO guidelines on hand hygiene in health care. World alliance for patient safety. Geneva (Switzerland): WHO Press Geneva; 2009.
37. Beggs CB, Shepherd SJ, Kerr KG. How does healthcare worker hand hygiene behaviour impact upon the transmission of MRSA between patients? an analysis using a Monte Carlo model. BMC Infect Dis 2009;9:64.
38. Robicsek A, Beaumont JL, Paule SM, et al. Universal surveillance for methicillin-resistant Staphylococcus aureus in 3 affiliated hospitals. Ann Intern Med 2008; 148(6):409–18.
39. Davis KA, Stewart JJ, Crouch HK, et al. Methicillin-resistant Staphylococcus aureus (MRSA) nares colonization at hospital admission and its effect on subsequent MRSA infection. Clin Infect Dis 2004;39(6):776–82.
40. Albrich WC, Harbarth S. Health-care workers: source, vector, or victim of MRSA? Lancet Infect Dis 2008;8(5):289–301.
41. Harbarth S, Masuet-Aumatell C, Schrenzel J, et al. Evaluation of rapid screening and pre-emptive contact isolation for detecting and controlling methicillin-resistant Staphylococcus aureus in critical care: an interventional cohort study. Crit Care 2006;10(1):R25.
42. Jernigan JA, Titus MG, Groschel DH, et al. Effectiveness of contact isolation during a hospital outbreak of methicillin-resistant Staphylococcus aureus. Am J Epidemiol 1996;143(5):496–504.
43. Huang SS, Yokoe DS, Hinrichsen VL, et al. Impact of routine intensive care unit surveillance cultures and resultant barrier precautions on hospital-wide methicillin-resistant Staphylococcus aureus bacteremia. Clin Infect Dis 2006; 43(8):971–8.
44. Chaberny IF, Schwab F, Ziesing S, et al. Impact of routine surgical ward and intensive care unit admission surveillance cultures on hospital-wide nosocomial methicillin-resistant Staphylococcus aureus infections in a university hospital: an interrupted time-series analysis. J Antimicrob Chemother 2008;62(6):1422–9.
45. Harbarth S, Fankhauser C, Schrenzel J, et al. Universal screening for methicillin-resistant Staphylococcus aureus at hospital admission and nosocomial infection in surgical patients. JAMA 2008;299(10):1149–57.
46. Jeyaratnam D, Whitty CJ, Phillips K, et al. Impact of rapid screening tests on acquisition of meticillin resistant Staphylococcus aureus: cluster randomised crossover trial. BMJ 2008;336(7650):927–30.
47. Hardy K, Price C, Szczepura A, et al. Reduction in the rate of methicillin-resistant Staphylococcus aureus acquisition in surgical wards by rapid screening for colonization: a prospective, cross-over study. Clin Microbiol Infect 2010;16(4):333–9.
48. McGinigle KL, Gourlay ML, Buchanan IB. The use of active surveillance cultures in adult intensive care units to reduce methicillin-resistant Staphylococcus aureus-related morbidity, mortality, and costs: a systematic review. Clin Infect Dis 2008;46(11):1717–25.
49. Tacconelli E, De Angelis G, de Waure C, et al. Rapid screening tests for methicillin-resistant Staphylococcus aureus at hospital admission: systematic review and meta-analysis. Lancet Infect Dis 2009;9(9):546–54.
50. Farr BM, Jarvis WR. Methicillin-resistant Staphylococcus aureus: misinterpretation and misrepresentation of active detection and isolation. Clin Infect Dis 2008; 47(9):1238–9 [author reply: 1239–40].
51. Wagenvoort JH, De Brauwer EI, Gronenschild JM, et al. Active surveillance cultures for methicillin-resistant Staphylococcus aureus in an intensive care unit. Clin Infect Dis 2008;47(9):1237–8.

52. Dancer SJ. Considering the introduction of universal MRSA screening. J Hosp Infect 2008;69(4):315–20.
53. Millar M. Should we screen low risk patients for methicillin resistant Staphylococcus aureus? BMJ 2009;339:b4035.
54. Edmond MB, Ober JF, Bearman G. Active surveillance cultures are not required to control MRSA infections in the critical care setting. Am J Infect Control 2008; 36(6):461–3.
55. Wenzel RP, Bearman G, Edmond MB. Screening for MRSA: a flawed hospital infection control intervention. Infect Control Hosp Epidemiol 2008;29(11):1012–8.
56. Farr BM, Jarvis WR. Why we disagree with the analysis of Wenzel et al. Infect Control Hosp Epidemiol 2009;30(5):497–9, author reply 499–500.
57. McCaughey B. Screening for methicillin-resistant Staphylococcus aureus. Infect Control Hosp Epidemiol 2009;30(9):927–8.
58. Muto CA, Jernigan JA, Ostrowsky BE, et al. SHEA guideline for preventing nosocomial transmission of multidrug-resistant strains of Staphylococcus aureus and enterococcus. Infect Control Hosp Epidemiol 2003;24(5):362–86.
59. Siegel JD, Rhinehart E, Jackson M, et al, Healthcare infection control practices advisory committee. Management of multidrug resistant organisms in healthcare settings. 2006. Available at: http://www.cdc.gov/ncidod/dhqp/pdf/ar/mdroGuideline2006.pdf. Accessed November 3, 2010.
60. Strausbaugh LJ, Siegel JD, Weinstein RA. Preventing transmission of multidrug-resistant bacteria in health care settings: a tale of 2 guidelines. Clin Infect Dis 2006;42(6):828–35.
61. Muto CA, Jarvis WR, Farr BM. Another tale of two guidelines. Clin Infect Dis 2006;43(6):796–7 [author reply: 797–8].
62. Diekema DJ, Edmond MB. Look before you leap: active surveillance for multidrug-resistant organisms. Clin Infect Dis 2007;44(8):1101–7.
63. Farr BM, Jarvis WR. Searching many guidelines for how best to control methicillin-resistant Staphylococcus aureus healthcare-associated spread and infection. Infect Control Hosp Epidemiol 2009;30(8):808–9.
64. Calfee DP, Salgado CD, Classen D, et al. Strategies to prevent transmission of methicillin-resistant Staphylococcus aureus in acute care hospitals. Infect Control Hosp Epidemiol 2008;29(Suppl 1):S62–80.
65. Weber SG, Huang SS, Oriola S, et al. Legislative mandates for use of active surveillance cultures to screen for methicillin-resistant Staphylococcus aureus and vancomycin-resistant enterococci: position statement from the Joint SHEA and APIC Task Force. Infect Control Hosp Epidemiol 2007;28(3):249–60.
66. Fraser V, Murphy D, Brennan PJ, et al. Politically incorrect: legislation must not mandate specific healthcare epidemiology and infection prevention and control practices. Infect Control Hosp Epidemiol 2007;28(5):594–5.
67. Farr BM. Political versus epidemiological correctness. Infect Control Hosp Epidemiol 2007;28(5):589–93.
68. Klein BS, Perloff WH, Maki DG. Reduction of nosocomial infection during pediatric intensive care by protective isolation. N Engl J Med 1989;320(26):1714–21.
69. Grant J, Ramman-Haddad L, Dendukuri N, et al. The role of gowns in preventing nosocomial transmission of methicillin-resistant Staphylococcus aureus (MRSA): gown use in MRSA control. Infect Control Hosp Epidemiol 2006;27(2):191–4.
70. Coia JE, Duckworth GJ, Edwards DI, et al. Guidelines for the control and prevention of meticillin-resistant Staphylococcus aureus (MRSA) in healthcare facilities. J Hosp Infect 2006;63(Suppl 1):S1–44.

71. Bracco D, Dubois MJ, Bouali R, et al. Single rooms may help to prevent noso-comial bloodstream infection and cross-transmission of methicillin-resistant Staphylococcus aureus in intensive care units. Intensive Care Med 2007; 33(5):836–40.
72. Cepeda JA, Whitehouse T, Cooper B, et al. Isolation of patients in single rooms or cohorts to reduce spread of MRSA in intensive-care units: prospective two-centre study. Lancet 2005;365(9456):295–304.
73. Morgan DJ, Diekema DJ, Sepkowitz K, et al. Adverse outcomes associated with Contact Precautions: a review of the literature. Am J Infect Control 2009;37(2): 85–93.
74. Kirkland KB. Taking off the gloves: toward a less dogmatic approach to the use of contact isolation. Clin Infect Dis 2009;48(6):766–71.
75. Santos RP, Mayo TW, Siegel JD. Healthcare epidemiology: active surveillance cultures and contact precautions for control of multidrug-resistant organisms: ethical considerations. Clin Infect Dis 2008;47(1):110–6.
76. Kluytmans J, Struelens M. Methicillin resistant Staphylococcus aureus in the hospital. BMJ 2009;338:b364.
77. Ammerlaan HS, Kluytmans JA, Wertheim HF, et al. Eradication of methicillin-resistant Staphylococcus aureus carriage: a systematic review. Clin Infect Dis 2009;48(7):922–30.
78. Simor AE, Daneman N. Staphylococcus aureus decolonization as a prevention strategy. Infect Dis Clin North Am 2009;23(1):133–51.
79. Loveday HP, Pellowe CM, Jones SR, et al. A systematic review of the evidence for interventions for the prevention and control of meticillin-resistant Staphylo-coccus aureus (1996–2004): report to the joint MRSA working party (Subgroup A). J Hosp Infect 2006;63(Suppl 1):S45–70.
80. Loeb M, Main C, Walker-Dilks C, et al. Antimicrobial drugs for treating methi-cillin-resistant *Staphylococcus aureus* colonization. Cochrane Database Syst Rev 2003;4:CD003340.
81. Sandri AM, Dalarosa MG, Ruschel de Alcantara L, et al. Reduction in incidence of nosocomial methicillin-resistant Staphylococcus aureus (MRSA) infection in an intensive care unit: role of treatment with mupirocin ointment and chlorhexi-dine baths for nasal carriers of MRSA. Infect Control Hosp Epidemiol 2006; 27(2):185–7.
82. Ridenour G, Lampen R, Federspiel J, et al. Selective use of intranasal mupirocin and chlorhexidine bathing and the incidence of methicillin-resistant Staphylo-coccus aureus colonization and infection among intensive care unit patients. Infect Control Hosp Epidemiol 2007;28(10):1155–61.
83. van Rijen M, Bonten M, Wenzel R, et al. Mupirocin ointment for preventing Staphylococcus aureus infections in nasal carriers. Cochrane Database Syst Rev 2008;4:CD006216.
84. Robicsek A, Beaumont JL, Thomson RB Jr, et al. Topical therapy for methicillin-resistant Staphylococcus aureus colonization: impact on infection risk. Infect Control Hosp Epidemiol 2009;30(7):623–32.
85. Kluytmans J, Harbarth S. Methicillin-resistant Staphylococcus aureus decoloni-zation: "yes, we can," but will it help? Infect Control Hosp Epidemiol 2009;30(7): 633–5.
86. Upton A, Lang S, Heffernan H. Mupirocin and Staphylococcus aureus: a recent paradigm of emerging antibiotic resistance. J Antimicrob Chemother 2003; 51(3):613–7.

87. Walker ES, Levy F, Shorman M, et al. A decline in mupirocin resistance in methicillin-resistant Staphylococcus aureus accompanied administrative control of prescriptions. J Clin Microbiol 2004;42(6):2792–5.

88. Patel JB, Gorwitz RJ, Jernigan JA. Mupirocin resistance. Clin Infect Dis 2009; 49(6):935–41.

89. Simor AE, Phillips E, McGeer A, et al. Randomized controlled trial of chlorhexidine gluconate for washing, intranasal mupirocin, and rifampin and doxycycline versus no treatment for the eradication of methicillin-resistant Staphylococcus aureus colonization. Clin Infect Dis 2007;44(2):178–85.

90. Mody L, Kauffman CA, McNeil SA, et al. Mupirocin-based decolonization of Staphylococcus aureus carriers in residents of 2 long-term care facilities: a randomized, double-blind, placebo-controlled trial. Clin Infect Dis 2003; 37(11):1467–74.

91. Milstone AM, Passaretti CL, Perl TM. Chlorhexidine: expanding the armamentarium for infection control and prevention. Clin Infect Dis 2008;46(2):274–81.

92. Popovich KJ, Hota B, Hayes R, et al. Effectiveness of routine patient cleansing with chlorhexidine gluconate for infection prevention in the medical intensive care unit. Infect Control Hosp Epidemiol 2009;30(10):959–63.

93. Climo MW, Sepkowitz KA, Zuccotti G, et al. The effect of daily bathing with chlorhexidine on the acquisition of methicillin-resistant Staphylococcus aureus, vancomycin-resistant Enterococcus, and healthcare-associated bloodstream infections: results of a quasi-experimental multicenter trial. Crit Care Med 2009;37(6):1858–65.

94. Batra R, Cooper BS, Whiteley C, et al. Efficacy and limitation of a chlorhexidine-based decolonization strategy in preventing transmission of methicillin-resistant Staphylococcus aureus in an intensive care unit. Clin Infect Dis 2010;50(2): 210–7.

95. Dancer SJ. The effect of antibiotics on methicillin-resistant Staphylococcus aureus. J Antimicrob Chemother 2008;61(2):246–53.

96. Denis O, Jans B, Deplano A, et al. Epidemiology of methicillin-resistant Staphylococcus aureus (MRSA) among residents of nursing homes in Belgium. J Antimicrob Chemother 2009;64(6):1299–306.

97. Tacconelli E, De Angelis G, Cataldo MA, et al. Does antibiotic exposure increase the risk of methicillin-resistant Staphylococcus aureus (MRSA) isolation? A systematic review and meta-analysis. J Antimicrob Chemother 2008;61(1): 26–38.

98. Vernaz N, Sax H, Pittet D, et al. Temporal effects of antibiotic use and hand rub consumption on the incidence of MRSA and Clostridium difficile. J Antimicrob Chemother 2008;62(3):601–7.

99. Kaier K, Hagist C, Frank U, et al. Two time-series analyses of the impact of antibiotic consumption and alcohol-based hand disinfection on the incidences of nosocomial methicillin-resistant Staphylococcus aureus infection and Clostridium difficile infection. Infect Control Hosp Epidemiol 2009;30(4):346–53.

100. Harbarth S, Samore MH. Interventions to control MRSA: high time for time-series analysis? J Antimicrob Chemother 2008;62(3):431–3.

101. Gould IM. Comment on: Interventions to control MRSA: high time for time-series analysis? J Antimicrob Chemother 2009;63(1):224.

102. Charbonneau P, Parienti JJ, Thibon P, et al. Fluoroquinolone use and methicillin-resistant Staphylococcus aureus isolation rates in hospitalized patients: a quasi experimental study. Clin Infect Dis 2006;42(6):778–84.

103. Tacconelli E. Antimicrobial use: risk driver of multidrug resistant microorganisms in healthcare settings. Curr Opin Infect Dis 2009;22(4):352–8.
104. Dellit TH, Owens RC, McGowan JE Jr, et al. Infectious Diseases Society of America and the Society for Healthcare Epidemiology of America guidelines for developing an institutional program to enhance antimicrobial stewardship. Clin Infect Dis 2007;44(2):159–77.
105. Sexton T, Clarke P, O'Neill E, et al. Environmental reservoirs of methicillin-resistant Staphylococcus aureus in isolation rooms: correlation with patient isolates and implications for hospital hygiene. J Hosp Infect 2006;62(2):187–94.
106. Chang S, Sethi AK, Eckstein BC, et al. Skin and environmental contamination with methicillin-resistant Staphylococcus aureus among carriers identified clinically versus through active surveillance. Clin Infect Dis 2009;48(10):1423–8.
107. Dancer SJ. Importance of the environment in methicillin-resistant Staphylococcus aureus acquisition: the case for hospital cleaning. Lancet Infect Dis 2008;8(2):101–13.
108. Kramer A, Schwebke I, Kampf G. How long do nosocomial pathogens persist on inanimate surfaces? A systematic review. BMC Infect Dis 2006;6:130.
109. Bhalla A, Pultz NJ, Gries DM, et al. Acquisition of nosocomial pathogens on hands after contact with environmental surfaces near hospitalized patients. Infect Control Hosp Epidemiol 2004;25(2):164–7.
110. Huang SS, Datta R, Platt R. Risk of acquiring antibiotic-resistant bacteria from prior room occupants. Arch Intern Med 2006;166(18):1945–51.
111. Goodman ER, Platt R, Bass R, et al. Impact of an environmental cleaning intervention on the presence of methicillin-resistant Staphylococcus aureus and vancomycin-resistant enterococci on surfaces in intensive care unit rooms. Infect Control Hosp Epidemiol 2008;29(7):593–9.
112. Dancer SJ, White LF, Lamb J, et al. Measuring the effect of enhanced cleaning in a UK hospital: a prospective cross-over study. BMC Med 2009;7:28.
113. Humphreys H. Can we do better in controlling and preventing methicillin-resistant Staphylococcus aureus (MRSA) in the intensive care unit (ICU)? Eur J Clin Microbiol Infect Dis 2008;27(6):409–13.
114. Keshtgar MR, Khalili A, Coen PG, et al. Impact of rapid molecular screening for meticillin-resistant Staphylococcus aureus in surgical wards. Br J Surg 2008;95(3):381–6.
115. Aldeyab MA, Kearney MP, Hughes CM, et al. Can the use of a rapid polymerase chain screening method decrease the incidence of nosocomial methicillin-resistant Staphylococcus aureus? J Hosp Infect 2009;71(1):22–8.

Common Approaches to the Control of Multidrug-resistant Organisms Other Than Methicillin-resistant *Staphylococcus aureus* (MRSA)

Courtney Hebert, MD, Stephen G. Weber, MD, MS*

KEYWORDS

- Multidrug-resistant organisms
- Vancomycin-resistant enterococcus
- Multidrug-resistant gram-negative infection
- *Clostridium difficile*

Curbing the spread of antibiotic resistance is one of the greatest challenges in health care today. Infections caused by multidrug-resistant organisms (MDRO) such as methicillin-resistant *Staphylococcus aureus* (MRSA), *Clostridium difficile*, and vanco-mycin-resistant enterococci (VRE) are estimated to result in 12,000 deaths and 3.5 billion dollars in excess health care costs in the United States each year.[1] Multi-drug-resistant bacterial infections are a growing problem. Surveillance studies of infections in intensive care units (ICU) demonstrate a 47% increase in *Klebsiella* species resistant to third-generation cephalosporin and a 12% increase in VRE from 1999 to 2003.[2] However, drug resistance in human pathogens is by no means new; penicillin-resistant *S aureus* was first isolated only 4 years after the drug became widely available. In the last half century as new antibiotics have been developed, bacteria continue to express new resistance mechanisms to escape them. With this in mind, it is clear that new drug development alone is no panacea. Effective and sustainable strategies to prevent the spread of these potentially lethal pathogens are urgently needed, especially in hospitals and other health care facilities. Although

Section of Infectious Diseases and Global Health, University of Chicago, 5841 South Maryland Avenue, MC 5065, Chicago, IL 60637, USA
* Corresponding author.
E-mail address: sgweber@medicine.bsd.uchicago.edu

Infect Dis Clin N Am 25 (2011) 181–200
doi:10.1016/j.idc.2010.11.006
0891-5520/11/$ – see front matter © 2011 Elsevier Inc. All rights reserved.

a great deal of the literature has focused largely on just 1 pathogen, MRSA, there are several other clinically and epidemiologically significant pathogens for which practical and systematic infection control strategies have been examined.

Resistant strains of Enterococcus are a relatively recent discovery, but these strains are now widespread and are associated with significant morbidity and mortality.[3] VRE accounts for 28.5% of ICU isolates of Enterococcus in the United States.[2] VRE infection has been associated with increased mortality compared with infection with vancomycin-susceptible strains.[4] Some VRE strains have demonstrated resistance to even the newest antimicrobial options, including linezolid, thus complicating management.[5]

Gram-negative bacterial resistance is a growing problem in American hospitals.[6] Although gram-negative resistance is not new, there has been increased concern recently for multidrug-resistant gram-negative (MDRGN) isolates, specifically those harboring genes for extended spectrum β-lactamases (ESBLs), inducible β-lactamases (AmpC), and carbapenemases. Some of the broadest spectrum antibiotics are rendered ineffective by these resistance mechanisms and unfortunately, few antibiotics to treat gram-negative infections are in development.[7] The results of studies that examine the consequences of MDRGN infections are somewhat conflicting; however in general these infections seem to be associated with increased length of stay, hospital cost, and mortality.[8,9]

C difficile is also an important health care–associated pathogen. Although not usually considered to be an MDRO, it has been suggested that the proliferation of this organism may be partly a result of the development of resistance to multiple classes of antibiotics.[10] C difficile infection was first reported in the 1970s, and was initially believed to be associated with clindamycin use, however it is now well known that most antibiotics can precipitate C difficile disease.[11] C difficile is currently the leading cause of infectious diarrhea in hospitalized patients[12] and the incidence is increasing.[13] The mortality associated with C difficile infection has also been increasing.[14] More recently, an epidemic strain of C difficile has emerged that has increased virulence, adding to the difficulty of controlling this serious infection.[15]

This article focuses on relevant infection control measures for VRE, MDRGN, and C difficile. The rationale and available evidence for common control strategies specifically targeting these pathogens are reviewed and opportunities for new research and more effective deployment of existing tools are highlighted. When there is less extensive evidence available from the published literature, the experience with MRSA is discussed as it might apply to these other pathogens. (MRSA control is discussed separately elsewhere in this issue).

RATIONALE FOR COMMONLY USED MDRO CONTROL STRATEGIES

To best appreciate the general approach to MDRO control, it is useful to first review the epidemiologic and biologic underpinnings that inform the strategies that have been developed in the past half century. MDRO prevention measures generally fall into 2 categories: control of transmission and antimicrobial stewardship. Transmission control is focused on preventing the spread of clinically significant pathogens, principally via the contaminated hands of health care workers (HCWs) and the environment (particularly contaminated surfaces and equipment). In 1938 a landmark paper categorized the microflora of human skin into transient and resident flora.[16] Resident flora are found mostly on nonexposed skin, and represent a fairly stable population of low virulence organisms. Resident flora are difficult to remove through hand washing and are generally not spread through routine contact with patients or the environment. In contrast, transient flora tend to be found on exposed skin and have been associated with health care–associated infections. These transient bacteria are generally picked up through contact with contaminated surfaces and are much more easily removed by hand hygiene. The hands of HCWs have been implicated in the spread of hospital-acquired infections, including those caused by MDRO, in several reports including point prevalence surveys, laboratory models, and particularly in epidemics and clusters.[17] Even in cases in which HCW are colonized with resistant pathogens (including those from whom MRSA can be isolated from nasal swabs), the hands represent the most common and potentially most effective means by which to transfer such pathogens to vulnerable patients.

Although hand hygiene is the cornerstone of transmission control, additional measures are necessary for many serious health care–associated pathogens. An increasing number of well-designed studies have demonstrated a potentially important role for the transmission of such pathogens on inanimate objects, including the clothing and personal equipment of HCWs. In these studies, pathogens have been recovered from physicians' white coats, pagers, and cell phones.[18–20] In addition, MDRO have been cultured from environmental surfaces such as sinks, bedrails, and ventilator water (**Table 1**).[21] Health care–associated pathogens have been found to persist for months on inanimate surfaces.[22] The consequence of contamination of inanimate surfaces was highlighted in a recent retrospective study by Huang and colleagues.[23] They showed that a patient admitted to a hospital room previously occupied by a patient with MRSA or VRE were themselves at increased risk for MRSA or VRE infection. With this in mind, it is recommended that patients with MDRO be isolated and their health care providers use barrier protection with gowns and gloves. This is necessary to prevent the HCW from contaminating hands and clothing by coming in contact with an infected or colonized patient and to decrease the potential for the HCW to come in contact with contaminated surfaces in the patient's rooms.

Complimenting transmission prevention as a tool for MDRO control is antimicrobial stewardship. Fundamentally, it has been recognized that antibiotic use, and particularly misuse and abuse, is the primary precipitant to the emergence of antimicrobial resistance. Exposure to antibiotics has been shown in animal models to increase the risk of colonization with resistant bacteria including VRE and ESBL-producing organisms.[24,25] Given that at least one-third of patients admitted to the hospital will be treated with a course of antibiotics, opportunities for inappropriate use abound.[26] One study documented antibiotic misuse in 37.4% of hospital prescriptions.[27] The effect of antimicrobial exposure does not just affect the individual taking the drug but also has been shown to increase the risk of MDRO colonization among close contacts.[28] By addressing these issues, stewardship programs that promote judicious antimicrobial use can have a major effect on MDRO control. Antimicrobial stewardship is discussed in detail elsewhere in this issue.

Table 1
Environmental sampling

Inanimate Objects from Which MDRO have been Recovered			
MRSA	VRE	MDRGN	*C difficile*
Pagers[18]	Stethoscopes[58]	Bedrails, sinks, ventilator water[21]	Bed frames[108]
White coats[19]		Computer keyboards[109]	
Blood pressure cuffs[110]			

EVIDENCE OF EFFECTIVENESS FOR SPECIFIC MDRO CONTROL STRATEGIES
Hand Hygiene

Hand hygiene has been recognized as an essential element of infection control for more than a century. The potential benefit of hand hygiene was first documented by Semmelweis in his initial reports on childbed fever in 1846.[29] As is true for many of the strategies discussed in this article, some of the best evidence for the effectiveness of hand hygiene in MDRO control comes from the experience with MRSA. In 2000 Pittet and colleagues[30] instituted a multidisciplinary hospital-wide program to improve hand hygiene. They documented an improvement in hand hygiene adherence from 48% to 66%, but most impressively they demonstrated a 50% reduction in the incidence of MRSA transmission.

More recently, alcohol-based hand rubs (ABHR) have been promoted for hand hygiene. In some studies they have been found to be more effective than soap and water and have been definitively shown to increase HCW adherence to hand hygiene standards.[31,32] Although there is not an extensive body of literature on ABHR for control of all MDRO, it is reasonable to believe that they would be as effective for these organisms as for other pathogens (with the exception of C difficile, discussed later). Consequently, ABHR promotion should have a role in any comprehensive infection control program. Hand hygiene is discussed in detail elsewhere in this issue.

VRE

VRE can easily pass onto HCW hands and then contaminate another environmental surface or the patient, sustaining the cycle of transmission.[33] In a recent study, VRE was found on 52% of those HCWs who touched only the environment and 70% of those who touched the environment and the patient.[34] In epidemiologic studies, VRE has been documented on the hands HCWs between 13% and 41% of the time[35] and can persist on the hands for at least 60 minutes.[36] VRE is successfully removed from hands with soap and water and with ABHRs.[36,37]

The specific effect of hand hygiene on VRE transmission has been examined in mathematical models and has been suggested to be an essential element of a comprehensive infection control program.[38] However, according to at least 1 model, the effect is dependent on compliance rates greater than 50% which, unfortunately, may be difficult to sustain in many centers. The effect of hand hygiene on VRE transmission was measured in a 2-hospital observational study completed in 2000.[39] Interventions at the study hospital focused on changing organizational culture to increase hand hygiene adherence. The other hospital served as a control. During the study period, hand hygiene adherence increased at the intervention hospital significantly. Simultaneously, the incidence of VRE infections decreased by 85% at the intervention hospital compared with a decrease of 44% at the control hospital.

MDRGN

Like VRE, gram-negative organisms can commonly be found on environmental surfaces as well as on the hands of HCWs. Gram-negative pathogens seem to survive longer on inanimate objects than on hands.[40] However, they have been shown to be carried persistently on the hands of 21% of HCWs.[41] Wearing artificial fingernails has also been shown to increase the risk of carriage of gram-negative organisms among HCWs.[42]

The specific role of hand hygiene in controlling the incidence of MDRGN infections has not been as extensively studied as for the other pathogens discussed here. An outbreak of multidrug-resistant Pseudomonas aeruginosa in Germany was controlled with the implementation of strict hand hygiene, together with enhanced deployment of isolation precautions.[43] In contrast, an improvement in hand hygiene adherence did not result in a decrease in MDRGN infection or colonization among neonatal ICU patients in a resource-poor setting with very high rates of MDRGN colonization.[44]

C difficile

Like VRE and MDRGN, *C difficile* has been recovered from the hands of HCWs and can transfer between HCW hands and patients.[45] *C difficile* can be distinguished from the other pathogens discussed in this article by its capacity to form spores. This has significant implications for transmission control strategies in general and for hand hygiene in particular. Antiseptic hand rubs and antimicrobial soaps are not effective against *C difficile* because they lack sporocidal activity.[46] Physical removal of spores by washing with soap and water has been shown to be the best way to clean hands after caring for a patient with *C difficile*.[47] Not surprisingly, studies have shown little effect on *C difficile* infection rates after the introduction of ABHRs even when they decrease the rate of other health care–associated pathogens.[48,49] However, it is equally important to note that the widespread use of ABHRs does not seem to increase the incidence of *C difficile* infection.[50] This could be because increased awareness of the importance of hand hygiene through promotion of ABHR might also enhance the likelihood of using soap and water.

An effective hand hygiene campaign against *C difficile* should include an intervention to educate HCWs on the importance of using soap and water when caring for those patients with *C difficile* infection. This was illustrated in a study by Abbett and colleagues[51] in which a central element of the intervention program was promotion of soap and water as primary hand hygiene after care of a patient with *C difficile*. Implementation of the program was accompanied by a significant decrease in the incidence of *C difficile* infection. Recent guidelines have recommended hand hygiene with soap and water for *C difficile* particularly in epidemic settings.[52]

Isolation Precautions and Personal Protective Equipment

Isolating people with serious infections from healthy individuals is one of the oldest forms of infection control. The Old Testament documents the practice of isolating those with leprosy from the general population and more recently, in the late nineteenth and early twentieth centuries, isolation of patients with tuberculosis was viewed as one of the few effective methods to curb spread.[53] Modern medicine has moved away from isolating patients from society and instead isolation precautions have been integrated into routine hospital care to prevent propagation of resistant or highly infectious pathogens. One key element of isolation precautions in the hospital is the use of personal protective equipment. It has been shown that HCWs who don gloves during patient encounters have a significantly decreased risk of hand contamination.[54] Jernigan and colleagues[55] showed that when patients were not placed in precautions (gowns and gloves), the transmission rate of MRSA to uncolonized patients was 0.14 transmissions per day. In contrast, when patients were cared for using isolation precautions the transmission rate was significantly lower (0.009 per day). Although these methods have been widely applied and endorsed by expert authorities, the overall evidence in support of isolation precautions remains somewhat lacking. A 2004 systematic review of the literature concluded that there was insufficient evidence supporting a benefit of isolation precautions in controlling MRSA, largely as a result of a lack of well-designed studies.[56] Isolation precautions and specifically the use of personal protective equipment for control of VRE, MDGRN, and *C difficile* are discussed in detail later.

VRE

Current guidelines recommend contact isolation for patients with VRE.[26,57] However, as was the case for MRSA, there are few large, well-executed, controlled trials of VRE and contact isolation. Nonetheless, there is a significant amount of circumstantial evidence in favor of wearing gowns and gloves to prevent VRE transmission. One study documents contamination of gloves, gowns, or stethoscopes after 67% of encounters with a patient with VRE[58] and gloves have been shown to reduce the risk of contamination of hands with VRE by 71%.[59] As has already been noted, VRE contamination of a patient's room can also be an important risk for transmission.[23]

Most specific evidence for the effectiveness of contact precautions to prevent VRE acquisition comes from intervention studies and particularly from the experience with outbreaks. However, nearly all successful intervention studies enforced contact precautions along with active surveillance and antibiotic restriction, which makes it difficult to determine the specific contribution of contact isolation to overall effectiveness.[60–63]

The relative contribution of gowns versus gloves in preventing the transmission of VRE has also been evaluated separately. Srinivasan and colleagues[64] examined the incidence of hospital-acquired VRE in an ICU. There was a significant increase in the acquisition of VRE when HCWs were encouraged to wear only gloves and not gowns. In the same year Puzniak and colleagues[65] also showed that acquisition of VRE in a medical ICU was higher during a no gown period. Overall the evidence suggests that the use of both gowns and gloves are important in the prevention and control of VRE.

MDRGN

There are a relatively few studies that specifically support the use of contact precautions in decreasing the incidence of MDRGN. French investigators demonstrated an increase in the incidence of infection with *Acinetobacter* spp during a period in which the use of contact isolation was discontinued.[66] After reinstituting the practice, the incidence of *Acinetobacter* infections returned to baseline. When infection control measures, including isolation and contact precautions, were instituted at a Canadian hospital, the incidence of health care–associated infections caused by ESBL-producing organisms remained stable despite an increase in ESBL-producing organisms in the surrounding region.[67] In contrast with these findings, a Belgian study showed that instituting contact precautions during an outbreak of infections with ESBL-producing *Klebsiella* spp had little effect.[68] The outbreak was only contained once additional measures were instituted, including room decontamination, restriction of broad-spectrum antibiotics, and creation of patient cohorts with dedicated nursing.

Despite the uncertainly of the relative effectiveness of contact precautions for controlling the spread of MDRGN, the continued application of these measures is likely justified by the lack of alternatives. As has already been noted, antibiotic treatment options are limited for MDRGN, and as new resistance mechanisms emerge these options will continue to dwindle. A conservative approach that attempts to limit the spread of these potentially lethal pathogens is appropriate, even while additional confirmation of effectiveness is sought.

C difficile

Current guidelines recommend that patients with diarrhea who are known or suspected to have *C difficile* infection should be placed under contact precautions.[69] Several studies support this approach. A before-after intervention study in 1998 showed that with institution of infection control measures including contact precautions, the incidence of C difficile dropped significantly, by 60%.[70] Unfortunately without a control group it is difficult to separate the effect of contact precautions from other concurrent interventions. In 1990 a prospective controlled trial evaluated the effect of universal glove use while caring for all patients on the incidence of C difficile. On wards where glove use was instituted, incidence fell significantly from 7.7 C difficile infection cases per 1000 discharges to 1.5 per 1000 but remained unchanged on the control wards.[71] More recently, Salgado and colleagues[72] described their experience with an outbreak of C difficile. By instituting several infection control strategies including isolation for patients with suspected C difficile and targeted hand hygiene with soap and water, they observed a decrease in incidence of C difficile infection of 45.3%.

Although randomized controlled trials regarding the specific benefit of contact isolation for C difficile are for the most part lacking, the available evidence still generally supports barrier precautions for reducing horizontal spread. However, it remains to be seen which measures are the most important at reducing transmission.

Limitations to isolation and contact precautions
Even when successful at preventing the spread of disease, the isolation of patients should not be viewed as an entirely benign procedure. Several studies have highlighted the potentially negative effects of patient isolation. Stelfox and colleagues[73] found that several quality of care measures for patients who are in isolation precautions are significantly worse than for those who are not. In addition, patients on precautions may be more likely to experience signs and symptoms of depression and anxiety.[74] These are serious consequences that must be weighed against the potential benefit of isolation precautions and carefully considered when formulating hospital-wide infection control policies.

Active Surveillance

Recently, considerable attention has been focused on the usefulness of active surveillance, in which patients are screened for carriage of MDRO, as an important adjunct to the transmission control strategies already introduced. What remains uncertain is the relative benefit of this approach for the range of MDRO commonly encountered in the hospital setting. Ultimately, the overall effectiveness of these basic measures is limited by the ability to detect all those patients who are colonized or infected with MDRO. One useful way to examine this limitation is by calculating the undetected ratio, which is the proportion of patients not identified by routine clinical cultures among all those who are colonized or infected.[75] The greater the proportion, the greater usefulness of active surveillance to detect colonized individuals who could be a reservoir for transmission. For MRSA, studies have found this proportion to be as low as 30% and as high as 90%.[75] Despite the wide range of these estimates, targeted surveillance for MRSA has been successful in helping to control this organism in many settings (**Table 2**). Routine surveillance in the ICU accompanied by the implementation of appropriate precautions has been shown to effectively reduce MRSA bacteremia by 75%.[76] Universal hospital surveillance of MRSA has also been shown to decrease overall incidence.[77] Although the effectiveness of surveillance has largely been confirmed for MRSA (and is discussed in detail elsewhere in this issue), this is not the case for all MDROs, as is summarized in the following sections.

VRE
VRE poses a unique challenge because of the very high undetected ratio associated with the organism.[78] Put another way, many more patients are colonized than clinical

Table 2 Evidence for efficacy of active surveillance		
	MDRO	Level of Surveillance
Ostrowsky et al[62]	VRE	Region
Bode et al[111]	MRSA	Patient
Robicsek et al[77]	MRSA	Single hospital
Calderwood et al[112]	VRE	Single hospital ward
Huang et al[76]	MRSA	Single intensive care unit

cultures would detect. Finding and isolating those colonized patients may be an important part of VRE control. Byers and colleagues[79] found that unprotected proximity to a patient with VRE was a significant risk factor for VRE acquisition but proximity to a patient colonized with VRE who was isolated was not.

Price and colleagues[80] compared the incidence of VRE at 2 hospitals, 1 that used active surveillance and 1 that did not, and showed that VRE bacteremia was significantly less common in the surveillance hospital. Ostrowsky and colleagues[62] documented an initiative to control VRE in a 3-state area through active surveillance and isolation. They were successful at decreasing incidence of VRE from 2.2% to less than 1% in only 2 years. Because of the strong evidence in support of active surveillance for VRE, organizations such as the Society for Healthcare Epidemiology of America (SHEA) recommend active surveillance for those at high risk for colonization.[26] The decision whether or not to deploy an active surveillance program for VRE should be primarily influenced by the overall burden of disease (in terms of incidence and clinical consequences) at a given institution.

MDRGN

Although most hospitals have not used active surveillance as a routine control strategy for MDRGNs, some studies have tested the feasibility of this approach. One obstacle to screening for MDRGNs is the heterogeneity of the various organisms involved in terms of microbiological characteristics and even the epidemiology of colonization and infection. Strategies such as the use of selective media for screening surveillance specimens have been used to try to isolate only relevant organisms.[81] Another approach is to use molecular testing. There are polymerase chain reaction (PCR) protocols for Klebsiella pneumoniae carbapenemase (KPC)- and ESBL-producing organisms but these are each specific for one type of MDRGN. Deciding which MDRGN to address and how to target it is a daunting first step in the surveillance of MDRGN. Specific MDRGNs can be targeted individually. For example, the Centers for Disease Control has suggested point prevalence surveillance if a single case of a KPC-producing organism is detected at a hospital.[82]

As with VRE, many studies of MDRGN surveillance have been performed to better understand the epidemiology so that appropriate infection control strategies can be implemented. Other studies have been specifically designed to determine if MDRGN surveillance can help clinicians choose appropriate empirical antibiotic therapy. Papadomichaelakis and colleagues[81] performed biweekly surveillance cultures of ICU patients and found that there was good concordance between MDRGN detected by active surveillance and the causal organisms in ventilator-associated pneumonia and blood stream infections. There was a significantly increased rate of appropriate empirical antibiotic therapy in those who underwent active surveillance screening.

Other studies of active surveillance for MDRGN have provided mixed results. Gardam and colleagues[83] instituted an active surveillance program for

Enterobacteriaceae only to find that almost all isolates were genotypically unique and it was unlikely that there was any horizontal spread. They concluded that the costs of such a program outweighed any potential benefit. Currently there are no specific recommendations to survey for MDRGN on a routine basis, only in the case of an outbreak.

C difficile

The epidemiology of colonization with C difficile remains an area of intense study and considerable uncertainty. At least 1 study has found that colonization may actually be associated with a decreased risk of symptomatic disease.[84] Nonetheless, carriers of C difficile can still serve as a reservoir for health care–associated spread of C difficile and prevalence of asymptomatic carriage can be as high as 20% of inpatients.[85] Given these conflicting findings, and the challenges of interpreting and acting on the results of such an active surveillance program, active surveillance has not been recommended for C difficile in any recent guidelines.

Limitations to active surveillance

Because the effectiveness of active surveillance for MDRO control depends on more stringent deployment of basic practices such as isolation precautions, even an effective program may be associated with the same issues regarding patient safety and satisfaction associated with isolation precautions that were discussed in the preceding section. However, there are also several potential downsides that are unique to active surveillance. Patients may believe that they are being unfairly labeled, especially if without routine active surveillance they would not have been put in isolation.[86] Other practical concerns exist. For example, implementation of precautions for a large number of patients may disrupt patient flow between units and facilities, and could conceivably strain the capacity of some institutions in terms of staffing, laboratory resources, and patient bed spaces.

Antimicrobial Stewardship

Considering the growing number and incidence of antimicrobial-resistant pathogens and the increasingly limited range of antibiotic agents available to treat them, one of the most crucial MDRO control strategies is the rational use of currently available antibiotics. The fundamental goal of antimicrobial stewardship is to promote the selection of antimicrobial therapy that will treat infection, at the same time avoiding toxicity as well as the risk of emerging resistance.[87] Considerable economic benefits have also been reported in many cases as a result of decreased drug acquisition and administration costs as well as the avoidance of expenses related to monitoring and adverse events. Two of the most basic approaches to antimicrobial stewardship, prospective auditing/feedback and preauthorization, are discussed here in the context of MDRO control. A more detailed discussion of the subject is provided elsewhere in this issue.

Antimicrobial stewardship has been used in the hospital setting for decades.[88] In a 1988 study of streamlining therapy, the investigators found that for 54% of cases for which narrower coverage was recommended, the change was adopted by providers more than 80% of the time. This led to total cost savings of about 40,000 dollars. As early as 1974, McGowan and Finland[89] described a system of restricting new and costly antibiotics. They showed that by requiring physicians to contact an infectious diseases consultant before prescribing restricted agents they were able to substantially decrease the use of these drugs. A more recent addition to these approaches uses computerized decision support. By moving the stewardship function to the computerized record, it becomes easier to reach the physician at the time the clinical decision is being made. These programs have been shown to decrease costs associated with antimicrobials and decrease excess antibiotic use.[90]

In the subsections that follow, the specific rationale and evidence for the usefulness of stewardship in curbing the spread of VRE, MDGNR, and *C difficile* are discussed.

VRE

Not surprisingly, exposure to vancomycin has been commonly linked to subsequent VRE acquisition. However, a meta-analysis of epidemiologic studies found that although there was a small effect of vancomycin on infection or colonization with VRE, the association was not statistically significant once adjusted for confounding factors.[91] It is not at all clear that limiting vancomycin use alone will decrease VRE incidence. A review of the literature in 2007 examined all randomized controlled trials or quasi-experimental studies that documented a decrease in vancomycin use.[92] The investigators concluded that it was impossible to determine the specific role of vancomycin usage in preventing VRE colonization or infection as a result of conflicting data. Vancomycin is not the only antibiotic that has been linked with VRE. In a study by Smith,[93] a decrease in VRE was observed after the institution of a hospital-wide initiative to decrease cephalosporin use. In another study, third-generation cephalosporin use was found to be significantly associated with risk of VRE acquisition.[94] However, in this same study, when the prevalence of VRE colonization was greater than 50%, the effect of cephalosporin use on time to VRE acquisition was negligible. Restricting the use of certain antimicrobials is certainly part of a comprehensive infection control strategy for control of VRE infection, however in hospitals where colonization rates for VRE run high, antibiotic stewardship may not be as effective in curbing the spread of VRE.

MDRGN

Several studies show the benefit of restricting antibiotic use to help decrease the incidence of MDRGNs. In 2000, a cross-over study performed in 2 neonatal ICUs showed that when empirical sepsis coverage with amoxicillin + cefotaxime was enforced, rates of resistant gram-negative colonization were significantly higher than when penicillin + tobramycin was used.[95] Another study looked at an outbreak of ceftazidime-resistant *Klebsiella* spp, which was believed to be associated with increased ceftazidime use.[96] By implementing ceftazidime restriction and other infection control measures the investigators documented a 60% reduction in resistant isolates.

The experience with antimicrobial stewardship in control of MDRGN has highlighted the difficulty in controlling resistance in the hospital setting. Although restricting 1 class of antibiotics can decrease the incidence of bacteria resistant to that class it often results in an increase in resistance to the alternative agent. A study by Rahal and colleagues[97] highlighted this difficulty. A program intended to decrease cephalosporin resistance in *Klebsiella* spp by restricting cephalosporins had the unintended consequence of increasing carbapenem resistance by indirectly encouraging the use of this class of antibiotic. Despite these challenges, antimicrobial stewardship can be important for MDRGN control. With dwindling therapeutic options, it is prudent to try to limit use of broad-spectrum antibiotics whenever possible to retain those antibiotics for use when others have failed.

C difficile

Because *C difficile* in the hospital is usually associated with antibiotic use, one of the most important strategies to decrease the incidence of *C difficile* is to limit unnecessary use of antibiotics. The most convincing evidence for stewardship in general is probably for the control of *C difficile*. Several reports highlight the potential importance of limiting unnecessary antibiotic use, even without regard to the restriction of specific classes. In a report of a severe outbreak of C difficile Polgreen and colleagues[98] found that of the patients with C difficile who had been given antibiotics for pneumonia, 50% did not have evidence of lung infection. In this case, excessive antibiotic use may have contributed to avoidable infection and death.

Although an overall decrease in antibiotic exposure might be of greatest benefit, limiting the use of specific classes of antibiotics, such as third-generation cephalosporins, has also been shown to decrease C difficile incidence. In 2002, Khan and Cheesbrough[99] tracked the incidence of C difficile infection when empirical pneumonia treatment was changed from ceftriaxone to levofloxacin. They demonstrated a decrease in the proportion of positive C difficile tests from 14.5% to 8.6%. McNulty and colleagues[100] reported on an outbreak of C difficile that could not be controlled with transmission control measures. However, when broad-spectrum cephalosporin use was limited and narrower spectrum antibiotics were used, the incidence of C difficile decreased significantly. A more recent study by Valiquette and colleagues[101] instituted a nonrestrictive antimicrobial stewardship program to control an outbreak of the hypervirulent strain of C difficile, NAP1/027. Their policy included recommendations to decrease the use of second- and third-generation cephalosporins, ciprofloxacin, clindamycin, and macrolides. They found that there was a reduction in the use of targeted antibiotics and, in addition, C difficile incidence decreased by 60%. More specific associations between exposure to particular antimicrobial agents and epidemic C difficile infection continue to be explored. For example, the NAP1 strain is more likely to demonstrate resistance to certain fluoroquinolones than non-NAP1 strains.[15] A recent study described an intervention to decrease fluoroquinolone use in an outbreak involving the NAP1 strain.[102] By decreasing fluoroquinolone use by 66% the investigators demonstrated a 22% decrease in the percentage of NAP1 C difficile isolates. In addition, there was a nonsignificant decrease in the incidence of all C difficile strains after this intervention was undertaken.

Limitations to antimicrobial stewardship

Antimicrobial stewardship programs are effective in curbing costs, medical errors, and unnecessary antibiotic use,[88,103] but there have been relatively fewer studies that have convincingly demonstrated a meaningful and sustained decrease in the overall burden of antimicrobial resistance at hospitals that have deployed such programs. In part this limitation is a result of the difficulty in separating out the benefit of antimicrobial stewardship from other interventions initiated concurrently, especially in the setting of an outbreak. In addition, it is possible that limiting antibiotic use in a hospital without simultaneously addressing community antibiotic misuse may fail to have an overall effect on the resistance of isolates in the hospital.[104] It can also be difficult to predict which antibiotics should be restricted to decrease the incidence of a particular targeted organism. For example, prior fluoroquinolone exposure has been found to be a significant risk factor for MRSA acquisition,[105] an association that may not be intuitively clear to many providers. Similarly, as has been noted, cephalosporin use may be more closely associated with the emergence of VRE than even exposure to vancomycin itself. These unexpected relationships may come about through as yet unappreciated molecular phenomena or a more complex interaction between drug, host, and pathogen. However, whatever the cause, the development of rational stewardship recommendations to predictably influence the epidemiology of antimicrobial resistance remains elusive.

CHALLENGES AND OPPORTUNITIES

The measures described in the previous sections offer considerable promise to clinicians and other stakeholders committed to the control of pathogens such as VRE,

MDRGN, and *C difficile* in the hospital setting. However, it is important to acknowledge several limitations to the interpretation of the evidence that has been presented in support of the effectiveness of the various prevention strategies (**Table 3**). These limitations undoubtedly present a challenge to those responsible for formulating and deploying a rational and cost-effective MDRO control program in both small and large facilities. Simultaneously, recognition of these limitations allows for a more focused and rigorous approach to future investigations to ensure that the beneficial effects of these strategies are maximized across the spectrum of care.

One serious limitation to the available evidence for various MDRO control strategies relates to the design and execution of the studies in which these measures have been tested. One principle issue is that many reports describing the effect of control measures were conducted in the setting of outbreaks and clusters. Fundamentally, the epidemiology (and in some cases the biology and pathogenicity) of a microbe is altered in the setting of an epidemic. As such, it is difficult to know for certain the extent to which the findings of interventions tested in this context can be applied to the control of endemic disease in other settings. MDRO control measures are often deployed (particularly in the setting of an outbreak) in a multimodal fashion in which several separate interventions are implemented simultaneously. Because of this, it is impossible for those reporting the experience to quantify the relative contribution of any 1 specific measure to a successful outcome. Partially as a result of this phenomenon, control measures have frequently been promoted as bundles leaving clinicians to guess as to which elements of the intervention are truly effective and which are no more than a waste of resources. In general, the design and analysis of the intervention studies on which the entire discipline of MDRO control is based remains somewhat lacking. Many investigators continue to rely on relatively unsophisticated study designs (most typically, before-and-after studies) that limit the interpretability and generalizability of findings. Moreover, more sophisticated statistical methods have not yet come into widespread use by many in the infection control field, further hindering definitive analysis and conclusions.

There are more practical and everyday limitations to the available evidence as well. One of the most common (and uncomfortable) challenges to the application of the control strategies described here relates to the continued failure of HCWs to adhere to even basic measures to prevent the spread of infection. This shortcoming has largely been accepted and even acknowledged in the scientific examination of these

Table 3
Limitations to infection control strategies

MDRO Control Method	Limitations
Hand hygiene	Poor adherence by providers
Isolation precautions	Poor adherence by providers Psychological stress for patients Diminished quality of care and safety Diminished patient satisfaction
Active surveillance	Psychological stress for patients caused by isolation precautions Disruption in patient and laboratory flow Lack of standardized methods and analysis
Antimicrobial stewardship	Poor adherence to policies and standards by prescribers Unintended increase in the incidence of antimicrobial resistance among nontarget MDRO

strategies. For example, many reports of the effectiveness of hand hygiene in preventing the spread of antimicrobial resistance describe adherence rates of less than 70% after the deployment of an intervention. The lack of adherence to basic measures is compounded when more intensive and sophisticated methods are studied or deployed. For example, although active surveillance programs in part rely on the timely availability of the results of microbiological sampling (often through the use of PCR or other rapid testing methods), the entire effectiveness of this approach absolutely depends on the adherence of providers to more basic practices such as hand hygiene and the use of personal protective equipment. Shortcomings in adherence to these standards will ultimately limit the overall effectiveness of even the most sophisticated control strategy.

Fortunately, these limitations are not unavoidable and there is already ample and growing evidence that the study and practice of MDRO control is moving to a higher level of sophistication. Several investigators and methodologists have championed the use of more rigorous study design and statistical analysis,[106] including the use of more sophisticated measures to determine the cost-effectiveness of MDRO control interventions.[107] Similarly, collaborative studies are pooling the resources and expertise across centers to allow for more rigorous investigation of the epidemiology (and prevention) of endemic disease. It is likely that competition for enhanced federal and private support for investigation into the control of MDRO will promote even greater improvements.

Unfortunately, improvement in adherence to control practices will not come about simply through the use of more sophisticated statistical techniques and multicenter collaborations. However, the opportunity exists to apply the same level and intensity of sophisticated, rigorous, and well-designed investigations to a greater understanding of the barriers that limit the adherence of bedside providers to these critical measures. Reliable research into the diffusion, dissemination, and adoption of best practices will rely on collaboration from many other disciplines than microbiology and clinical infectious diseases including behavioral science, economics, and psychology. Only when the gap between actual and ideal adherence is closed will we be able to truly measure the effectiveness of the tools at our disposal.

SUMMARY

Antibiotic resistance will continue to be a problem as long as selective antibiotic pressure gives a competitive advantage to resistant strains and contaminated hands pass these strains along to new and vulnerable hosts. Comprehensive infection control strategies are vital. Despite a relative dearth of prospective randomized studies of transmission prevention measures and antimicrobial stewardship for the control of VRE, MDRGN, and *C difficile*, there is a growing amount of evidence supporting specific interventions. It is imperative that the rigorous examination of the performance and consequences of these strategies continue to determine which are the most influential. Given the limits of the available evidence, clinicians and other leaders must continue to balance the benefit of these potentially life-saving strategies against any unintended consequences and the expenses that are associated with their implementation.

REFERENCES

1. Zell BL, Goldmann DA. Healthcare-associated infection and antimicrobial resistance: moving beyond description to prevention. Infect Control Hosp Epidemiol 2007;28(3):261–4.

2. National Nosocomial Infections Surveillance System. National Nosocomial Infections Surveillance (NNIS) system report, data summary from January 1992 through June 2004, issued October 2004. Am J Infect Control 2004;32(8): 470–85.

3. Leclercq R, Derlot E, Duval J, et al. Plasmid-mediated resistance to vancomycin and teicoplanin in *Enterococcus faecium*. N Engl J Med 1988;319(3):157–61.

4. Vergis EN, Hayden MK, Chow JW, et al. Determinants of vancomycin resistance and mortality rates in enterococcal bacteremia. A prospective multicenter study. Ann Intern Med 2001;135(7):484–92.

5. Rahim S, Pillai SK, Gold HS, et al. Linezolid-resistant, vancomycin-resistant *Enterococcus faecium* infection in patients without prior exposure to linezolid. Clin Infect Dis 2003;36(11):E146–8.

6. Gaynes R, Edwards JR, National Nosocomial Infections Surveillance System. Overview of nosocomial infections caused by gram-negative bacilli [see comment]. Clin Infect Dis 2005;41(6):848–54.

7. Boucher HW, Talbot GH, Bradley JS, et al. Bad bugs, no drugs: no ESKAPE! An update from the Infectious Diseases Society of America. Clin Infect Dis 2009; 48(1):1–12.

8. Shorr AF. Review of studies of the impact on Gram-negative bacterial resistance on outcomes in the intensive care unit. Crit Care Med 2009;37(4):1463–9.

9. Peralta G, Sanchez MB, Garrido JC, et al. Impact of antibiotic resistance and of adequate empirical antibiotic treatment in the prognosis of patients with *Escherichia coli* bacteraemia. J Antimicrob Chemother 2007;60(4):855–63.

10. Gerding DN. Editorial commentary: clindamycin, cephalosporins, fluoroquinolones, and *Clostridium difficile*-associated diarrhea: this is an antimicrobial resistance problem. Clin Infect Dis 2004;38(5):646–8.

11. Hoberman LJ, Eigenbrodt EH, Kilman WJ, et al. Colitis associated with oral clindamycin therapy. A clinical study of 16 patients. Am J Dig Dis 1976; 21(1):1–17.

12. Kelly CP, LaMont JT. *Clostridium difficile*–more difficult than ever. N Engl J Med 2008;359(18):1932–40.

13. McDonald LC, Owings M, Jernigan DB. *Clostridium difficile* infection in patients discharged from US short-stay hospitals, 1996–2003. Emerg Infect Dis 2006; 12(3):409–15.

14. Salazar M, Baskin L, Garey KW, et al. *Clostridium difficile*-related death rates in Texas 1999–2005. J Infect 2009;59(5):303–7.

15. McDonald LC, Killgore GE, Thompson A, et al. An epidemic, toxin gene-variant strain of *Clostridium difficile*. N Engl J Med 2005;353(23):2433–41.

16. Price PB. The bacteriology of normal skin, a new quantitative test applied to a study of the bacterial flora and the disinfectant action of mechanical cleansing. J Infect Dis 1938;63:301–18.

17. Lin YC, Lauderdale TL, Lin HM, et al. An outbreak of methicillin-resistant *Staphylococcus aureus* infection in patients of a pediatric intensive care unit and high carriage rate among health care workers. J Microbiol Immunol Infect 2007;40(4): 325–34.

18. Singh D, Kaur H, Gardner WG, et al. Bacterial contamination of hospital pagers. Infect Control Hosp Epidemiol 2002;23(5):274–6.

19. Treakle AM, Thom KA, Furuno JP, et al. Bacterial contamination of health care workers' white coats. Am J Infect Control 2009;37(2):101–5.

20. Borer A, Gilad J, Smolyakov R, et al. Cell phones and *Acinetobacter* transmission. Emerg Infect Dis 2005;11(7):1160–1.

21. Podnos YD, Cinat ME, Wilson SE, et al. Eradication of multi-drug resistant *Acine-tobacter* from an intensive care unit. Surg Infect (Larchmt) 2001;2(4):297–301.
22. Kramer A, Schwebke I, Kampf G. How long do nosocomial pathogens persist on inanimate surfaces? A systematic review. BMC Infect Dis 2006;6:130.
23. Huang SS, Datta R, Platt R. Risk of acquiring antibiotic-resistant bacteria from prior room occupants. Arch Intern Med 2006;166(18):1945–51.
24. Stiefel U, Pultz NJ, Donskey CJ. Effect of carbapenem administration on establish-ment of intestinal colonization by vancomycin-resistant enterococci and *Klebsiella pneumoniae* in mice. Antimicrob Agents Chemother 2007;51(1):372–5.
25. Pultz NJ, Stiefel U, Donskey CJ. Effects of daptomycin, linezolid, and vancomycin on establishment of intestinal colonization with vancomycin-resis-tant enterococci and extended-spectrum-beta-lactamase-producing *Klebsiella pneumoniae* in mice. Antimicrob Agents Chemother 2005;49(8):3513–6.
26. Muto CA, Jernigan JA, Ostrowsky BE, et al. SHEA guideline for preventing noso-comial transmission of multidrug-resistant strains of *Staphylococcus aureus* and enterococcus. Infect Control Hosp Epidemiol 2003;24(5):362–86.
27. Willemsen I, Groenhuijzen A, Bogaers D, et al. Appropriateness of antimicrobial therapy measured by repeated prevalence surveys. Antimicrob Agents Chemo-ther 2007;51(3):864–7.
28. Miller YW, Eady EA, Lacey RW, et al. Sequential antibiotic therapy for acne promotes the carriage of resistant staphylococci on the skin of contacts. J Antimicrob Chemother 1996;38(5):829–37.
29. Noakes TD, Borresen J, Hew-Butler T, et al. Semmelweis and the aetiology of puerperal sepsis 160 years on: an historical review. Epidemiol Infect 2008; 136(1):1–9.
30. Pittet D, Hugonnet S, Harbarth S, et al. Effectiveness of a hospital-wide programme to improve compliance with hand hygiene. Infection Control Programme. Lancet 2000;356(9238):1307–12.
31. Boyce JM, Pittet D. Guideline for hand hygiene in health-care settings: recom-mendations of the Healthcare Infection Control Practices Advisory Committee and the HICPAC/SHEA/APIC/IDSA Hand Hygiene Task Force. Infect Control Hosp Epidemiol 2002;23(Suppl 12):S3–40.
32. Rupp ME, Fitzgerald T, Puumala S, et al. Prospective, controlled, cross-over trial of alcohol-based hand gel in critical care units. Infect Control Hosp Epidemiol 2008;29(1):8–15.
33. Lankford MG, Collins S, Youngberg L, et al. Assessment of materials commonly utilized in health care: implications for bacterial survival and transmission. Am J Infect Control 2006;34(5):258–63.
34. Hayden MK, Blom DW, Lyle EA, et al. Risk of hand or glove contamination after contact with patients colonized with vancomycin-resistant enterococcus or the colonized patients' environment. Infect Control Hosp Epidemiol 2008;29(2): 149–54.
35. Bonilla HF, Zervos MA, Lyons MJ, et al. Colonization with vancomycin-resistant *Enterococcus faecium*: comparison of a long-term-care unit with an acute-care hospital. Infect Control Hosp Epidemiol 1997;18(5):333–9.
36. Noskin GA, Stosor V, Cooper I, et al. Recovery of vancomycin-resistant entero-cocci on fingertips and environmental surfaces. Infect Control Hosp Epidemiol 1995;16(10):577–81.
37. Gaonkar TA, Geraldo I, Caraos L, et al. An alcohol hand rub containing a syner-gistic combination of an emollient and preservatives: prolonged activity against transient pathogens. J Hosp Infect 2005;59(1):12–8.

38. Austin DJ, Bonten MJM, Weinstein RA, et al. Vancomycin-resistant enterococci in intensive-care hospital settings: transmission dynamics, persistence, and the impact of infection control programs. Proc Natl Acad Sci U S A 1999;96(12): 6908–13.

39. Larson EL, Early E, Cloonan P, et al. An organizational climate intervention associated with increased handwashing and decreased nosocomial infections. Behav Med 2000;26(1):14–22.

40. Fryklund B, Tullus K, Burman LG. Survival on skin and surfaces of epidemic and nonepidemic strains of enterobacteria from neonatal special care units. J Hosp Infect 1995;29(3):201–8.

41. Larson EL. Persistent carriage of gram-negative bacteria on hands. Am J Infect Control 1981;9(4):112–9.

42. Pottinger J, Burns S, Manske C. Bacterial carriage by artificial versus natural nails. Am J Infect Control 1989;17(6):340–4.

43. Pitten FA, Panzig B, Schröder G, et al. Transmission of a multiresistant *Pseudomonas aeruginosa* strain at a German University Hospital. J Hosp Infect 2001; 47(2):125–30.

44. Gill CJ, Mantaring JB, Macleod WB, et al. Impact of enhanced infection control at 2 neonatal intensive care units in the Philippines. Clin Infect Dis 2009;48(1): 13–21.

45. Bacon AE, Fekety R, Schaberg DR, et al. Epidemiology of *Clostridium difficile* colonization in newborns: results using a bacteriophage and bacteriocin typing system. J Infect Dis 1988;158(2):349–54.

46. Boyce JM, Pittet D. Guideline for hand hygiene in health-care settings. Recommendations of the Healthcare Infection Control Practices Advisory Committee and the HICPAC/SHEA/APIC/IDSA Hand Hygiene Task Force. Society for Healthcare Epidemiology of America/Association for Professionals in Infection Control/Infectious Diseases Society of America. MMWR Recomm Rep 2002; 51(RR-16):1–45 [quiz: CE1–4].

47. Oughton MT, Loo VG, Dendukuri N, et al. Hand hygiene with soap and water is superior to alcohol rub and antiseptic wipes for removal of *Clostridium difficile*. Infect Control Hosp Epidemiol 2009;30(10):939–44.

48. Gordin FM, Schultz ME, Huber RA, et al. Reduction in nosocomial transmission of drug-resistant bacteria after introduction of an alcohol-based handrub. Infect Control Hosp Epidemiol 2005;26(7):650–3.

49. Vernaz N, Sax H, Pittet D, et al. Temporal effects of antibiotic use and hand rub consumption on the incidence of MRSA and *Clostridium difficile*. J Antimicrob Chemother 2008;62(3):601–7.

50. Boyce JM, Ligi C, Kohan C, et al. Lack of association between the increased incidence of *Clostridium difficile*-associated disease and the increasing use of alcohol-based hand rubs. Infect Control Hosp Epidemiol 2006;27(5):479–83.

51. Abbett SK, Yokoe DS, Lipsitz SR, et al. Original article: proposed checklist of hospital interventions to decrease the incidence of healthcare-associated *Clostridium difficile* infection. Infect Control Hosp Epidemiol 2009;30(11):1062–9.

52. Dubberke ER, Gerding DN, Classen D, et al. Strategies to prevent *Clostridium difficile* infections in acute care hospitals. Infect Control Hosp Epidemiol 2008; 29(Suppl 1):S81–92.

53. Gensini GF, Yacoub MH, Conti AA. The concept of quarantine in history: from plague to SARS. J Infect 2004;49(4):257–61.

54. Olsen RJ, Lynch P, Coyle MB, et al. Examination gloves as barriers to hand contamination in clinical practice. JAMA 1993;270(3):350–3.

55. Jernigan JA, Titus MG, Groschel DH, et al. Effectiveness of contact isolation during a hospital outbreak of methicillin-resistant *Staphylococcus aureus*. Am J Epidemiol 1996;143(5):496–504.

56. Cooper BS, Stone SP, Kibbler CC, et al. Isolation measures in the hospital management of methicillin resistant *Staphylococcus aureus* (MRSA): systematic review of the literature. BMJ 2004;329(7465):533.

57. Siegel JD, Rhinehart E, Jackson M, et al. 2007 Guideline for isolation precautions: preventing transmission of infectious agents in health care settings. Am J Infect Control 2007;35(10 Suppl 2):S65–164.

58. Zachary KC, Bayne PS, Morrison VJ, et al. Contamination of gowns, gloves, and stethoscopes with vancomycin-resistant enterococci. Infect Control Hosp Epidemiol 2001;22(9):560–4.

59. Tenorio Allan R, Badri Sheila M, Sahgal Nishi B, et al. Effectiveness of gloves in the prevention of hand carriage of vancomycin-resistant enterococcus species by health care workers after patient care. Clin Infect Dis 2001; 32(5):826–9.

60. Kurup A, Chlebicki MP, Ling ML, et al. Control of a hospital-wide vancomycin-resistant enterococci outbreak. Am J Infect Control 2008;36(3):206–11.

61. Aumeran C, Baud O, Lesens O, et al. Successful control of a hospital-wide vancomycin-resistant *Enterococcus faecium* outbreak in France. Eur J Clin Microbiol Infect Dis 2008;27(11):1061–4.

62. Ostrowsky BE, Trick WE, Sohn AH, et al. Control of vancomycin-resistant enterococcus in health care facilities in a region. N Engl J Med 2001; 344(19):1427–33.

63. Servais A, Mercadal L, Brossier F, et al. Rapid curbing of a vancomycin-resistant *Enterococcus faecium* outbreak in a nephrology department. Clin J Am Soc Nephrol 2009;4(10):1559–64.

64. Srinivasan A, Song X, Ross T, et al. A prospective study to determine whether cover gowns in addition to gloves decrease nosocomial transmission of vancomycin-resistant enterococci in an intensive care unit. Infect Control Hosp Epidemiol 2002;23(8):424–8.

65. Puzniak LA, Leet T, Mayfield J, et al. To gown or not to gown: the effect on acquisition of vancomycin-resistant enterococci. Clin Infect Dis 2002;35(1):18–25.

66. Gbaguidi-Haore H, Legast S, Thouverez M, et al. Ecological study of the effectiveness of isolation precautions in the management of hospitalized patients colonized or infected with *Acinetobacter baumannii*. Infect Control Hosp Epidemiol 2008;29(12):1118–23.

67. Conterno LO, Shymanski J, Ramotar K, et al. Impact and cost of infection control measures to reduce nosocomial transmission of extended-spectrum [beta]-lactamase-producing organisms in a non-outbreak setting. J Hosp Infect 2007;65(4):354–60.

68. Laurent C, Rodriguez-Villalobos H, Rost F, et al. Intensive care unit outbreak of extended-spectrum beta-lactamase-producing *Klebsiella pneumoniae* controlled by cohorting patients and reinforcing infection control measures. Infect Control Hosp Epidemiol 2008;29(6):517–24.

69. Yokoe DS, Mermel LA, Anderson DJ, et al. A compendium of strategies to prevent healthcare-associated infections in acute care hospitals. Infect Control Hosp Epidemiol 2008;29(Suppl 1):S12–21.

70. Zafar AB, Gaydos LA, Furlong WB, et al. Effectiveness of infection control program in controlling nosocomial *Clostridium difficile*. Am J Infect Control 1998;26(6):588–93.

71. Johnson S, Gerding DN, Olson MM, et al. Prospective, controlled study of vinyl glove use to interrupt *Clostridium difficile* nosocomial transmission. Am J Med 1990;88(2):137–40.
72. Salgado CD, Mauldin PD, Fogle PJ, et al. Analysis of an outbreak of *Clostridium difficile* infection controlled with enhanced infection control measures. Am J Infect Control 2009;37(6):458–64.
73. Stelfox HT, Bates DW, Redelmeier DA. Safety of patients isolated for infection control. JAMA 2003;290(14):1899–905.
74. Catalano G, Houston SH, Catalano MC, et al. Anxiety and depression in hospitalized patients in resistant organism isolation. South Med J 2003; 96(2):141–5.
75. Harris AD, McGregor JC, Furuno JP. What infection control interventions should be undertaken to control multidrug-resistant gram-negative bacteria? Clin Infect Dis 2006;43(Suppl 2):S57–61.
76. Huang SS, Yokoe DS, Hinrichsen VL, et al. Impact of routine intensive care unit surveillance cultures and resultant barrier precautions on hospital-wide methicillin-resistant *Staphylococcus aureus* bacteremia. Clin Infect Dis 2006;43(8): 971–8.
77. Robicsek A, Beaumont JL, Paule SM, et al. Universal surveillance for methicillin-resistant *Staphylococcus aureus* in 3 affiliated hospitals. Ann Intern Med 2008; 148(6):409–18.
78. Ostrowsky BE, Venkataraman L, D'Agata EM, et al. Vancomycin-resistant enterococci in intensive care units: high frequency of stool carriage during a non-outbreak period. Arch Intern Med 1999;159(13):1467–72.
79. Byers KE, Anglim AM, Anneski CJ, et al. A hospital epidemic of vancomycin-resistant *Enterococcus*: risk factors and control. Infect Control Hosp Epidemiol 2001;22(3):140–7.
80. Price CS, Paule S, Noskin GA, et al. Active surveillance reduces the incidence of vancomycin-resistant enterococcal bacteremia. Clin Infect Dis 2003;37(7): 921–8.
81. Papadomichelakis E, Kontopidou F, Antoniadou A, et al. Screening for resistant gram-negative microorganisms to guide empiric therapy of subsequent infection. Intensive Care Med 2008;34(12):2169–75.
82. Centers for Disease Control and Prevention (CDC). Guidance for control of infections with carbapenem-resistant or carbapenemase-producing Enterobacteriaceae in acute care facilities. MMWR Morb Mortal Wkly Rep 2009;58(10): 256–60.
83. Gardam MA, Burrows LL, Kus JV, et al. Is surveillance for multidrug-resistant Enterobacteriaceae an effective infection control strategy in the absence of an outbreak? J Infect Dis 2002;186(12):1754–60.
84. Shim JK, Johnson S, Samore MH, et al. Primary symptomless colonisation by *Clostridium difficile* and decreased risk of subsequent diarrhoea. Lancet 1998;351(9103):633–6.
85. Clabots CR, Johnson S, Olson MM, et al. Acquisition of *Clostridium difficile* by hospitalized patients: evidence for colonized new admissions as a source of infection. J Infect Dis 1992;166(3):561–7.
86. Santos RP, Mayo TW, Siegel JD. Healthcare epidemiology: active surveillance cultures and contact precautions for control of multidrug-resistant organisms: ethical considerations. Clin Infect Dis 2008;47(1):110–6.
87. Owens RC Jr. Antimicrobial stewardship: concepts and strategies in the 21st century. Diagn Microbiol Infect Dis 2008;61(1):110–28.

88. Briceland LL, Nightingale CH, Quintiliani R, et al. Antibiotic streamlining from combination therapy to monotherapy utilizing an interdisciplinary approach. Arch Intern Med 1988;148(9):2019–22.
89. McGowan JE Jr, Finland M. Usage of antibiotics in a general hospital: effect of requiring justification. J Infect Dis 1974;130(2):165–8.
90. Evans RS, Pestotnik SL, Classen DC, et al. A computer-assisted management program for antibiotics and other antiinfective agents. N Engl J Med 1998; 338(4):232–8.
91. Carmeli Y, Samore MH, Huskins C. The association between antecedent vancomycin treatment and hospital-acquired vancomycin-resistant enterococci: a meta-analysis. Arch Intern Med 1999;159(20):2461–8.
92. de Bruin MA, Riley LW. Does vancomycin prescribing intervention affect vancomycin-resistant enterococcus infection and colonization in hospitals? A systematic review. BMC Infect Dis 2007;7:24.
93. Smith DW. Decreased antimicrobial resistance after changes in antibiotic use. Pharmacotherapy 1999;19(8 Pt 2):129S–32S [discussion: 33S–7S].
94. Bonten MJM, Slaughter S, Ambergen AW, et al. The role of "colonization pressure" in the spread of vancomycin-resistant enterococci: an important infection control variable. Arch Intern Med 1998;158(10):1127–32.
95. de Man P, Verhoeven BA, Verbrugh HA, et al. An antibiotic policy to prevent emergence of resistant bacilli. Lancet 2000;355(9208):973–8.
96. Meyer KS, Urban C, Eagan JA, et al. Nosocomial outbreak of *Klebsiella* infection resistant to late-generation cephalosporins. Ann Intern Med 1993;119(5):353–8.
97. Rahal JJ, Urban C, Horn D, et al. Class restriction of cephalosporin use to control total cephalosporin resistance in nosocomial *Klebsiella*. JAMA 1998; 280(14):1233–7.
98. Polgreen PM, Chen YY, Cavanaugh JE, et al. An outbreak of severe *Clostridium difficile*-associated disease possibly related to inappropriate antimicrobial therapy for community-acquired pneumonia. Infect Control Hosp Epidemiol 2007;28(2):212–4.
99. Khan R, Cheesbrough J. Impact of changes in antibiotic policy on *Clostridium difficile*-associated diarrhoea (CDAD) over a five-year period in a district general hospital. J Hosp Infect 2003;54(2):104–8.
100. McNulty C, Logan M, Donald IP, et al. Successful control of *Clostridium difficile* infection in an elderly care unit through use of a restrictive antibiotic policy. J Antimicrob Chemother 1997;40(5):707–11.
101. Valiquette L, Cossette B, Garant MP, et al. Impact of a reduction in the use of high-risk antibiotics on the course of an epidemic of *Clostridium difficile*-associated disease caused by the hypervirulent NAP1/027 strain. Clin Infect Dis 2007; 45(s2):S112–21.
102. Kallen Alexander J, Thompson A, Ristaino P, et al. Complete restriction of fluoroquinolone use to control an outbreak of *Clostridium difficile* infection at a community hospital. Infect Control Hosp Epidemiol 2009;30(3):264–72.
103. Gross R, Morgan AS, Kinky DE, et al. Impact of a hospital-based antimicrobial management program on clinical and economic outcomes. Clin Infect Dis 2001; 33(3):289–95.
104. Fishman N. Antimicrobial stewardship. Am J Infect Control 2006;34(5 Suppl 1): S55–63 [discussion: S4–73].
105. Weber SG, Gold HS, Hooper DC, et al. Fluoroquinolones and the risk for methicillin-resistant *Staphylococcus aureus* in hospitalized patients. Emerg Infect Dis 2003;9(11):1415–22.

106. Harris AD, Lautenbach E, Perencevich E. A systematic review of quasi-experimental study designs in the fields of infection control and antibiotic resistance. Clin Infect Dis 2005;41(1):77–82.

107. Perencevich EN, Stone PW, Wright SB, et al. Raising standards while watching the bottom line: making a business case for infection control. Infect Control Hosp Epidemiol 2007;28(10):1121–33.

108. Verity P, Wilcox MH, Fawley W, et al. Prospective evaluation of environmental contamination by *Clostridium difficile* in isolation side rooms. J Hosp Infect 2001;49(3):204–9.

109. Lu PL, Siu LK, Chen TC, et al. Methicillin-resistant *Staphylococcus aureus* and *Acinetobacter baumannii* on computer interface surfaces of hospital wards and association with clinical isolates. BMC Infect Dis 2009;9:164.

110. Boyce JM, Potter-Bynoe G, Chenevert C, et al. Environmental contamination due to methicillin-resistant *Staphylococcus aureus*: possible infection control implications. Infect Control Hosp Epidemiol 1997;18(9):622–7.

111. Bode LGM, Kluytmans JAJW, Wertheim HFL, et al. Preventing surgical-site infections in nasal carriers of *Staphylococcus aureus*. N Engl J Med 2010; 362(1):9–17.

112. Calderwood MS, Mauer A, Tolentino J, et al. Epidemiology of vancomycin-resistant enterococci among patients on an adult stem cell transplant unit: observations from an active surveillance program. Infect Control Hosp Epidemiol 2008; 29(11):1019–25.

Nosocomial Fungal Infections: Epidemiology, Infection Control, and Prevention

George J. Alangaden, MD

KEYWORDS

• Nosocomial • Fungal infection • *Candida* • *Aspergillus*

Fungal infections are an increasing cause of morbidity and mortality in hospitalized patients. This article reviews the current epidemiology of nosocomial fungal infections in adult patients, with an emphasis on invasive candidiasis and aspergillosis. Recently published recommendations and guidelines for the control and prevention of these nosocomial fungal infections are summarized.

IMPACT OF NOSOCOMIAL FUNGAL INFECTIONS

There has been an overall increase in fungal health care–associated infections (HAIs) in the last few decades, which is likely a consequence of the advances in medical and surgical therapies. The wider use of more aggressive modalities of treatments, such as hematopoietic stem cell transplantation (HSCT), solid organ transplantation (SOT), new chemotherapeutic agents, and immunomodulatory agents, has increased the population of immunocompromised patients at risk for invasive fungal infection.[1] The predisposing risk factors for opportunistic invasive fungal infections, particularly candidiasis and aspergillosis, in these immunocompromised hosts include neutropenia, qualitative neutrophil dysfunction, cell-mediated immune dysfunction, and disruption of mucosal integrity.[2] Moreover, the prevalence of invasive devices, especially intravascular central lines, has resulted in an increase in nosocomial catheter-related bloodstream infections (CRBSIs), candidemia, and disseminated candidiasis.[3,4] Exposure to airborne fungal pathogens such as *Aspergillus* spp within the hospital environment, especially during construction, has caused outbreaks of nosocomial aspergillosis in severely immunocompromised patients such as patients who underwent HSCT.[5]

Division of Infectious Diseases, Wayne State University, 3990 John R, Suite 5930, Detroit, MI 48201, USA
E-mail address: galangaden@med.wayne.edu

Infect Dis Clin N Am 25 (2011) 201–225
doi:10.1016/j.idc.2010.11.003
0891-5520/11/$ – see front matter © 2011 Elsevier Inc. All rights reserved.

Candida spp are the most common fungal pathogens causing serious HAIs, especially in patients admitted to intensive care units (ICUs).[3,6–9] A recent study using the National Hospital Discharge Survey estimated the incidence rate of invasive candidiasis to have increased from 23 per 100,000 US population in 1996 to 29 per 100,000 in 2003.[10] The corresponding incidence rate of invasive candidiasis per 10,000 hospital discharges increased from 20 in 1996 to 24 in 2003.[10] Among invasive candidiasis, candidemia is estimated to account for 2 to 8 infections per 10,000 hospital discharges in recent studies from the United States and Europe.[11–14] The true incidence of health care–associated candidemia is likely to be higher because of the relatively poor diagnostic yield (approximately 50%) of positive blood culture results in patients with disseminated candidiasis with implicit candidemia. Matched cohort and case-control studies in various hospitalized patient populations, including those in the ICU and those who have undergone a transplant, report attributable mortality rates for candidemia ranging from 5% to 71%.[15] A recent case-control study based on hospital discharge diagnosis estimated the mortality from candidemia to be age-related, 15% to 25% for adults and 10% to 15% for children.[16] The excess health care cost, primarily related to an increased length of stay, is projected to be $29,000 to as high as $39,000 for each episode of candidemia.[16–18] The estimated annual cost in the United States for the treatment of systemic fungal infections was $2.8 billion in 1998, of which $1.7 billion was for the treatment of candidiasis.[19]

Based on hospital discharge data, there were an estimated 10,190 aspergillosis-related hospitalizations and 1970 deaths during 1996 in the United States.[20] Unlike invasive candidiasis, the incidence rate of invasive aspergillosis per 100,000 US population declined from 3.4 in 1996 to 2.2 in 2003, with a decrease in the incidence rate from 3 to 2 per 10,000 hospital discharges.[10] The reasons for this decline are unclear. However, in severely immunocompromised patients, such as HSCT recipients, invasive aspergillosis remains the most important cause of infection-related mortality.[21] In a large prospective registry of 234 HSCT recipients with invasive fungal infection, aspergillosis accounted for 59% of all invasive fungal infections and was associated with a 6-week mortality rate of 22%.[21] This mortality rate is lower than previously reported rates and may be related to the increasing use of nonmyeloablative HSCT, early diagnosis, and use of broad-spectrum antifungals such as voriconazole.[22] The average length of stay for a hospitalization related to *Aspergillus* infection was 17 days at a cost of $62,426, resulting in an overall estimated cost of $633.1 million.[20]

The overall burden of disease caused by nosocomial fungal infections is substantial. Limitations of the current diagnostic tests available to establish an early diagnosis of fungal infection and the emergence of fungal pathogens that are resistant to antifungal agents make the prevention of fungal HAIs increasingly important. Infection control strategies targeted to reduce nosocomial CRBSIs caused by *Candida* spp emphasize hand hygiene[23] and adherence to guidelines for prevention of intravascular catheter-related infections.[24,25] Prevention of exposure to airborne *Aspergillus* spp and molds in the hospital environment can be minimized by implementing recommendations on environmental controls[26] and specific preventive measures targeting high-risk HSCT recipients.[27]

COMMON NOSOCOMIAL INFECTIONS CAUSED BY YEASTS
Candida spp

Certain *Candida* spp, especially *Candida albicans*, are part of the human microbial flora; hence, most candidal infections are endogenous in origin. Invasive candidiasis, namely, candidemia, disseminated hematogenous infections, or deep-seated infections in normally sterile body sites, can occur in immunocompromised patients, such as those with neutropenia, and in critically ill patients. In patients with cancer and chemotherapy-induced neutropenia and mucositis, candidemia may originate from the gastrointestinal tract.[28] However, in critically ill patients, the source of candidemia is most likely the intravascular catheters colonized by Candida spp from the patient's endogenous microflora or Candida spp acquired from the health care environment.[29] Candida spp have been isolated from environmental cultures of the floor, countertops, and other inanimate surfaces in the hospital.[30,31] Patient acquisition and colonization with Candida spp found in the hospital environment and food has been demonstrated.[30–32] The propensity of Candida spp, especially Candida parapsilosis, to cause CRBSIs is likely related to this pathogen's ability to form biofilms on catheters.[33,34] The true incidence of nosocomial candidemia is likely underestimated. This fact was highlighted in a recent molecular epidemiologic study of candidemia over a 16-year period in Iceland, which identified previously unrecognized smoldering nosocomial clusters in a third of a patient population with candidemia.[35]

Overall, Candida spp were the fourth most common pathogen accounting for 11% of 28,502 HAIs reported to the National Healthcare Safety Network at the Centers for Disease Control and Prevention (CDC) between 2006 and 2007.[3] Candida spp were the second most common pathogen causing 21% of catheter-associated urinary tract infections and the third most common pathogen accounting for 11% of CRBSIs.[3] In a prospective nationwide surveillance study (surveillance and control of pathogens of epidemiological importance [SCOPE]) of 24,179 nosocomial bloodstream infections (BSIs) in 49 US hospitals (ICU and non-ICU patients) conducted between 1995 and 2002, the incidence rate of BSIs caused by Candida spp was 4.6 per 10,000 hospital admissions.[4] Candida spp were the fourth most common pathogen isolated and accounted for 9% of BSIs. There was a significant increase in the proportion of Candida spp isolated in blood cultures, from 8% in 1995 to 12% in 2002. Although Candida spp accounted for 10% of BSIs among patients in ICUs, they also caused 8% of BSIs in patients in non-ICU settings. Other studies have also noted the increasing proportion of patients with candidemia in non-ICU settings, possibly because of the presence of long-term indwelling central venous lines.[11,12,36] In population-based studies, the factors associated with candidemia have included extremes of age, African American population, underlying cancer or diabetes, and the presence of indwelling intravascular catheters.[11,12,36] Additional risk factors for nosocomial candidemia in hospitalized patients include ICU stay; major surgery (especially abdominal surgery); renal failure; dialysis; use of broad-spectrum antibiotics, corticosteroids, or immunosuppressive agents; total parenteral nutrition; and colonization with Candida spp.[29,37,38]

In the ARTEMIS DISK global antifungal surveillance project, of the 197,000 Candida spp isolated from patients with invasive candidiasis between 1997 and 2005, 90% of infections were caused by 5 species, C albicans, Candida glabrata, C parapsilosis, and Candida tropicalis.[39] Similarly, the Candida spp isolated from patients with nosocomial candidemia in the SCOPE study were C albicans (54%), C glabrata (19%), C parapsilosis (11%), and C tropicalis (11%).[4] The overall crude mortality rate associated with candidemia was 47%, with the lowest rate of 30% for BSIs caused by C parapsilosis and the highest rate of 59% for Candida krusei fungemias.[4] The relative frequencies of the nonalbicans Candida spp causing candidemia varies across the world and among types of health care centers. Overall, there has been a recent increase in the proportion of infections caused by nonalbicans Candida spp.[3,10,40] In a recent study from the United States, nonalbicans Candida spp were reported to cause most of the candidemias.[41] Most of the nonalbicans species, particularly C glabrata, seem to be reported from specialized cancer centers in the United States.[40,42] In contrast, there are low rates of *C glabrata* and high rates of *C parapsilosis* and *C tropicalis* reported from Latin America.[10] The clinical significance of the isolation of nonalbicans *Candida* spp is the increased likelihood of resistance to fluconazole and other azoles. In particular, of the commonly isolated nonalbicans *Candida* spp, fluconazole resistance was noted in 16% of *C glabrata*, 78% of *C krusei*, and 11% of *Candida guilliermondii*.[10]

Although most cases of candidemia and invasive candidiasis are caused by endogenous patient microflora, exogenous transmission of *Candida* spp may occur particularly in neonatal ICUs. In a prospective study of candidemias in surgical and neonatal ICUs, 33% of surgical ICU and 29% of neonatal ICU medical personnel had *Candida* spp recovered from their hands.[43] Candida colonization of artificial nails of a health care worker (HCW) has also been implicated as a cause of postoperative candidal osteomyelitis.[44]

Characteristics of specific *Candida* spp may influence the risk for exogenous transmission and nosocomial infections in certain patient populations.[45] In molecular epidemiologic studies, *C albicans* has been implicated in nosocomial transmission among patients in burn units.[46,47] Person-to-person transmission has also been reported from geriatric short-stay units.[48]

C glabrata seems to be more frequently isolated from older patients,[49] patients with cancer and prior exposure to fluconazole,[42,50] and patients treated with piperacillin-tazobactam or vancomycin.[51]

C parapsilosis has emerged as an important cause of candidemia in the neonatal population[52–55] and transplant recipients.[55] *C parapsilosis* is the most common *Candida* spp isolated from the hands of HCWs. In a prospective multicenter study of neonatal candidiasis, *C parapsilosis* was isolated from 19% of 2 989 cultures obtained from the hands of HCWs.[56] Colonization with *C parapsilosis* was also found on the hands of 7 of 21 neonatal ICU HCWs.[57] A recent review of molecular epidemiologic studies of outbreaks of *C parapsilosis* suggests horizontal transmission from HCWs to neonates.[58] The ability of *C parapsilosis* to produce biofilms[34,59] may explain its propensity to cause outbreaks of nosocomial candidemias associated with central venous catheters (CVCs).[60,61] In addition, outbreaks of *C parapsilosis* candidemia have been associated with the use of parenteral nutrition,[61] which may be because of the selective growth advantage of *C parapsilosis* in glucose-rich hyperalimentation solutions.[62] Hence, the frequent isolation of *C parapsilosis* should prompt measures to enhance hand hygiene and appropriate care of intravascular catheters.

C tropicalis is increasingly isolated from patients with hematologic malignancies in the setting of mucositis and neutropenia,[63] and colonization in these patients is predictive of subsequent infection.[41,64]

C krusei was the fifth most common *Candida* spp isolated and accounted for 2.5% of 137,487 *Candida* isolates in a global antifungal surveillance program.[65] *C krusei,* intrinsically resistant to fluconazole, has often been reported in patients with hematologic malignancies and HSCT recipients with prior fluconazole and antifungal exposure and is associated with the highest mortality of all *Candida* spp.[41,42,63,66,67] In nonneutropenic patients, risk factors for *C krusei* nosocomial candidemias include recent gastrointestinal surgery and exposure to fluconazole.[68]

Emerging *Candida* spp that are relatively resistant to fluconazole, such as *C guilliermondii*[69] and *C rugosa*,[70,71] have also been associated with nosocomial outbreaks, some involving intravascular catheters.

Other Yeasts

Malassezia spp are lipophilic yeasts that are frequent colonizers of the skin and are the cause of pityriasis. Few outbreaks of *Malassezia* fungemia have been reported in low-birth-weight neonates and in immunocompromised adults.[72–74] The prolonged use of intravascular catheters and parenteral lipid formulations were important predisposing conditions identified.[72,74] Investigation of a group of 8 neonates with *Malassezia pachydermatis* fungemia reported colonization of the hands and pet dogs of HCWs, suggesting possible transmission from HCWs to patients.[73]

Trichosporon spp are the cause of white piedra, a superficial infection of the hair shaft. Fungemia has been reported in immunocompromised patients, primarily those with hematologic malignancies, and HSCT and SOT recipients.[75–77] Systemic disease has also been reported in nonneutropenic ICU and burn patients.[78–80] One of the common risk factors in cases of nosocomial trichosporonosis is the presence of an indwelling intravascular catheter and exposure to prior antibiotics.[75,76,80] The reported all-cause mortality rate is high and ranges from 42% to 83%, with the highest rates in patients with hematologic malignancies.[75–77,80]

Most outbreaks of nosocomial invasive candidiasis and invasive infections with other yeasts have been associated with intravascular catheters. Hence, infection control strategies targeted to improve adherence to hand hygiene recommendations, including avoidance of long nails and artificial nails, and guidelines for care of intravascular catheters are important in the prevention of these infections.

NOSOCOMIAL INFECTIONS CAUSED BY MOLDS

Unlike invasive candidiasis, which can affect relatively noncompromised patients, invasive disease caused by *Aspergillus* spp and molds generally involves severely immunocompromised patients. Although several outbreaks of environmental airborne fungal infection within hospital settings have been reported, most cases of invasive aspergillosis are sporadic. At present, there is no uniform definition of what constitutes nosocomial aspergillosis.[81] One of the primary reasons for the difficulty in defining hospital-acquired aspergillosis is that the incubation period of invasive aspergillosis is unknown. Moreover, the prolonged period of immunosuppression in high-risk patients such as HSCT recipients and frequent hospital admissions and discharges makes it difficult to determine if exposure to *Aspergillus* spores occurred during hospitalization or within the community. One definition that is frequently used considers nosocomial aspergillosis as invasive disease that occurs after 1 week of hospitalization or within 2 weeks of hospital discharge.[82] Although most hospital outbreaks have been caused by *Aspergillus* spp, other airborne molds have also been implicated, including *Zygomycetes* spp,[83] *Fusarium* spp,[84] *Scedosporium* spp,[85,86] and *Penicillium* spp.[87]

Aspergillus spp

Aspergillus spp are ubiquitous molds found widely in the environment; they reproduce by means of asexual propagules termed conidia or spores. Exposure to airborne spores of *Aspergillus* occurs frequently in the environment, especially near decaying organic matter. Although these conidia (2.5–3.0 μm in diameter) are frequently inhaled, invasive pulmonary disease is rare in immunocompetent persons. Opportunistic invasive aspergillosis occurs primarily in severely immunocompromised patients. *Aspergillus fumigatus* is the species most often associated with disease, although other species, including *Aspergillus flavus*[88–90] *Aspergillus niger*, *Aspergillus terreus*, *Aspergillus nidulans*, and *Aspergillus ustus*, have also been isolated from patients with invasive disease.

Aspergillosis is an important cause of morbidity and mortality, particularly in allogeneic HSCT recipients and neutropenic patients with hematologic malignancies.[91–96]

Immunocompromised patients at a lower risk for invasive aspergillosis include SOT recipients,[93,97,98] patients with AIDS,[99–102] and those with chronic granulomatous disease.[103] There are increasing reports of invasive aspergillosis being described in critically ill patients in the ICU without the traditional risk factors, including patients with *chronic obstructive pulmonary disease*, liver cirrhosis, and those receiving corticosteroids.[104–110]

Aspergillus outbreaks

Although most cases of invasive aspergillosis are sporadic, the information on the environmental exposures and the association with infection has been derived from investigations of outbreaks of aspergillosis in hospital settings. A recent extensive review of nosocomial aspergillosis identified 53 reported outbreaks involving 458 patients.[5] Of these, 33 outbreaks involving 299 patients (65%) occurred in HSCT recipients or patients with hematologic malignancies. Other patient populations involved in these outbreaks were SOT recipients (10%), predominately renal transplant recipients; other severely immunocompromised patients (13%); patients without severe immunodeficiency (8%); and patients on high-dose steroids (3%).[5] Aspergillosis was associated with mortality greater than 50% in patients with hematologic malignancies, HSCT and SOT recipients, and patients with severe immunodeficiency. The most common site of infection was the lungs in 77% of cases, with about 5% involving surgical site or skin infections. A fumigatus and A flavus were the most commonly identified *Aspergillus* spp. Volumetric air sampling performed during the course of epidemiologic investigations in 24 of the outbreaks noted spore counts ranging from 0 to 100 spores per cubic meter. Outbreaks were primarily attributed to airborne infections related to construction or renovation activities in about 50% of cases and to compromised air quality in 17%.[5] The various environmental vehicles implicated in the transmission of *Aspergillus* spp and other molds have also been detailed in the CDC guidelines for environmental infection control in health care facilities (HCFs). These vehicles include improperly functioning ventilation systems, poorly maintained air filters, contamination of false ceilings and insulation material, construction within and around the hospital, water leaks, food, and ornamental plants.[26]

The most frequent nosocomial source of *Aspergillus* infection seems be contaminated air, but *Aspergillus* has also been recovered from the hospital water supply and plumbing systems.[111–113] The highest airborne *Aspergillus* spore counts were detected in patient's bathrooms, suggesting possible aerosolization of *Aspergillus* spores from the shower facilities.[112] The clinical implications of this finding remain to be defined.

Clusters of cutaneous aspergillosis have occurred in burn wounds as a result of the use of dressings contaminated with *Aspergillus* spores during hospital construction.[114] Cutaneous aspergillosis has also occurred at intravenous (IV) insertion sites because of contaminated dressings used to secure arm boards that provided support for IV lines in children undergoing treatment of leukemia.[115]

Although the association between construction and invasive aspergillosis has often been reported, there is poor correlation of the *Aspergillus* spp recovered from the hospital environment and species isolated from patients with aspergillosis.[112,116,117] One explanation for this discordance between hospital and patient strains of *Aspergillus* might relate to the lack of a clearly defined incubation period for aspergillosis and the relationship to exposure within the hospital environment and subsequent infection.[81] Other factors include the methods of air sampling used,[118] the broad diversity of *Aspergillus* spp in the environment,[119] and the various methods used for typing of *Aspergillus* and other pathogenic molds.[120,121]

Zygomycetes

Zygomycetes are ubiquitous molds and, like *Aspergillus* spp, are found in the soil and decaying organic matter in the environment. Although infection caused by Zygomycetes is uncommon, it is often a fatal disease. Population-based studies estimate an annual incidence of 0.43 to 1.7 cases per million persons.[122,123] In a recent review of 929 patients with zygomycosis, the underlying conditions were diabetes (36%), malignancy (17%), SOT (7%), desferrioxamine therapy (6%), injection drug use (5%), and bone marrow transplantation (5%).[124] The overall mortality was 54%, with the mortality exceeding 80% in HSCT recipients, patients with renal failure, patients on desferrioxamine therapy, and patients with systemic lupus erythematosus. Mortality was 76% with pulmonary zygomycosis and 100% with disseminated and central nervous system diseases.[124] Infection often occurs via inhalation of fungal spores, resulting in sinopulmonary disease, but systemic infection can result from inoculation of the skin or gastrointestinal mucosa.[124] The treatment of localized infections is often surgical, and antifungal therapeutic options are limited to amphotericin B or posaconazole.[125]

Nosocomial infections caused by Zygomycetes have been recently reviewed.[83] Clusters of cutaneous infections have occurred in orthopedic and cardiothoracic patients, children with leukemia, and burn patients. These infections were associated with Elastoplast adhesive dressings possibly contaminated with *Rhizopus* and *Absidia* spp.[83,126] Outbreaks in patients with hematologic malignancies have resulted from airborne transmission associated with contamination of hospital ventilation systems.[127–129] Unusual routes of transmission have been traced to the use of contaminated wooden tongue depressors[130,131] and nonsterile karaya (plant-derived adhesive) for securing ostomy bags.[132] A recent outbreak of gastrointestinal zygomycosis caused by *Rhizopus* in 12 patients with hematologic malignancies was traced to contaminated cornstarch used as an excipient in the manufacture of allopurinol and ready-to-eat foods.[133]

Fusarium spp

Fusarium is a soil saprophyte and causes keratitis and onychomycosis in humans. Outbreaks of keratitis caused by possible contamination of contact lens solutions have been described.[134,135] Invasive disease has generally been reported in patients with prolonged neutropenia, especially in HSCT recipients,[84,136] and to a lesser extent in SOT recipients.[137] The incidence of fusariosis has been estimated to be 4 to 5 cases per 1000 HLA antigen–matched allogeneic HSCT recipients to as high as 20 cases per 1000 HLA antigen–mismatched recipients. Fusariosis in HSCT recipients has a bimodal distribution, with a peak before engraftment and later during the period of graft-versus-host disease (GVHD), and is associated with an actuarial survival of 13%.[136] Most infections are believed to be caused by airborne transmission; however, contamination of the water system in the hospital has been reported to result in dispersal of airborne conidia.[84] DNA sequencing has demonstrated evidence of widespread distribution of clones that were similar to isolates recovered from nosocomial infections in patients.[138]

Other Molds

Several other pathogenic molds have been associated with HAIs. Outbreaks caused by *Scedosporium* spp have been reported in patients with leukemia undergoing chemotherapy.[85,86,139] *Paecilomyces* spp have a propensity to cause intraocular implant infections and have been associated with possible contamination of the air in the operating room.[140] Cutaneous inoculation of *Paecilomyces* spp from contaminated skin lotion has resulted in cutaneous and invasive infections in HSCT recipients.[141] *Phialemonium* spp have been linked to outbreaks of intravascular infections in patients undergoing hemodialysis resulting from contamination of water distribution systems.[142–144] Outbreak of infections caused by *Phialemonium* has also been linked to contaminated prefilled syringes of vasoactive agents used for injection of penile implants.[145] *Curvularia* spp have been isolated from saline-filled breast implants, resulting from contamination of saline stored beneath a water-damaged ceiling.[146]

Pneumocystis jiroveci

Opportunistic pneumonia caused by *Pneumocystis jiroveci*, now classified as a fungus, is believed to be because of the reactivation of latent infection during periods of severe T-cell–mediated immunosuppression, as in transplant recipients and patients with AIDS. However, recent reports suggest possible person-to-person airborne transmission of infection.[147–153] Polymerase chain reaction (PCR) testing identified *P jiroveci* DNA in close contacts of patients with HIV infection and *Pneumocystis* pneumonia, including HCWs.[147,148] Molecular evidence has also identified person-to-person transmission of *P jiroveci* to be the likely cause of outbreaks of *Pneumocystis* pneumonia, particularly among renal transplant recipients.[149–156] Most of the renal transplant recipients were not receiving anti–*Pneumocystis* pneumonia prophylaxis. However, population-based studies have not detected an increased risk of *P jiroveci* infections in the contacts of HIV-seropositive persons.[157,158] Current guidelines do not recommend specific isolation measures for the care of hospitalized patients with *Pneumocystis* pneumonia.[27,159]

STRATEGIES FOR PREVENTION OF NOSOCOMIAL CANDIDIASIS
Prevention of Intravascular Catheter-related Candidemia

Guidelines for the prevention of intravascular CRBSIs have been published.[24,25] Evidenced-based recommendations emphasize (1) education and training of HCWs who insert and maintain catheters, (2) use of maximal sterile-barrier precautions during CVC insertion, (3) use of 2% chlorhexidine for skin antisepsis, (4) avoiding routine replacement of CVCs, and (5) use of antibiotic/antiseptic-impregnated CVCs if there are high rates of infection despite implementation of recommendations.[24] The measures strongly recommended for implementation as described in the Society for Healthcare Epidemiology of America and the Infectious Diseases Society of America guidelines for the prevention of CRBSIs are discussed in detail by Drs David J. Weber and William A. Rutala elsewhere in this issue.

The effectiveness of these strategies, using the 5 processes, namely, appropriate hand hygiene, chlorhexidine antisepsis, full-barrier precautions, the preferred use of the subclavian site, and removal of unnecessary CVCs for the prevention of CRBSIs, was examined in 103 ICUs in Michigan.[160] The median rate of CRBSIs during the 18 months after implementation declined 66% from 2.7 to 0 per 1000 catheter-days.[160] A similar reduction in CRBSIs has been reported in surgical ICUs after implementation of these guidelines.[161]

STRATEGIES FOR PREVENTION OF NOSOCOMIAL ASPERGILLOSIS AND MOLD INFECTIONS

Aspergillosis is primarily acquired by inhalation of fungal spores and subsequent invasive disease in immunocompromised patients with prolonged neutropenia or those on high-dose corticosteroid therapy. Hence, the primary infection control strategy is to minimize exposure to airborne environmental fungal spores within HCFs during the high-risk period. Exposure to fungal spores of *Aspergillus* spp and other pathogenic molds after hospital discharge may occur in high-risk patients, such as the allogeneic HSCT recipient with chronic GVHD who is administered steroids. Patient education to minimize exposures to fungal spores and chemoprophylaxis with antifungal agents may be necessary. Guidelines for the use of antifungal agents for prophylaxis against invasive aspergillosis have been recently published.[27,162]

The CDC and the Healthcare Infection Control Practices Advisory Committee have published recommendations regarding environmental infection control measures in HCFs.[26] These recommendations include infection control strategies and engineering controls directed primarily for the prevention of exposure of immunocompromised patients to environmental airborne fungal spores of *Aspergillus* and other molds. Additional recommendations to prevent HCF-associated pulmonary aspergillosis have also been published.[159]

Because opportunistic *Aspergillus* and airborne mold infections occur primarily in severely immunocompromised patients such as HSCT recipients, one of the main components of these prevention strategies is the provision of a protected environment (PE) for these patients within the HCF.

Protected Environment

A PE is a specialized patient care environment in acute care hospitals for the care of allogeneic HSCT recipients.[26,27] The benefit of a PE for other immunocompromised patients, such as autologous HSCT or SOT recipients, remains undefined.[159] A PE is designed to minimize HSCT patient exposure to airborne environmental *Aspergillus* spores. The essential features of a PE are shown in **Box 1**. Additional infection control measures for patients housed in a PE include (1) daily monitoring and maintenance of a positive pressure in PE areas, (2) minimizing exposures to activities that can cause aerosolization of fungal spores (eg, vacuuming), (3) minimizing the length of time that the patients are outside the PE for procedures, and (4) provision of high-efficiency respiratory protection (eg, N95 respirators; 3M, St Paul, MN, USA) when outside the PE if there is ongoing construction activity in the HCF.[159] The effectiveness of respirators in the absence of construction or the use of surgical masks to prevent fungal infection has not been evaluated.

Box 1
Protective environment

Requirements of protective environment rooms

- Central or point-of-use high-efficiency particulate air (HEPA) filters with 99.97% efficiency for removing particles 0.3 μm or larger

- Directed airflow, air intake occurs at 1 side and air exhaust occurs at the opposite side of the room

- Positive air pressure differential between room and corridor ($\geq$2.5 Pa)

- Maintenance of 12 or more air changes per hour

- Well sealed patient rooms

Data from Sehulster L, Chinn RY. Guidelines for environmental infection control in health-care facilities. Recommendations of CDC and the Healthcare Infection Control Practices Advisory Committee (HICPAC). MMWR Recomm Rep 2003;52(RR–10):1–42.

The other infection control strategies and engineering controls recommendations that reduce exposure to environmental airborne *Aspergillus* and other fungal spores emphasize the provision of safe air during routine care and importantly during hospital construction.[26,159] These strategies are outlined in **Box 2**.

Infection Control Risk Assessment

ICRA is a multistep process that determines the potential effect of construction within an HCF on the environment and exposure of at-risk patients to infectious agents, particularly fungal spores.[163,164] The members of the ICRA include the infection control team, construction engineers, and hospital administration. The steps in the ICRA process before start of any construction activity are the following:

1. Categorize the type of construction activity (types A–D) based on the degree of dust generated. Type A activities are those that produce no dust (eg, electrical trim work or minor plumbing), and type D activities are major demolition or construction.
2. Identify the patients who will be affected by the construction activity and determine the level of infection risk: low risk (eg, office areas), medium risk (eg, physical therapy), high risk (eg, emergency department), and highest risk (eg, immunocompromised patient areas).
3. Match the patient risk group with the type of construction activity and determine the class of infection control precautions necessary. The classes of infection control precautions range from class 1 (minimal precautions) to class 4 (major precautions, including barriers and safe air handling).

Implementation of recommended infection control strategies during hospital construction has been successful in the prevention of fungal contamination of air in patient care areas in prospective environmental surveillance studies using cultures and PCR assays for detection of airborne fungi.[165–167] Newer mobile nonfiltration-based air treatment systems that use exposure to electric fields and electrostatic nanofiltration to destroy airborne organisms have also been effective in preventing fungal contamination during construction.[168,169]

Additional recommendations for the prevention and control of nosocomial aspergillosis are included in **Box 3**.

STRATEGIES FOR PREVENTION OF FUNGAL INFECTION IN HSCT RECIPIENTS

The term severely immunocompromised patient often refers to the allogeneic HSCT recipient. To implement strategies to prevent fungal infections in this population, it is important to define the high-risk periods after HSCT. In the allogeneic HSCT recipient, the risk of infections is related to the time from transplant.[27] The post-HSCT period is generally divided into 3 phases:

- Phase I: the preengraftment period (<15–45 days post-HSCT). Risk of infection is related to prolonged neutropenia and disruption of the mucocutaneous barriers because of cytotoxic chemotherapy. Infections during this period are generally caused by bacteria, *herpes simplex virus*, *Candida*, and *Aspergillus* spp.
- Phase II: the postengraftment phase (30–100 days post-HSCT). Risk of infection is related to impaired cell-mediated immunity based on the severity of GVHD and the intensity of immunosuppressive therapy used for treatment. Infections during this period are caused by cytomegalovirus (CMV), *Aspergillus* spp, and *P jiroveci*.

Box 2
Environmental infection control measures in healthcare facilities to minimize exposure to fungal spores

Recommendations	Rating Category[a]
Air handling systems	
• Use the American Institute of Architects (AIA) guidelines or state regulations for design and construction of ventilations systems[164]	IC
• Conduct ICRA and provide adequate number of PE rooms for the HSCT population	IA, IC
• Monitor ventilation systems for removal of particulates and excess moisture	IB, IC
Proper location and maintenance of air intake and exhaust outlets, for example, removal of bird roosts from near air intake outlets to prevent entry of fungal spores	
Appropriate installation, maintenance, and disposal of HVAC filters	
Monitor PE areas for ACH, filtration, and pressure differentials	
• Develop a contingency plan for backup capacity in case of a power failure	IC
• Coordinate HVAC system shutdowns with infection control staff to allow for safe air handling to PE areas and to relocate immunocompromised patients if necessary	IC
Infection control measures during construction projects	
• Set up a multidisciplinary team that includes infection control staff to coordinate proactive preventive measures to reduce exposure to fungal spores and monitor adherence	IB,IC
• Provide education to HCWs and the construction crew in immunocompromised patient care areas regarding airborne infections	IB
• Perform an ICRA to assess potential exposure of high-risk patients to high ambient air fungal spore count	IB, IC
• Develop and implement measures to keep airborne spores from construction areas away from patient care units	IB, IC
Dust control measures (eg, dust barriers, safe air handling, negative pressure in construction work zones)	
Water damage response plan to prevent fungal growth	
• Maintain surveillance for cases of HCF-associated aspergillosis and mold infections in immunocompromised patients	IB
• Undertake an epidemiologic investigation if a case of nosocomial *Aspergillus* or other mold infection is detected	IB
Surveillance for additional cases	
Determine appropriate air handling in the PE and in construction areas	
Conduct environmental assessment to identify the source	
Take corrective action to improve deficiencies identified and to eliminate the source of fungal spores	

Environmental services recommendations to minimize exposure to fungal spores

- Avoid carpeting and upholstered furniture and furnishings in areas housing immunocompromised patients   IB

- Avoid cleaning methods that disperse dust   IB

  Wet dust horizontal surfaces using EPA-registered hospital disinfectant

  Equip vacuums with HEPA filters

  Close the doors of rooms of immunocompromised patients when cleaning

  Dry carpeting immediately if wet to prevent growth of fungi, replace if wet after 72 hours

- Avoid fresh flowers and potted plants in areas housing   II
  immunocompromised patients

Abbreviations: ACH, air changes per hour; EPA, environmental protection agency; HSCT, hematopoeitic stem cell transplantation HVAC, heating ventilation air conditioning; ICRA, infection control risk assessment; PE, protected environment.
[a] Ratings category: IA, strongly recommended for all hospitals and supported by well-designed experimental or epidemiologic evidence; IB, strongly recommended for all hospitals and viewed as effective by experts because of strong rationale and suggestive evidence; IC, required by state or federal regulation or representing an established association standard; II, suggested for implementation in many hospitals, supported by suggestive clinical or epidemiologic studies with a strong theoretical rationale or definitive studies applicable to some but not all hospitals.
Data from Sehulster L, Chinn RY. Guidelines for environmental infection control in health-care facilities. Recommendations of CDC and the Healthcare Infection Control Practices Advisory Committee (HICPAC). MMWR Recomm Rep 2003;52(RR–10):1–42; and Tablan OC, Anderson LJ, Besser R, et al. Guidelines for preventing health-care–associated pneumonia, 2003: recommendations of CDC and the Healthcare Infection Control Practices Advisory Committee. MMWR Recomm Rep 2004;53(RR–3):1–36.

- Phase III: the late phase (>100 days post-HSCT). Risk of infection is dictated by chronic GVHD and it treatment. Pathogens are primarily CMV, varicella-zoster virus, encapsulated bacteria, and *Aspergillus* spp.

As a general measure, avoidance of certain foods has been recommended to reduce exposure to fungi, primarily during the high-risk period of neutropenia (such as during receipt of conditioning therapy).[27] These foods include unpasteurized dairy products, cheeses made from mold cultures, uncooked eggs, meat, fish, tofu, unwashed vegetables, and fruits.[27]

Invasive aspergillosis displays a bimodal distribution, with increasing number of cases of late-onset disease (>40 days post-HSCT) that is associated with immunosuppression for chronic GVHD.[22,170,171] A similar pattern of late-onset disease has also been noted with invasive infection with Zygomycetes and *Fusarium* spp in HSCT recipients.[136,172] Educating the patient in minimizing exposure to *Aspergillus* spp and pathogenic molds outside the hospital is important. However, because the risk of exposure within the hospital and community settings cannot be eliminated, novel strategies such as the use of antifungal prophylaxis may be necessary.

Chemoprophylaxis for Fungal Infection in HSCT Patients

Prevention of invasive candidiasis

Antifungal chemoprophylaxis during the preengraftment period of neutropenia and mucositis can prevent the dissemination of endogenous *Candida* spp from the

Box 3
Recommendations for prevention and control of health care–associated pulmonary aspergillosis

Recommendations	Rating Category[a]
Staff education	
• Educate HCWs about infection control procedures to reduce HCA-PA	II
Surveillance	
• Conduct surveillance for HCA-PA in patients in severely immunocompromised patients[b]	IA
• Monitor for HCA-PA by surveillance and periodic review of microbiologic and histopathologic data	II
• Do not perform routine surveillance cultures of patients or devices	IB
• Monitor ventilation status of PE and maintain appropriate standards	IB
Specialized care units for high-risk patients	
• Provide a PE for care of allogeneic HSCT recipients	IB
• Do not routinely use LAF in the PE	IB
• No recommendation for a PE for autologous HSCT and SOT recipients	UR
• Minimize the time high-risk patients are outside the PE for procedures	II
High-risk patients to wear N95 respirators outside the PE during ongoing construction	
No recommendation for type of mask outside the PE when no construction	
When case of aspergillosis occurs	
• Assess if health care related or community acquired	II
Determine if there is an increase in the number of cases of HCA-PA and length of hospital stay	IB
Determine if there is ventilation deficiency in the PE	IB
• If not health care related, continue routine maintenance as mentioned earlier	IB
• If health care related, conduct epidemiologic investigation to identify and eliminate source	IB
• Use EPA-registered antifungal biocide for decontamination of structural materials	IB

Abbreviations: EPA, environmental protection agency; HCA-PA, health care–associated pulmonary aspergillosis; HCW, healthcare worker; HSCT, hematopoeitic stem cell transplantation; LAF, laminar airflow; PE, protective environment; SOT, solid organ transplantation.
[a] Ratings category: IA, strongly recommended for all hospitals and supported by well-designed experimental or epidemiologic evidence; IB, strongly recommended for all hospitals and viewed as effective by experts because of strong rationale and suggestive evidence; II, suggested for implementation in many hospitals, supported by suggestive clinical or epidemiologic studies with a strong theoretical rationale or definitive studies applicable to some but not all hospitals; UR, unresolved, practices for which insufficient evidence or consensus regarding efficacy exists.
[b] Severely immunocompromised patients, those with absolute neutrophil counts <500/mm^3 × 2 weeks or <100/mm^3 × 1 week, eg, HSCT and SOT recipients and patients on prolonged high-dose steroids.
Data from Sehulster L, Chinn RY. Guidelines for environmental infection control in health-care facilities. Recommendations of CDC and the Healthcare Infection Control Practices Advisory Committee (HICPAC). MMWR Recomm Rep 2003;52(RR-10):1–42; and Tablan OC, Anderson LJ, Besser R, et al. Guidelines for preventing health-care–associated pneumonia, 2003: recommendations of CDC and the Healthcare Infection Control Practices Advisory Committee. MMWR Recomm Rep 2004;53(RR-3):1–36.

gastrointestinal tract of patients. Fluconazole started with the conditioning regimen and continued till resolution of neutropenia is effective in the prevention of invasive candidiasis and is recommended.[27,173,174] Other agents shown to be effective in the prophylaxis of candidiasis in HSCT recipients are micafungin,[175] posaconazole,[176] and itraconazole.[177] Chemoprophylaxis of invasive candidiasis in nonneutropenic patients may be effective in carefully selected ICU patients,[178,179] including liver[180] and pancreas[181] transplant recipients and patients with a gastrointestinal leak.[182] Clinical variables that are predictive of identifying ICU patients at high risk for invasive candidiasis, and thus potential candidates for prophylaxis, include patients receiving systemic antibiotic steroids, immunosuppressive agents, or *total parenteral nutrition*; patients undergoing dialysis; patients with a CVC; patients with pancreatitis; and patients who have had recent major surgery.[38]

Prevention of Aspergillosis

Given the prolonged duration of the risk for aspergillosis in HSCT recipients with chronic GVHD, recent guidelines recommend the use of an antimold prophylaxis.[27,162] Antifungal agents that have demonstrated efficacy in the prevention of mold infections in HSCT recipients include posaconazole,[176] itraconazole,[177,183] and aerosolized liposomal amphotericin B.[184] The duration of prophylaxis is not clearly defined but is generally dictated by the severity of GVHD and the intensity of immunosuppression used to treat GVHD.[162] The use of antiaspergillus prophylaxis has also been recommended for patients with acute myelogenous leukemia and myelodysplastic syndromes during periods of prolonged neutropenia.

Prevention of Pneumocystis pneumonia

Pneumocystis pneumonia prophylaxis is recommended for HSCT and SOT recipients during high-risk periods of immunosuppression, especially the first 100 days after transplantation. The preferred regimen is trimethoprim-sulfamethoxazole, with alternative agents being aerosolized pentamidine, oral dapsone, and oral atovaquone.[27]

SUMMARY

Nosocomial fungal infections, especially candidemias and invasive aspergillosis, can result in significant morbidity and mortality in the critically ill and severely immunocompromised patients. Implementation of recommended infection control strategies can prevent catheter-related candidemia and minimize exposure of severely immunocompromised patients to airborne *Aspergillus* spores within the hospital environment. In select patient populations at high risk for invasive fungal infections, antifungal prophylaxis should be considered.

REFERENCES

1. Fridkin SK. The changing face of fungal infections in health care settings. Clin Infect Dis 2005;41(10):1455–60.
2. Segal BH, Kwon-Chung J, Walsh TJ, et al. Immunotherapy for fungal infections. Clin Infect Dis 2006;42(4):507–15.
3. Hidron AI, Edwards JR, Patel J, et al. NHSN annual update: antimicrobial-resistant pathogens associated with healthcare-associated infections: annual summary of data reported to the National Healthcare Safety Network at the Centers for Disease Control and Prevention, 2006–2007. Infect Control Hosp Epidemiol 2008;29(11):996–1011.

4. Wisplinghoff H, Bischoff T, Tallent SM, et al. Nosocomial bloodstream infections in US hospitals: analysis of 24,179 cases from a prospective nationwide surveillance study. Clin Infect Dis 2004;39(3):309–17.

5. Vonberg RP, Gastmeier P. Nosocomial aspergillosis in outbreak settings. J Hosp Infect 2006;63(3):246–54.

6. Bouza E, Munoz P. Epidemiology of candidemia in intensive care units. Int J Antimicrob Agents 2008;32(Suppl 2):S87–91.

7. Tortorano AM, Caspani L, Rigoni AL, et al. Candidosis in the intensive care unit: a 20-year survey. J Hosp Infect 2004;57(1):8–13.

8. Trick WE, Fridkin SK, Edwards JR, et al. Secular trend of hospital-acquired candidemia among intensive care unit patients in the United States during 1989–1999. Clin Infect Dis 2002;35(5):627–30.

9. Pappas PG, Rex JH, Lee J, et al. A prospective observational study of candidemia: epidemiology, therapy, and influences on mortality in hospitalized adult and pediatric patients. Clin Infect Dis 2003;37(5):634–43.

10. Pfaller MA, Diekema DJ. Epidemiology of invasive candidiasis: a persistent public health problem. Clin Microbiol Rev 2007;20(1):133–63.

11. Almirante B, Rodriguez D, Park BJ, et al. Epidemiology and predictors of mortality in cases of *Candida* bloodstream infection: results from population-based surveillance, Barcelona, Spain, from 2002 to 2003. J Clin Microbiol 2005;43(4):1829–35.

12. Hajjeh RA, Sofair AN, Harrison LH, et al. Incidence of bloodstream infections due to *Candida* species and in vitro susceptibilities of isolates collected from 1998 to 2000 in a population-based active surveillance program. J Clin Microbiol 2004;42(4):1519–27.

13. Marchetti O, Bille J, Fluckiger U, et al. Epidemiology of candidemia in Swiss tertiary care hospitals: secular trends, 1991–2000. Clin Infect Dis 2004;38(3):311–20.

14. Richet HM, McNeil MM, Edwards MC, et al. Cluster of *Malassezia furfur* pulmonary infections in infants in a neonatal intensive-care unit. J Clin Microbiol 1989;27(6):1197–200.

15. Falagas ME, Apostolou KE, Pappas VD. Attributable mortality of candidemia: a systematic review of matched cohort and case-control studies. Eur J Clin Microbiol Infect Dis 2006;25(7):419–25.

16. Zaoutis TE, Argon J, Chu J, et al. The epidemiology and attributable outcomes of candidemia in adults and children hospitalized in the United States: a propensity analysis. Clin Infect Dis 2005;41(9):1232–9.

17. Morgan J, Meltzer MI, Plikaytis BD, et al. Excess mortality, hospital stay, and cost due to candidemia: a case-control study using data from population-based candidemia surveillance. Infect Control Hosp Epidemiol 2005;26(6):540–7.

18. Smith PB, Morgan J, Benjamin JD, et al. Excess costs of hospital care associated with neonatal candidemia. Pediatr Infect Dis J 2007;26(3):197–200.

19. Wilson LS, Reyes CM, Stolpman M, et al. The direct cost and incidence of systemic fungal infections. Value Health 2002;5(1):26–34.

20. Dasbach EJ, Davies GM, Teutsch SM. Burden of aspergillosis-related hospitalizations in the United States. Clin Infect Dis 2000;31(6):1524–8.

21. Neofytos D, Horn D, Anaissie E, et al. Epidemiology and outcome of invasive fungal infection in adult hematopoietic stem cell transplant recipients: analysis of Multicenter Prospective Antifungal Therapy (PATH) Alliance registry. Clin Infect Dis 2009;48(3):265–73.

22. Upton A, Kirby KA, Carpenter P, et al. Invasive aspergillosis following hemato-poietic cell transplantation: outcomes and prognostic factors associated with mortality. Clin Infect Dis 2007;44(4):531–40.

23. Boyce JM, Pittet D. Guideline for hand hygiene in health-care settings. Recom-mendations of the Healthcare Infection Control Practices Advisory Committee and the HICPAC/SHEA/APIC/IDSA Hand Hygiene Task Force. Society for Healthcare Epidemiology of America/Association for Professionals in Infection Control/Infectious Diseases Society of America. MMWR Recomm Rep 2002; 51(RR–16):1–45 [quiz: CE41–4].

24. O'Grady NP, Alexander M, Dellinger EP, et al. Guidelines for the prevention of intravascular catheter-related infections. Centers for Disease Control and Prevention. MMWR Recomm Rep 2002;51(RR–10):1–29.

25. Marschall J, Mermel LA, Classen D, et al. Strategies to prevent central line-asso-ciated bloodstream infections in acute care hospitals. Infect Control Hosp Epi-demiol 2008;29(Suppl 1):S22–30 [Erratum in: Infect Control Hosp Epidemiol 2009;30:815].

26. Sehulster L, Chinn RY. Guidelines for environmental infection control in health-care facilities. Recommendations of CDC and the Healthcare Infection Control Practices Advisory Committee (HICPAC). MMWR Recomm Rep 2003; 52(RR–10):1–42.

27. Tomblyn M, Chiller T, Einsele H, et al. Guidelines for preventing infectious complications among hematopoietic cell transplantation recipients: a global perspective. Biol Blood Marrow Transplant 2009;15(10):1143–238.

28. Nucci M, Anaissie E. Revisiting the source of candidemia: skin or gut? Clin Infect Dis 2001;33(12):1959–67.

29. Blumberg HM, Jarvis WR, Soucie JM, et al. Risk factors for candidal blood-stream infections in surgical intensive care unit patients: the NEMIS prospective multicenter study. The National Epidemiology of Mycosis Survey. Clin Infect Dis 2001;33(2):177–86.

30. Vazquez JA, Sanchez V, Dmuchowski C, et al. Nosocomial acquisition of Candida albicans: an epidemiologic study. J Infect Dis 1993;168(1):195–201.

31. Vazquez JA, Dembry LM, Sanchez V, et al. Nosocomial Candida glabrata colo-nization: an epidemiologic study. J Clin Microbiol 1998;36(2):421–6.

32. Berger C, Frei R, Gratwohl A, et al. Bottled lemon juice – a cryptic source of inva-sive Candida infections in the immunocompromised host. J Infect Dis 1988; 158(3):654–5.

33. Kuhn DM, Ghannoum MA. Candida biofilms: antifungal resistance and emerging therapeutic options. Curr Opin Investig Drugs 2004;5(2):186–97.

34. Kuhn DM, Chandra J, Mukherjee PK, et al. Comparison of biofilms formed by Candida albicans and Candida parapsilosis on bioprosthetic surfaces. Infect Immun 2002;70(2):878–88.

35. Asmundsdottir LR, Erlendsdottir H, Haraldsson G, et al. Molecular epidemiology of candidemia: evidence of clusters of smoldering nosocomial infections. Clin Infect Dis 2008;47(2):e17–24.

36. Kao AS, Brandt ME, Pruitt WR, et al. The epidemiology of candidemia in two United States cities: results of a population-based active surveillance. Clin Infect Dis 1999;29(5):1164–70.

37. Leon C, Ruiz-Santana S, Saavedra P, et al. A bedside scoring system ("Candida score") for early antifungal treatment in nonneutropenic critically ill patients with Candida colonization. Crit Care Med 2006;34(3):730–7.

38. Ostrosky-Zeichner L, Sable C, Sobel J, et al. Multicenter retrospective development and validation of a clinical prediction rule for nosocomial invasive candidiasis in the intensive care setting. Eur J Clin Microbiol Infect Dis 2007; 26(4):271–6.

39. Pfaller MA, Diekema DJ, Gibbs DL, et al. Results from the ARTEMIS DISK Global Antifungal Surveillance Study, 1997 to 2005: an 8.5-year analysis of susceptibilities of Candida species and other yeast species to fluconazole and voriconazole determined by CLSI standardized disk diffusion testing. J Clin Microbiol 2007;45(6):1735–45.

40. Abi-Said D, Anaissie E, Uzun O, et al. The epidemiology of hematogenous candidiasis caused by different Candida species. Clin Infect Dis 1997;24(6):1122–8.

41. Horn DL, Neofytos D, Anaissie EJ, et al. Epidemiology and outcomes of candidemia in 2019 patients: data from the prospective antifungal therapy alliance registry. Clin Infect Dis 2009;48(12):1695–703.

42. Hachem R, Hanna H, Kontoyiannis D, et al. The changing epidemiology of invasive candidiasis: Candida glabrata and Candida krusei as the leading causes of candidemia in hematologic malignancy. Cancer 2008;112(11):2493–9.

43. Rangel-Frausto MS, Wiblin T, Blumberg HM, et al. National epidemiology of mycoses survey (NEMIS): variations in rates of bloodstream infections due to Candida species in seven surgical intensive care units and six neonatal intensive care units. Clin Infect Dis 1999;29(2):253–8.

44. Parry MF, Grant B, Yukna M, et al. Candida osteomyelitis and diskitis after spinal surgery: an outbreak that implicates artificial nail use. Clin Infect Dis 2001;32(3): 352–7.

45. Pfaller MA. Nosocomial candidiasis: emerging species, reservoirs, and modes of transmission. Clin Infect Dis 1996;22(Suppl 2):S89–94.

46. Robert F, Lebreton F, Bougnoux ME, et al. Use of random amplified polymorphic DNA as a typing method for Candida albicans in epidemiological surveillance of a burn unit. J Clin Microbiol 1995;33(9):2366–71.

47. Gupta N, Haque A, Lattif AA, et al. Epidemiology and molecular typing of Candida isolates from burn patients. Mycopathologia 2004;158(4):397–405.

48. Fanello S, Bouchara JP, Jousset N, et al. Nosocomial Candida albicans acquisition in a geriatric unit: epidemiology and evidence for person-to-person transmission. J Hosp Infect 2001;47(1):46–52.

49. Malani A, Hmoud J, Chiu L, et al. Candida glabrata fungemia: experience in a tertiary care center. Clin Infect Dis 2005;41(7):975–81.

50. Marr KA. The changing spectrum of candidemia in oncology patients: therapeutic implications. Curr Opin Infect Dis 2000;13(6):615–20.

51. Lin MY, Carmeli Y, Zumsteg J, et al. Prior antimicrobial therapy and risk for hospital-acquired Candida glabrata and Candida krusei fungemia: a case-case-control study. Antimicrob Agents Chemother 2005;49(11):4555–60.

52. Levy I, Rubin LG, Vasishtha S, et al. Emergence of Candida parapsilosis as the predominant species causing candidemia in children. Clin Infect Dis 1998; 26(5):1086–8.

53. Lupetti A, Tavanti A, Davini P, et al. Horizontal transmission of Candida parapsilosis candidemia in a neonatal intensive care unit. J Clin Microbiol 2002;40(7): 2363–9.

54. Saiman L, Ludington E, Pfaller M, et al. Risk factors for candidemia in neonatal intensive care unit patients. The National Epidemiology of Mycosis Survey study group. Pediatr Infect Dis J 2000;19(4):319–24.

55. Almirante B, Rodriguez D, Cuenca-Estrella M, et al. Epidemiology, risk factors, and prognosis of *Candida parapsilosis* bloodstream infections: case-control population-based surveillance study of patients in Barcelona, Spain, from 2002 to 2003. J Clin Microbiol 2006;44(5):1681–5.

56. Saiman L, Ludington E, Dawson JD, et al. Risk factors for *Candida* species colonization of neonatal intensive care unit patients. Pediatr Infect Dis J 2001;20(12): 1119–24.

57. Bonassoli LA, Bertoli M, Svidzinski TI. High frequency of *Candida parapsilosis* on the hands of healthy hosts. J Hosp Infect 2005;59(2):159–62.

58. van Asbeck EC, Huang YC, Markham AN, et al. *Candida parapsilosis* fungemia in neonates: genotyping results suggest healthcare workers hands as source, and review of published studies. Mycopathologia 2007;164(6):287–93.

59. Kuhn DM, Mikherjee PK, Clark TA, et al. *Candida parapsilosis* characterization in an outbreak setting. Emerg Infect Dis 2004;10(6):1074–81.

60. Clark TA, Slavinski SA, Morgan J, et al. Epidemiologic and molecular characterization of an outbreak of *Candida parapsilosis* bloodstream infections in a community hospital. J Clin Microbiol 2004;42(10):4468–72.

61. Levin AS, Costa SF, Mussi NS, et al. *Candida parapsilosis* fungemia associated with implantable and semi-implantable central venous catheters and the hands of healthcare workers. Diagn Microbiol Infect Dis 1998;30(4):243–9.

62. Trofa D, Gacser A, Nosanchuk JD. *Candida parapsilosis*, an emerging fungal pathogen. Clin Microbiol Rev 2008;21(4):606–25.

63. Sipsas NV, Lewis RE, Tarrand J, et al. Candidemia in patients with hematologic malignancies in the era of new antifungal agents (2001–2007): stable incidence but changing epidemiology of a still frequently lethal infection. Cancer 2009; 115(20):4745–52.

64. Kontoyiannis DP, Vaziri I, Hanna HA, et al. Risk factors for *Candida tropicalis* fungemia in patients with cancer. Clin Infect Dis 2001;33(10):1676–81.

65. Pfaller MA, Diekema DJ, Gibbs DL, et al. *Candida krusei*, a multidrug-resistant opportunistic fungal pathogen: geographic and temporal trends from the ARTEMIS DISK Antifungal Surveillance Program, 2001 to 2005. J Clin Microbiol 2008;46(2):515–21.

66. Abbas J, Bodey GP, Hanna HA, et al. *Candida krusei* fungemia. An escalating serious infection in immunocompromised patients. Arch Intern Med 2000; 160(17):2659–64.

67. Hope W, Morton A, Eisen DP. Increase in prevalence of nosocomial non-*Candida albicans* candidaemia and the association of *Candida krusei* with fluconazole use. J Hosp Infect 2002;50(1):56–65.

68. Playford EG, Marriott D, Nguyen Q, et al. Candidemia in nonneutropenic critically ill patients: risk factors for non-albicans *Candida* spp. Crit Care Med 2008;36(7):2034–9.

69. Masala L, Luzzati R, Maccacaro L, et al. Nosocomial cluster of *Candida guillermondii* fungemia in surgical patients. Eur J Clin Microbiol Infect Dis 2003;22(11): 686–8.

70. Minces LR, Ho KS, Veldkamp PJ, et al. *Candida rugosa*: a distinctive emerging cause of candidaemia. A case report and review of the literature. Scand J Infect Dis 2009;41(11–12):892–7.

71. Colombo AL, Melo AS, Crespo Rosas RF, et al. Outbreak of *Candida rugosa* candidemia: an emerging pathogen that may be refractory to amphotericin B therapy. Diagn Microbiol Infect Dis 2003;46(4):253–7.

72. Barber GR, Brown AE, Kiehn TE, et al. Catheter-related *Malassezia furfur* fungemia in immunocompromised patients. Am J Med 1993;95(4):365–70.
73. Chang HJ, Miller HL, Watkins N, et al. An epidemic of *Malassezia pachydermatis* in an intensive care nursery associated with colonization of health care workers' pet dogs. N Engl J Med 1998;338(11):706–11.
74. Chryssanthou E, Broberger U, Petrini B. *Malassezia pachydermatis* fungaemia in a neonatal intensive care unit. Acta Paediatr 2001;90(3):323–7.
75. Krcmery V Jr, Mateicka F, Kunova A, et al. Hematogenous trichosporonosis in cancer patients: report of 12 cases including 5 during prophylaxis with itraconazol. Support Care Cancer 1999;7(1):39–43.
76. Kontoyiannis DP, Torres HA, Chagua M, et al. Trichosporonosis in a tertiary care cancer center: risk factors, changing spectrum and determinants of outcome. Scand J Infect Dis 2004;36(8):564–9.
77. Girmenia C, Pagano L, Martino B, et al. Invasive infections caused by *Trichosporon* species and *Geotrichum capitatum* in patients with hematological malignancies: a retrospective multicenter study from Italy and review of the literature. J Clin Microbiol 2005;43(4):1818–28.
78. Cawley MJ, Braxton GR, Haith LR, et al. *Trichosporon beigelii* infection: experience in a regional burn center. Burns 2000;26(5):483–6.
79. Wolf DG, Falk R, Hacham M, et al. Multidrug-resistant *Trichosporon asahii* infection of nongranulocytopenic patients in three intensive care units. J Clin Microbiol 2001;39(12):4420–5.
80. Ruan SY, Chien JY, Hsueh PR. Invasive trichosporonosis caused by *Trichosporon asahii* and other unusual *Trichosporon* species at a medical center in Taiwan. Clin Infect Dis 2009;49(1):e11–7.
81. Hajjeh RA, Warnock DW. Counterpoint: invasive aspergillosis and the environment – rethinking our approach to prevention. Clin Infect Dis 2001;33(9):1549–52.
82. Patterson JE, Zidouh A, Miniter P, et al. Hospital epidemiologic surveillance for invasive aspergillosis: patient demographics and the utility of antigen detection. Infect Control Hosp Epidemiol 1997;18(2):104–8.
83. Antoniadou A. Outbreaks of zygomycosis in hospitals. Clin Microbiol Infect 2009;15(Suppl 5):55–9.
84. Anaissie EJ, Kuchar RT, Rex JH, et al. Fusariosis associated with pathogenic *Fusarium* species colonization of a hospital water system: a new paradigm for the epidemiology of opportunistic mold infections. Clin Infect Dis 2001;33(11):1871–8.
85. Alvarez M, Lopez Ponga B, Rayon C, et al. Nosocomial outbreak caused by *Scedosporium prolificans* (*inflatum*): four fatal cases in leukemic patients. J Clin Microbiol 1995;33(12):3290–5.
86. Guerrero A, Torres P, Duran MT, et al. Airborne outbreak of nosocomial *Scedosporium prolificans* infection. Lancet 2001;357(9264):1267–8.
87. Fox BC, Chamberlin L, Kulich P, et al. Heavy contamination of operating room air by *Penicillium* species: identification of the source and attempts at decontamination. Am J Infect Control 1990;18(5):300–6.
88. Krishnan S, Manavathu EK, Chandrasekar PH. *Aspergillus flavus*: an emerging non-fumigatus *Aspergillus* species of significance. Mycoses 2009;52(3):206–22.
89. Pegues CF, Daar ES, Murthy AR. The epidemiology of invasive pulmonary aspergillosis at a large teaching hospital. Infect Control Hosp Epidemiol 2001;22(6):370–4.

90. Heinemann S, Symoens F, Gordts B, et al. Environmental investigations and molecular typing of *Aspergillus flavus* during an outbreak of postoperative infections. J Hosp Infect 2004;57(2):149–55.
91. Denning DW, Marinus A, Cohen J, et al. An EORTC multicentre prospective survey of invasive aspergillosis in haematological patients: diagnosis and therapeutic outcome. EORTC Invasive Fungal Infections Cooperative Group. J Infect 1998;37(2):173–80.
92. Lortholary O, Ascioglu S, Moreau P, et al. Invasive aspergillosis as an opportunistic infection in nonallografted patients with multiple myeloma: a European Organization for Research and Treatment of Cancer/Invasive Fungal Infections Cooperative Group and the Intergroupe Francais du Myelome. Clin Infect Dis 2000;30(1):41–6.
93. Paterson DL, Singh N. Invasive aspergillosis in transplant recipients. Medicine (Baltimore) 1999;78(2):123–38.
94. Williamson EC, Millar MR, Steward CG, et al. Infections in adults undergoing unrelated donor bone marrow transplantation. Br J Haematol 1999;104(3):560–8.
95. Marr KA, Carter RA, Boeckh M, et al. Invasive aspergillosis in allogeneic stem cell transplant recipients: changes in epidemiology and risk factors. Blood 2002;100(13):4358–66.
96. Barnes PD, Marr KA. Risks, diagnosis and outcomes of invasive fungal infections in haematopoietic stem cell transplant recipients. Br J Haematol 2007;139(4):519–31.
97. Singh N. Invasive aspergillosis in organ transplant recipients: new issues in epidemiologic characteristics, diagnosis, and management. Med Mycol 2005;43(Suppl 1):S267–70.
98. Singh N, Avery RK, Munoz P, et al. Trends in risk profiles for and mortality associated with invasive aspergillosis among liver transplant recipients. Clin Infect Dis 2003;36(1):46–52.
99. Woitas RP, Rockstroh JK, Theisen A, et al. Changing role of invasive aspergillosis in AIDS–a case control study. J Infect 1998;37(2):116–22.
100. Libanore M, Prini E, Mazzetti M, et al. Invasive Aspergillosis in Italian AIDS patients. Infection 2002;30(6):341–5.
101. Wallace JM, Lim R, Browdy BL, et al. Risk factors and outcomes associated with identification of *Aspergillus* in respiratory specimens from persons with HIV disease. Pulmonary Complications of HIV Infection Study Group. Chest 1998;114(1):131–7.
102. Wallace MR, Kanak RJ, Newton JA, et al. Invasive aspergillosis in patients with AIDS. Clin Infect Dis 1994;19(1):222.
103. Segal BH, Romani LR. Invasive aspergillosis in chronic granulomatous disease. Med Mycol 2009;47(Suppl 1):S282–90.
104. Meersseman W, Lagrou K, Maertens J, et al. Invasive aspergillosis in the intensive care unit. Clin Infect Dis 2007;45(2):205–16.
105. Meersseman W, Van Wijngaerden E. Invasive aspergillosis in the ICU: an emerging disease. Intensive Care Med 2007;33(10):1679–81.
106. Vandewoude KH, Blot SI, Benoit D, et al. Invasive aspergillosis in critically ill patients: attributable mortality and excesses in length of ICU stay and ventilator dependence. J Hosp Infect 2004;56(4):269–76.
107. Cornillet A, Camus C, Nimubona S, et al. Comparison of epidemiological, clinical, and biological features of invasive aspergillosis in neutropenic and nonneutropenic patients: a 6-year survey. Clin Infect Dis 2006;43(5):577–84.

108. Meersseman W, Vandecasteele SJ, Wilmer A, et al. Invasive aspergillosis in critically ill patients without malignancy. Am J Respir Crit Care Med 2004;170(6):621–5.
109. Garnacho-Montero J, Amaya-Villar R, Ortiz-Leyba C, et al. Isolation of *Aspergillus* spp. from the respiratory tract in critically ill patients: risk factors, clinical presentation and outcome. Crit Care 2005;9(3):R191–9.
110. Denning DW. Aspergillosis in "nonimmunocompromised" critically ill patients. Am J Respir Crit Care Med 2004;170(6):580–1.
111. Anaissie EJ, Costa SF. Nosocomial aspergillosis is waterborne. Clin Infect Dis 2001;33(9):1546–8.
112. Anaissie EJ, Stratton SL, Dignani MC, et al. Pathogenic *Aspergillus* species recovered from a hospital water system: a 3-year prospective study. Clin Infect Dis 2002;34(6):780–9.
113. Anaissie EJ, Stratton SL, Dignani MC, et al. Pathogenic molds (including *Aspergillus* species) in hospital water distribution systems: a 3-year prospective study and clinical implications for patients with hematologic malignancies. Blood 2003;101(7):2542–6.
114. Bryce EA, Walker M, Scharf S, et al. An outbreak of cutaneous aspergillosis in a tertiary-care hospital. Infect Control Hosp Epidemiol 1996;17(3):170–2.
115. McCarty JM, Flam MS, Pullen G, et al. Outbreak of primary cutaneous aspergillosis related to intravenous arm boards. J Pediatr 1986;108(5 Pt 1):721–4.
116. Leenders A, van Belkum A, Janssen S, et al. Molecular epidemiology of apparent outbreak of invasive aspergillosis in a hematology ward. J Clin Microbiol 1996;34(2):345–51.
117. Leenders AC, van Belkum A, Behrendt M, et al. Density and molecular epidemiology of *Aspergillus* in air and relationship to outbreaks of *Aspergillus* infection. J Clin Microbiol 1999;37(6):1752–7.
118. Morris G, Kokki MH, Anderson K, et al. Sampling of *Aspergillus* spores in air. J Hosp Infect 2000;44(2):81–92.
119. Debeaupuis JP, Sarfati J, Chazalet V, et al. Genetic diversity among clinical and environmental isolates of *Aspergillus fumigatus*. Infect Immun 1997;65(8):3080–5.
120. Kidd SE, Ling LM, Meyer W, et al. Molecular epidemiology of invasive aspergillosis: lessons learned from an outbreak investigation in an Australian hematology unit. Infect Control Hosp Epidemiol 2009;30(12):1223–6.
121. Balajee SA, Borman AM, Brandt ME, et al. Sequence-based identification of *Aspergillus, Fusarium*, and *Mucorales* species in the clinical mycology laboratory: where are we and where should we go from here? J Clin Microbiol 2009;47(4):877–84.
122. Rees JR, Pinner RW, Hajjeh RA, et al. The epidemiological features of invasive mycotic infections in the San Francisco Bay Area, 1992–1993: results of population-based laboratory active surveillance. Clin Infect Dis 1998;27(5):1138–47.
123. Torres-Narbona M, Guinea J, Martinez-Alarcon J, et al. Impact of zygomycosis on microbiology workload: a survey study in Spain. J Clin Microbiol 2007;45(6):2051–3.
124. Roden MM, Zaoutis TE, Buchanan WL, et al. Epidemiology and outcome of zygomycosis: a review of 929 reported cases. Clin Infect Dis 2005;41(5):634–53.
125. Rogers TR. Treatment of zygomycosis: current and new options. J Antimicrob Chemother 2007;61:I35–9.
126. Christiaens G, Hayette MP, Jacquemin D, et al. An outbreak of *Absidia corymbifera* infection associated with bandage contamination in a burns unit. J Hosp Infect 2005;61(1):88.

127. Garner D, Machin K. Investigation and management of an outbreak of mucormycosis in a paediatric oncology unit. J Hosp Infect 2008;70(1):53–9.
128. Abzug MJ, Gardner S, Globe MP, et al. Heliport-associated nosocomial mucormycoses. Infect Control Hosp Epidemiol 1992;13(6):325–6.
129. Levy V, Rio B, Bazarbachi A, et al. Two cases of epidemic mucormycosis infection in patients with acute lymphoblastic leukemia. Am J Hematol 1996;52(1):64–5.
130. Mitchell SJ, Gray J, Morgan ME, et al. Nosocomial infection with *Rhizopus microsporus* in preterm infants: association with wooden tongue depressors. Lancet 1996;348(9025):441–3.
131. Maravi-Poma E, Rodriguez-Tudela JL, de Jalon JG, et al. Outbreak of gastric mucormycosis associated with the use of wooden tongue depressors in critically ill patients. Intensive Care Med 2004;30(4):724–8.
132. LeMaile-Williams M, Burwell LA, Salisbury D, et al. Outbreak of cutaneous *Rhizopus arrhizus* infection associated with karaya ostomy bags. Clin Infect Dis 2006;43(9):E83–8.
133. Cheng VCC, Chan JFW, Ngan AHY, et al. Outbreak of intestinal infection due to *Rhizopus microsporus*. J Clin Microbiol 2009;47(9):2834–43.
134. Chang DC, Grant GB, O'Donnell K, et al. Multistate outbreak of *Fusarium* keratitis associated with use of a contact lens solution. JAMA 2006;296(8):953–63.
135. Saw SM, Ooi PL, Tan DTH, et al. Risk factors for contact lens-related *Fusarium* keratitis – a case-control study in Singapore. Arch Ophthalmol 2007;125(5):611–7.
136. Nucci M, Marr KA, Queiroz-Telles F, et al. *Fusarium* infection in hematopoietic stem cell transplant recipients. Clin Infect Dis 2004;38(9):1237–42.
137. Sampathkumar P, Paya CV. *Fusarium* infection after solid-organ transplantation. Clin Infect Dis 2001;32(8):1237–40.
138. O'Donnell K, Sutton DA, Rinaldi MG, et al. Genetic diversity of human pathogenic members of the *Fusarium oxysporum* complex inferred from multilocus DNA sequence data and amplified fragment length polymorphism analyses: evidence for the recent dispersion of a geographically widespread clonal lineage and nosocomial origin. J Clin Microbiol 2004;42(11):5109–20.
139. Ruiz-Diez B, Martin-Diez F, Rodriguez-Tudela JL, et al. Use of random amplification of polymorphic DNA (RAPD) and PCR-fingerprinting for genotyping a *Scedosporium prolificans* (*inflatum*) outbreak in four leukemic patients. Curr Microbiol 1997;35(3):186–90.
140. Tarkkanen A, Raivio V, Anttila VJ, et al. Fungal endophthalmitis caused by *Paecilomyces variotii* following cataract surgery: a presumed operating room air-conditioning system contamination. Acta Ophthalmol Scand 2004;82(2):232–5.
141. Orth B, Frei R, Itin PH, et al. Outbreak of invasive mycoses caused by *Paecilomyces lilacinus* from a contaminated skin lotion. Ann Intern Med 1996;125(10):799–806.
142. Proia LA, Hayden MK, Kammeyer PL, et al. *Phialemonium*: an emerging mold pathogen that caused 4 cases of hemodialysis-associated endovascular infection. Clin Infect Dis 2004;39(3):373–9.
143. Clark T, Huhn GD, Conover C, et al. Outbreak of bloodstream infection with the mold *Phialemonium* among patients receiving dialysis at a hemodialysis unit. Infect Control Hosp Epidemiol 2006;27(11):1164–70.
144. Rao CY, Pachucki C, Cali S, et al. Contaminated product water as the source of *Phialemonium curvatum* bloodstream infection among patients undergoing hemodialysis. Infect Control Hosp Epidemiol 2009;30(9):840–7.

145. Strahilevitz J, Rahav G, Schroers HJ, et al. An outbreak of *Phialemonium* infective endocarditis linked to intracavernous penile injections for the treatment of impotence. Clin Infect Dis 2005;40(6):781–6.

146. Kainer MA, Keshavarz H, Jensen BJ, et al. Saline-filled breast implant contamination with *Curvularia* species among women who underwent cosmetic breast augmentation. J Infect Dis 2005;192(1):170–7.

147. Vargas SL, Ponce CA, Gigliotti F, et al. Transmission of *Pneumocystis carinii* DNA from a patient with *P. carinii* pneumonia to immunocompetent contact health care workers. J Clin Microbiol 2000;38(4):1536–8.

148. Miller RF, Ambrose HE, Novelli V, et al. Probable mother-to-infant transmission of *Pneumocystis carinii f. sp. hominis* infection. J Clin Microbiol 2002;40(4): 1555–7.

149. Schmoldt S, Bader L, Huber I, et al. Molecular evidence of *Pneumocystis jirovecii* transmission among 16 patients after kidney transplantation. Int J Med Microbiol 2007;297:64–5.

150. Mueller NJ, Haeberli L, Joos B, et al. Molecular evidence of interhuman transmission in an outbreak of *Pneumocystis jirovecii* pneumonia in renal transplant recipients. Am J Transplant 2009;9:331.

151. Goto N, Yazaki H, Uchida K, et al. Major outbreak of *Pneumocystis jiroveci* pneumonia in a renal transplant unit. Am J Transplant 2009;9:640.

152. Hocker B, Wendt C, Nahimana A, et al. Molecular evidence of *Pneumocystis* transmission in pediatric transplant unit. Emerg Infect Dis 2005;11(2):330–2.

153. de Boer MG, Bruijnesteijn van Coppenraet LE, Gaasbeek A, et al. An outbreak of *Pneumocystis jiroveci* pneumonia with 1 predominant genotype among renal transplant recipients: interhuman transmission or a common environmental source? Clin Infect Dis 2007;44(9):1143–9.

154. Hughes WT. Transmission of *Pneumocystis* species among renal transplant recipients. Clin Infect Dis 2007;44(9):1150–1.

155. Rabodonirina L, Vanhems P, Couray-Targe S, et al. Molecular evidence of interhuman transmission of *Pneumocystis* pneumonia among renal transplant recipients hospitalized with HIV-infected patients. Emerg Infect Dis 2004;10(10): 1766–73.

156. Gianella S, Haeberli L, Joos B, et al. Molecular evidence of interhuman transmission in an outbreak of *Pneumocystis jirovecii* pneumonia in renal transplant recipients. Swiss Med Wkly 2009;139(9–10):5S.

157. Wohl AR, Simon P, Hu YW, et al. The role of person-to-person transmission in an epidemiologic study of *Pneumocystis carinii* pneumonia. AIDS 2002;16(13): 1821–5.

158. Manoloff ES, Francioli P, Taffe P, et al. Risk for *Pneumocystis carinii* transmission among patients with pneumonia: a molecular epidemiology study. Emerg Infect Dis 2003;9(1):132–4.

159. Tablan OC, Anderson LJ, Besser R, et al. Guidelines for preventing health-care–associated pneumonia, 2003: recommendations of CDC and the Healthcare Infection Control Practices Advisory Committee. MMWR Recomm Rep 2004; 53(RR–3):1–36.

160. Pronovost P, Needham D, Berenholtz S, et al. An intervention to decrease catheter-related bloodstream infections in the ICU. N Engl J Med 2006; 355(26):2725–32.

161. Berenholtz SM, Pronovost PJ, Lipsett PA, et al. Eliminating catheter-related bloodstream infections in the intensive care unit. Crit Care Med 2004;32(10): 2014–20.

162. Walsh TJ, Anaissie EJ, Denning DW, et al. Treatment of aspergillosis: clinical practice guidelines of the infectious diseases society of America. Clin Infect Dis 2008;46(3):327–60.
163. Mayhall C, editor. Hospital epidemiology and infection control. 3rd edition. Philadelphia: Lippincott Williams and Wilkins; 2004. p. 1549–75.
164. Guidelines for design and construction of hospital and health care facilities. Washington, DC: American Institute of Architects Facility Guidelines Institute AAoAfH, US Dept of Health & Human Services; 2006.
165. Goebes MD, Baron EJ, Mathews KL, et al. Effect of building construction on *Aspergillus* concentrations in a hospital. Infect Control Hosp Epidemiol 2008; 29(5):462–4.
166. Hansen D, Blahout B, Benner D, et al. Environmental sampling of particulate matter and fungal spores during demolition of a building on a hospital area. Int J Med Microbiol 2007;297:40.
167. Nihtinen A, Anttila VJ, Richardson M, et al. The utility of intensified environmental surveillance for pathogenic moulds in a stem cell transplantation ward during construction work to monitor the efficacy of HEPA filtration. Bone Marrow Transplant 2007;40(5):457–60.
168. Sautour M, Sixt N, Dalle F, et al. Prospective survey of indoor fungal contamination in hospital during a period of building construction. J Hosp Infect 2007; 67(4):367–73.
169. Sixt N, Dalle F, Lafon I, et al. Reduced fungal contamination of the indoor environment with the Plasmair (TM) system (Airinspace). J Hosp Infect 2007;65(2):156–62.
170. Grow WB, Moreb JS, Roque D, et al. Late onset of invasive *Aspergillus* infection in bone marrow transplant patients at a university hospital. Bone Marrow Transplant 2002;29(1):15–9.
171. Marr KA, Carter RA, Crippa F, et al. Epidemiology and outcome of mould infections in hematopoietic stem cell transplant recipients. Clin Infect Dis 2002;34(7): 909–17.
172. Nucci M, Marr KA, Queiroz-Telles F, et al. *Fusarium* infection in hematopoietic stem cell transplant (HSCT) recipients. Blood 2002;100(11):440b.
173. Goodman JL, Winston DJ, Greenfield RA, et al. A controlled trial of fluconazole to prevent fungal infections in patients undergoing bone marrow transplantation. N Engl J Med 1992;326(13):845–51.
174. Slavin MA, Osborne B, Adams R, et al. Efficacy and safety of fluconazole prophylaxis for fungal infections after marrow transplantation – a prospective, randomized, double-blind study. J Infect Dis 1995;171(6):1545–52.
175. van Burik JA, Ratanatharathorn V, Stepan DE, et al. Micafungin versus fluconazole for prophylaxis against invasive fungal infections during neutropenia in patients undergoing hematopoietic stem cell transplantation. Clin Infect Dis 2004;39(10):1407–16.
176. Ullmann AJ, Lipton JH, Vesole DH, et al. Posaconazole or fluconazole for prophylaxis in severe graft-versus-host disease. N Engl J Med 2007;356:335 [Erratum in: N Engl J Med. 2007;357(4):428].
177. Winston DJ, Maziarz RT, Chandrasekar PH, et al. Intravenous and oral itraconazole versus intravenous and oral fluconazole for long-term antifungal prophylaxis in allogeneic hematopoietic stem-cell transplant recipients. A multicenter, randomized trial. Ann Intern Med 2003;138(9):705–13.
178. Pappas PG, Rex JH, Sobel JD, et al. Guidelines for treatment of candidiasis. Clin Infect Dis 2004;38(2):161–89.

179. Playford EG, Webster AC, Sorrell TC, et al. Systematic review and meta-analysis of antifungal agents for preventing fungal infections in liver transplant recipients. Eur J Clin Microbiol Infect Dis 2006;25(9):549–61.
180. Winston DJ, Pakrasi A, Busuttil RW. Prophylactic fluconazole in liver transplant recipients. A randomized, double-blind, placebo-controlled trial. Ann Intern Med 1999;131(10):729–37.
181. Benedetti E, Gruessner AC, Troppmann C, et al. Intra-abdominal fungal infections after pancreatic transplantation: incidence, treatment, and outcome. J Am Coll Surg 1996;183(4):307–16.
182. Eggimann P, Francioli P, Bille J, et al. Fluconazole prophylaxis prevents intra-abdominal candidiasis in high-risk surgical patients. Crit Care Med 1999; 27(6):1066–72.
183. Marr KA, Crippa F, Leisenring W, et al. Itraconazole vs. fluconazole for antifungal prophylaxis in allogeneic HSCT recipients: results of a randomized trial. Blood 2002;100(11):215a.
184. Rijnders BJ, Cornelissen JJ, Slobbe L, et al. Aerosolized liposomal amphotericin B for the prevention of invasive pulmonary aspergillosis during prolonged neutropenia: a randomized, placebo-controlled trial. Clin Infect Dis 2008;46(9): 1401–8.

Health Care–Acquired Viral Respiratory Diseases

William P. Goins, MD, MPH[a], H. Keipp Talbot, MD, MPH[b],
Thomas R. Talbot, MD, MPH[b],*

KEYWORDS

- Influenza • Respiratory syncytial virus • Pandemic
- Nosocomial infection • Health care–acquired infection

Health care–associated viral respiratory infections, common among hospitalized children, also occur among adults and institutionalized persons and result in increased patient morbidity, mortality, and health care costs. Approximately 20% of patients with health care–associated pneumonia have viral respiratory infections, with 70% of these infections caused by adenovirus, influenza virus, parainfluenza virus, and respiratory syncytial virus (RSV).[1] These infections typically reflect the level of viral activity within the community.[1,2] This article focuses on the epidemiology, transmission, and control of health care–associated RSV and influenza virus.

RSV

Epidemiology

RSV is the most common cause of pneumonia and bronchiolitis in infants[3] and is a common pathogen in older and high-risk adults.[4] Outbreaks of RSV have occurred in a variety of pediatric and adult health care settings.[5–12] Secondary attack rates of

Funding support: H.K.T. received funding support from the National Institute of Allergy and Infectious Diseases grant K23 AI074863–03 and a T. Franklin Williams Scholarship Award, which is funded by Atlantic Philanthropies, Inc, the John A. Hartford Foundation, the Association of Specialty Professors, and the Infectious Diseases Society of America.

Disclosures: W.P.G. has no disclosures. H.K.T. has received funding from Protein Sciences Corporation, Wyeth, Sanofi Pasteur, VaxInnate, the National Institutes of Health, and the Centers for Disease Control and Prevention (CDC). T.R.T. has received influenza vaccine donated by Sanofi Pasteur for a study funded by the CDC and serves as a consultant for Joint Commission Resources.

[a] Division of Infectious Diseases, Department of Medicine, Baylor College of Medicine, 1709 Dryden Road, BCM 620, Suite 6.15, Houston, TX 77030, USA

[b] Division of Infectious Diseases, Department of Medicine, Vanderbilt University School of Medicine, 1161 21st Avenue South, A–2200 MCN, Nashville, TN 37232, USA

* Corresponding author.

E-mail address: tom.talbot@vanderbilt.edu

Infect Dis Clin N Am 25 (2011) 227–244
doi:10.1016/j.idc.2010.11.010
0891-5520/11/$ – see front matter © 2011 Elsevier Inc. All rights reserved.

19% to 45% have been reported among patients when limited or no infection control measures are implemented.[6,7,13] Similarly, 34% to 56% of personnel on infant wards may become infected.[6,7,13] Most infected personnel are symptomatic, and many may be absent from work.[14] However, many symptomatic personnel continue to work, and asymptomatic shedding of RSV occurs in 15% to 20% of infected personnel.[14] Therefore, these infected personnel may play a role in transmission to hospitalized patients.[7,15]

Transmission

Transmission of RSV occurs via inoculation of the eye and nose[16] and through close contact via direct inoculation of large droplets or self-inoculation after touching contaminated fomites.[17] RSV has been recovered on countertops for up to 6 hours, rubber gloves for up to 2 hours, and on cloth gowns and hands for 15 to 60 minutes after contamination with infected nasal secretions.[18] The duration of viral shedding among hospitalized infants averages 6.7 days but can be as long as 21 days.[19] Infants with a lower respiratory tract disease and a compromised immune status have more prolonged shedding and shed greater quantities of the virus.[19] Finally, because neonates may have atypical illness, the disease may be overlooked, thus facilitating transmission.[7]

Prevention and Control

Numerous studies have evaluated the effectiveness of various measures to prevent RSV transmission among patients and personnel. Studies evaluating the use of gowns and masks to prevent RSV transmission have shown mixed results. In a before-after design, the rate of health care–associated RSV infection among infants during the period when gowns and masks were routinely worn by staff was not statistically different from the rate during the period when gowns and masks were not used (32% vs 41%).[20] A second prospective randomized study failed to show that the use of gowns and masks prevented respiratory illness among personnel.[21] One possibility for the apparent ineffectiveness of gowns and masks to prevent health care–associated RSV transmission in earlier studies is the lack of adherence to the use of personal protective equipment (PPE) among staff. In another study, as compliance with the use of gowns and gloves increased from 39% to 95%, the incidence of health care–associated RSV decreased from 6.4 to 3.1 per 1000 patient-days.[22] However, others have expressed concerns that gowns and gloves may facilitate transmission by serving as fomites, particularly given the prolonged survival of RSV on rubber gloves compared to skin.[18] One study of 7 Canadian pediatric hospitals actually noted an increased risk of transmission with the use of gowns, thought to be because of the decreased adherence to other infection control measures related to the overuse of gowns.[23]

Another possibility for the lack of benefit from gowns and masks in RSV transmission may be the failure to protect against the eye as a portal of entry. Two studies suggested that wearing eye protection is beneficial.[24,25] In a before-after study, staff wore disposable eye-nose goggles during routine care of patients with RSV and the proportion of susceptible infants and staff developing the infection was 6% and 5%, respectively.[24] When the goggles were no longer used, the proportions increased to 43% and 34%. Similarly, only 5% of health care workers who wore goggles and masks when caring for RSV-infected children developed the infection compared with 61% of health care workers who did not wear PPE.[25]

Other studies have evaluated the effectiveness of a variety of measures in combination to prevent health care–associated RSV infection. A combination of both cohort nursing and routine use of gowns and gloves significantly reduced RSV transmission compared with either intervention alone.[26] An intervention consisting of education, hand washing, consistent use of gowns and gloves, isolating or cohorting patients, restriction of visitors, and cohort nursing was associated with a 39% reduction in health care–associated RSV.[27] Transmission of RSV in a special care nursery ended after instituting cohort nursing; active surveillance; patient cohorting; a strict policy limiting visitation in the winter; construction of segregate areas; and the use of gown, gloves, and masks during all patient contact.[28] A similar intervention that included isolation or cohorting infected infants, hand washing, use of gowns, cohort nursing, isolation of asymptomatic high-risk infants, and limitation of visitors seemed to be effective in reducing transmission among infants from 45% in the previous year to 19% following the intervention.[13]

Recommendations for RSV infection control

In addition to the standard precautions, the Centers for Disease Control and Prevention (CDC) recommend contact precautions to prevent health care–associated RSV (**Tables 1** and **2**).[1,29] Contact precautions should continue for the duration of illness but may be extended for immunocompromised patients because of prolonged viral shedding. Additional interventions to prevent health care–associated RSV include cohort nursing and the exclusion from the hospital of ill health care workers and visitors.

Rapid RSV antigen screening has also been proposed to prevent health care–associated RSV. Rapid screening of symptomatic children on admission resulted in a greater than 50% decrease in the proportion of health care–associated RSV infections.[30] Screening of all pediatric admissions, regardless of the presence of symptoms, with cohorting of infected patients reduced the incidence of health care–associated RSV from 7.2 to less than 1 per 1000 patient-days.[31] However, rapid antigen detection is an insensitive method for diagnosing RSV infection in adults.[32]

Several reports described the administration of palivizumab to susceptible infants to control outbreaks in neonatal intensive care units (ICU).[9,33] Palivizumab is a humanized mouse IgG monoclonal antibody that is effective in preventing hospitalizations caused by RSV infections.[34,35] Palivizumab is licensed for the prevention of RSV infection in infants born at 35 weeks' gestation or earlier, in infants with chronic lung disease of prematurity, or in infants with congenital heart disease. However, at present there are no guidelines for the use of this drug in controlling outbreaks of health care–associated RSV infections. Furthermore, use of palivizumab for controlling hospital outbreaks is limited to case reports, often with implementation of other infection control measures. There are no trials that have evaluated the individual effect of palivizumab in controlling nosocomial RSV transmission.

SEASONAL INFLUENZA
Epidemiology

Influenza infects approximately 5% to 20% of the US population annually, resulting in 226,000 hospitalizations and 36000 deaths.[36,37] Transmission of influenza has been reported in a variety of pediatric and adult health care settings, and health care workers may be often implicated in the outbreaks.[37] Health care workers are at an increased risk of acquiring influenza because of exposure to infection in both the health care and community settings,[38] and they often fail to recognize that they are infected. In one study, 23% of health care workers demonstrated serologic evidence of influenza infection during a single influenza season; however, 59% of those infected could not recall influenzalike illness (ILI) and 28% were asymptomatic.[39]

Table 1
Precautions for preventing transmission of respiratory infections

Precautions	Component	Recommendation
Standard	Hand hygiene	Wash hands with soap and water or use an alcohol-based hand rub: Before and after contact with a patient After contact with respiratory secretions After contact with potentially contaminated items in the patient's vicinity, including equipments and environmental surfaces
	Respiratory hygiene	Instruct staff and visitors with signs and symptoms of a respiratory infection to: Cover their mouth and nose when sneezing or coughing Perform hand hygiene after soiling hands with respiratory secretions Wear masks when tolerated Maintain spatial separation from others (>0.9 m) when in common waiting areas, if possible
	Gloves	Wear when contact with respiratory secretions could occur
	Gowns	Wear during procedures and activities when contact of clothing or exposed skin with respiratory secretions is anticipated
	Masks and eye protection	Wear during procedures and activities likely to generate splashes or sprays of respiratory secretions
Contact[a]	Patient placement	Place patient in a single-patient room, if possible, or cohort with other patients infected with the same organism Limit patient movement to medically necessary purposes
	Gloves and gowns	Wear upon entering room whenever contact is likely with the patient, patient's respiratory secretions, or potentially contaminated items in the patient's vicinity, including equipments and environmental surfaces
	Masks and eye protection	As per the standard precautions
Droplet[a]	Patient placement	Place patient in a single-patient room, if possible, or cohort with other patients infected with the same organism Limit patient movement to medically necessary purposes, and patients should wear a mask and follow respiratory hygiene during transport
	Gloves, gowns, and eye protection	As per the standard precautions.
	Masks	Wear a surgical mask on entering room if close contact (eg, <0.9 m) with the patient is anticipated

(continued on next page)

Table 1 (continued)		
Precautions	**Component**	**Recommendation**
Airborne[a]	Patient placement	Place infected patients in a single-patient airborne infection isolation room[b] Patient movement should be limited to medically necessary purposes, and patients should wear a mask and follow respiratory hygiene during transport
	Gloves, gowns, and eye protection	As per the standard precautions
	Masks	Wear a fit-tested N95 respirator before room entry

[a] Contact, droplet, and airborne precautions include hand hygiene and respiratory hygiene as per the standard precautions.
[b] Airborne infection isolation room consists of negative pressure relative to the surrounding area and 6 to 12 air changes per hour, and the air is exhausted directly to the outside or recirculated through high-efficiency particulate air filtration before return.
From Siegel JD, Rhinehart E, Jackson M, et al. 2007 guideline for isolation precautions: preventing transmission of infectious agents in health care settings. Available at: http://www.cdc.gov/hicpac/2007IP/2007isolationPrecautions.html.

Asymptomatic and mildly symptomatic health care workers may also shed influenza virus, potentially transmitting the infection to patients or other personnel.[40] Finally, ill health care workers often continue to work despite the presence of symptoms.[41,42]

Secondary attack rates as high as 50% have been reported among both health care workers and patients.[38] Such high attack rates can result in health care worker absenteeism and the subsequent disruption of patient care, particularly during periods of increased health care use. A 2003-2004 survey of 221 hospital epidemiologists from all regions in the United States indicated that a substantial number of hospitals experienced staffing shortages (34%), bed shortages (28%), ICU bed shortages (43%), and diversion of patients (9%) during the peak influenza activity.[43]

Transmission

The typical incubation period for influenza in healthy volunteers is 1 to 3 days.[40] Viral shedding begins before the appearance of symptoms and within the first 24 hours after inoculation, peaks on the second day after inoculation, and usually declines rapidly thereafter.[44,45] The virus is typically no longer detectable after 6 to 10 days after inoculation. However, prolonged viral shedding has been documented by culture for up to 21 days in children[46] and up to 44 days in immunocompromised adults.[47] Furthermore, the quantity of virus shed correlates with the severity of illness.[44,45] The potential for hospitalized children and immunocompromised or severely ill adults to shed greater amounts of virus and for prolonged durations has important implications on influenza transmission within the health care setting.

Transmission via contact with fomites has been also suggested by the recovery of influenza on porous surfaces (eg, cloth, paper, tissues) for 8 to 12 hours and on nonporous surfaces (eg, steel, plastic) for 24 to 48 hours after inoculation.[48] Transfer of virus from environmental surfaces to hands was also demonstrated. Likewise, influenza virus has been recovered from 23% and 53% of inanimate objects present in day care centers during fall and spring months, respectively.[49] Although no study has clearly documented infection resulting from contact with fomites, one nursing home outbreak suggested a link between the hands of health care workers and influenza transmission.[50] Nurses routinely had ungloved contact with patients' oral secretions

Table 2
Infection control recommendations for viral respiratory pathogens

Common measures for reducing transmission in the health care setting

Hand hygiene

Respiratory hygiene/cough etiquette

Standard precautions

Restrict ill visitors[a]

Restrict ill personnel for caring for patients at high risk for complications from infection

Cohort nursing

Prompt diagnosis of respiratory infections among patients by rapid diagnostic tests[b]

Restrict elective admissions of patients during outbreaks in the community and/or facility

Surveillance for an increase in activity of viral infections within the community

Measures for reducing transmission of specific pathogens in the health care setting

Intervention	RSV	Adenovirus	Parainfluenza Virus	Influenza Seasonal	2009 H1N1	H5N1
Precautions:						
Contact	•	•	•		•	•
Droplet	—	•	—	•	—	—
Airborne	—	—	—	○[c]	○[c]	•
Eye protection	—	—	—	—	—	•
Vaccination of personnel	—	—	—	•	•	—
Chemoprophylaxis	○[d]	—	—	○[e]	○[e]	•

Closed circles (•) denote recommended measures. Open circles (○) denote measures recommended in certain circumstances.

[a] Institutions may restrict only young children and/or screen all visitors for illness by using a trained health care worker to assess for signs and symptoms or by using an educational patient information list to advise ill visitors.

[b] To control outbreaks, institutions may perform preadmission screening of patients for infection.

[c] The CDC recommends health care workers wear respiratory protection such as an N95 respirator during aerosol-generating procedures.

[d] In addition to other infection control measures, palivizumab prophylaxis of high-risk infants has been used to control outbreaks in the neonatal intensive care unit.

[e] During a facility outbreak of influenza, administer antiviral chemoprophylaxis to all patients in the involved unit, regardless of the vaccination status, and to unvaccinated personnel working in the involved unit. If feasible, administer facility-wide chemoprophylaxis for all residents in long-term care facilities. Chemoprophylaxis may also be administered to personnel when the outbreak strain is not well matched by the vaccine.

while administering medications and tube feedings. Thirty-eight percent of patients who were tube fed or frequently suctioned contracted influenza compared to 13% of other patients ($P = .08$), and no illness was detected among personnel.

Several studies have suggested that influenza may be transmitted by droplet nuclei (<5 μm) or small particle aerosols between infected and noninfected animals. Transmission of influenza occurred among ferrets in wire mesh cages separated by at least 1.5 m despite the susceptible ferrets being placed at a higher elevation.[51] To control for air currents in the laboratory, additional experiments were conducted using cages connected by an S- or a U-shaped duct. Infection occurred at low air speeds using both types of ducts, which prevented transmission of coarse droplets. Murine experiments provided similar results on the effect of ventilation and physical separation. Twenty-four hours after their exposure to an aerosol spray of influenza, infected mice were placed in the same cage as noninfected mice in a closed chamber for 24 hours.[52] Transmission was not affected by physical separation with a wire screen. However, transmission was inversely correlated with airflow. Because transmission was affected by air currents rather than by separation, the investigators concluded that droplet nuclei are the principal means of influenza transmission. Recovery of infectious particles less than 10 μm from the air surrounding the infected mice provided additional support for droplet nuclei transmission.[53]

Studies have also examined the ability to infect humans with influenza via experimental aerosol. Twenty-three healthy men were exposed to various doses of influenza via aerosolized particles of 1 to 3 μm.[54] Half of the men with absent titers before inoculation became infected with a dose that was 40- to 500-fold lower than that required to cause disease when administered by nasal drops.[40] Albeit to a lesser extent, another study similarly demonstrated that smaller doses were required to cause illness among normal volunteers when administered as an aerosol rather than as nasal drops.[55] Although the lower respiratory tract seems to be a more efficient route of infection than the upper respiratory tract, the proportion of natural influenza infections acquired by aerosols remains unknown.

Several studies demonstrated that the size of particles produced during various activities is within the range in which deposition in the lower respiratory tract can occur. Loudon and Roberts[56] demonstrated that 8% and 50% of particles produced during talking and coughing, respectively, were less than 5 μm in diameter. Papineni and Rosenthal[57] similarly demonstrated that 36% of exhaled particles were less than or equal to 1 μm in diameter but 80% to 90% of the total particle concentration consisted of particles less than or equal to 1 μm in diameter. Furthermore, a recent sampling of aerosol particles in an emergency room demonstrated that 53% of influenza virus particles detected by polymerase chain reaction were less than or equal to 4 μm in diameter.[58]

Two commonly cited epidemiologic studies have suggested that influenza may be spread by droplet nuclei. During the 1957-1958 influenza outbreak, 150 patients with tuberculosis were housed in a building at a Veterans Administration Hospital with upper air ultraviolet radiation.[59] An additional 250 patients with tuberculosis were housed in a separate building with nonradiated air. Serologic evidence of influenza infection was found in only 2% of the patients in the radiated building compared with 19% of the patients in the nonradiated building and 18% of personnel. Patients in both radiated and nonradiated building were equally exposed to the infected personnel, and all patients were assumed susceptible because the influenza strain was new and antigenically distinct from the previous strains. Because upper air radiation would not disinfect large respiratory droplets, transmission of influenza via droplet nuclei was proposed. However, the possibility that influenza was not introduced into the radiated building cannot be excluded. The second outbreak occurred in 1977 when 54 persons aboard a commercial airliner were grounded for 3 hours during which time the ventilation system was inoperative.[60] A single index person became ill within 15 minutes after boarding. Within 72 hours, 72% of the remaining passengers developed ILI. The high illness rates and epidemic curve suggest airborne transmission from a single point source. However, passengers were allowed to move about the plane freely and the index patient sat immediately adjacent to the lavatory and galley areas, so droplet and contact transmission cannot be excluded.

Conversely, other observations have suggested that large respiratory droplets (>10 μm) play a more significant role in transmission than droplet nuclei. During the 1958-1959 pandemic, a single patient with influenza was hospitalized in a general medical ward before the appearance of influenza in the community[61] During the next 3 days 16 patients and staff became ill. The epidemic curve suggested an initial source with subsequent person-to-person spread. Furthermore, no patient in a single-occupancy room was infected as would have been expected of airborne transmission. Similarly, most health care–associated influenza cases at the University of Rochester Medical Center were reported in patients housed in the same room adjacent to the patients with the same infection.[62] Patients across the hall from infected patients were less likely to acquire influenza despite open doors and nonutilization of airborne infection isolation rooms (AIIR). Salgado and colleagues[38] reported that health care–associated influenza was rare, although most patients were placed in private, positive pressure rooms. Finally, the lack of reports of outbreak of health care–associated influenza during annual influenza seasons supports the lack of widespread airborne transmission in health care settings. Although transmission by droplet nuclei may play a role in certain conditions, large respiratory droplets are likely the primary mode of transmission within a health care setting, an environment in which frequent air changes and exhaust ventilation occur.

Prevention and Control

Guidelines for seasonal influenza infection control
In addition to the standard precautions, the CDC recommends implementation of droplet precautions to prevent health care–associated influenza (see **Tables 1** and **2**).[1,29] Droplet precautions should continue for at least 5 days but may be extended for immunocompromised patients because of prolonged viral shedding. In addition to vaccination and antiviral chemoprophylaxis, interventions to prevent health care–associated influenza include early identification of suspected patients with source control (ie wearing a mask), cohort nursing, exclusion of ill health care workers and visitors, and rapid diagnostic testing of symptomatic children. Similar to RSV infection, rapid antigen detection is an insensitive method for diagnosing influenza infection in most adults.[63]

Influenza vaccination of health care workers
Vaccination is the most effective strategy for preventing influenza and is recommended for health care workers for several reasons.[64] First, vaccination has been shown to be 88% effective in preventing laboratory-confirmed influenza in health care workers (**Fig. 1**).[65] Second, health care worker absenteeism can stress the health system during influenza epidemics, and influenza vaccination has resulted in a statistically significant 28% to 41% decrease in work days lost because of respiratory illness (see **Fig. 1**).[66,67] Third, health care workers have frequent contact with patients at high risk for complications from influenza and may transmit influenza to susceptible patients, resulting in increased patient morbidity and mortality. Improved health care worker vaccination rates have been linked with decreased health care–associated influenza among patients and personnel.[68] Three cluster randomized trials demonstrated that health care worker vaccination was associated with a statistically significant decrease in mortality among nursing home patients (see **Fig. 1**).[69–71] Similarly, health care worker vaccination led to a nonsignificant 13% decrease in patient mortality during a mild influenza season in a fourth cluster randomized trial.[72] However, the study was likely underpowered and the vaccination rate was higher than expected among patients in both arms (>80%) and among staff in the control arm (31%). Nevertheless, a multivariate analysis showed that staff vaccination was a significant independent predictor of patient mortality (odds ratio 0.80; 95% confidence interval, 0.67–0.97).

Despite recommendations for vaccination and evidence supporting its use, only 45% of health care workers were vaccinated during the 2007–2008 season.[73] Barriers

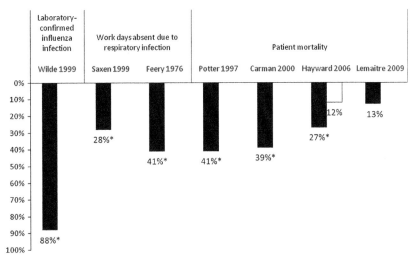

Fig. 1. Percentage reduction in noted outcomes in health care workers receiving influenza vaccination. Values marked by an asterisk were statistically significant (P<.05) compared to those of an unvaccinated control group. Patient mortality data from the study by Hayward and colleagues[71] was obtained in 2 different seasons. A multivariate analysis by Lemaitre and colleagues[72] showed that staff vaccination was a significant independent predictor of patient mortality. (*Adapted from* Talbot TR, Bradley SE, Cosgrove SE, et al. Influenza vaccination of healthcare workers and vaccine allocation for healthcare workers during vaccine shortages. Infect Control Hosp Epidemiol 2005;26(11):883; with permission.)

to vaccination include fear of needles and vaccine side effects, inconvenience, failure of the employer to pay for the vaccine, doubt about the risk of influenza, perceived lack of vaccine effectiveness, and failure to recognize the role of health care workers in transmission of influenza to patients.[37,74] Strategies for improving acceptance of vaccine by health care workers have been published.[37,74] Many health care organizations have adopted a policy requiring annual influenza vaccination of all health care workers as a condition of employment because of the patient safety ramifications of an unvaccinated workforce.[75] The state of New York and the US Department of Defense have adopted similar requirements.[75,76] However, mandatory vaccination programs should only be put into practice after careful planning and full assessment of the logistic barriers to successful implementation.

Chemoprophylaxis

Data from observational studies and controlled trials support recommendations to provide antiviral chemoprophylaxis to residents in long-term care facilities, regardless of their vaccination status, during an institutional influenza outbreak.[77] Moreover, because outbreaks may continue when prophylaxis is limited to residents of affected wards, facility-wide chemoprophylaxis is ideal.[78] Chemoprophylaxis may also be considered for unvaccinated staff or when the vaccine is likely to be ineffective because of strain mismatch; however, no studies have evaluated the effect of employee chemoprophylaxis on patient outcomes.[78] In the setting of an institutional outbreak, chemoprophylaxis should be continued for 14 days or for 7 to 10 days after the onset of symptoms in the last person infected, whichever is longer.[77,78]

After an unprotected exposure to someone with influenza, postexposure chemoprophylaxis can be considered for unvaccinated health care workers or for patients at high risk for complications from influenza.[79] Chemoprophylaxis is not recommended if more than 48 hours have elapsed since the last contact with the infectious person or if the exposure occurred outside that person's infectious period, defined as 1 day before symptom onset until 24 hours after fever resolution. Postexposure chemoprophylaxis should be continued for 10 days after the last known exposure. At present, the neuraminidase inhibitors, oseltamivir and zanamivir, are the recommended drugs for influenza chemoprophylaxis, but these recommendations may change depending on the antiviral resistance of circulating influenza strains.[79]

PANDEMIC INFLUENZA

Pandemic influenza results when a novel viral strain to which the population has little or no immunity achieves the ability to spread easily between humans, resulting in rapid spread across several continents. A novel virus emerges as a result of reassortment of human influenza genes with those of avian or swine strains. During the past century, there have been 4 major pandemics: 1918–1919 Spanish influenza (H1N1), 1957–1958 Asian influenza (H2N2), 1968–1969 Hong Kong influenza (H3N2), and 2009 H1N1 influenza A. Although there may be some differences between the seasonal and pandemic influenza strains, many of the basic infection control recommendations for the prevention of health care–associated seasonal influenza also apply for pandemic strains.

The 2009 Influenza A (H1N1) Pandemic

On April 21, 2009, the CDC reported that 2 children in California were infected with a novel influenza A (H1N1) virus of swine origin[80] and the virus subsequently spread rapidly across the globe. Transmission among health care workers has been reported.[81] According to the CDC's interim recommendations to prevent the transmission of 2009 H1N1 influenza in health care settings, contact precautions and eye protection should be used for all patient care activities in addition to the standard precautions (see **Tables 1** and **2**).[82] At the outset of the pandemic, the CDC also recommended that all health care workers entering the room should wear respiratory protection at least as protective as a fit-tested disposable N95 respirator. Patients should be placed in single-patient rooms. However, for aerosol-generating procedures (eg, bronchoscopy, intubation, open airway suctioning), patients should be placed in an AIIR with negative pressure air handling and 6 to 12 air changes per hour. These enhanced precautions (eg, use of N95 respirators during routine care) were the result of the lack of an effective vaccine for 2009 H1N1 influenza at the pandemic's outset, the increased susceptibility of patients to 2009 H1N1 influenza, and the limited knowledge of the severity and transmissibility of the novel virus. Transmission-based precautions should be continued for 7 days after onset of illness or until resolution of symptoms.[82] Similar to seasonal influenza, postexposure chemoprophylaxis for 10 days should be considered for patients at high risk for complications from influenza and health care workers exposed to a patient infected with 2009 H1N1 influenza.[79]

Following the CDC recommendations, the Society for Healthcare Epidemiology of America, the Healthcare Infection Control Practices Advisory Committee, and the World Health Organization released recommendations for infection control precautions for 2009 H1N1 influenza infections, endorsing the same practices as recommended for seasonal influenza, which did not include the use of N95 respirators by health care workers during routine patient care.[83–85] Use of an N95 respirator and an AIIR, however, were still recommended for aerosol-generating procedures because of an increased risk of transmission to health care workers during these procedures. To help resolve doubts about the optimal use of PPE for 2009 H1N1 influenza infections, an Institute of Medicine panel was convened in August 2009. The panel recommended that health care workers wear a fit-tested N95 respirator when caring for patients infected with 2009 H1N1 influenza because of experimental studies demonstrating droplet nuclei as a possible route of transmission and studies demonstrating the efficacy of respirators and masks.[86] However, the panel did not consider availability of respirators and other implementation issues when issuing the recommendation. Furthermore, a subsequent randomized controlled trial demonstrated that masks were noninferior to respirators in protecting health care workers from influenza.[87] Although a second randomized controlled trial initially reported a difference between respirators and surgical masks, adjustment for the clustered randomization and multiple outcomes yielded no statistical significance between the 2 types of respiratory protection.[88] In 2010 the CDC updated the interim guidance on infection control measures for 2009 H1N1 influenza. Similar to seasonal influenza, the CDC now recommends that health care workers should adhere to droplet precautions for routine patient care. However, airborne precautions are still recommended for aerosol-generating procedures.[89]

Avian Influenza

A highly pathogenic avian influenza A (H5N1) virus was first reported to cause human infections in 1997 in China.[90] However, no other human infections were reported until the virus reemerged in Hong Kong in 2003. Since then, this virus has caused several hundred infections worldwide with a case-fatality rate of 60%.[91] Several family clusters of disease suggest probable human-to-human transmission.[92,93] A study of the 1997 cluster indicated that 3.7% of exposed health care workers had serologic evidence of infection[94]; however, more recent serologic surveys have not identified any cases among exposed personnel despite the lack of appropriate infection control precautions.[95,96] The inefficient spread among humans may be explained by recent evidence showing a preferential binding of the H5N1 virus in the lower respiratory tract of humans.[97]

Avian influenza should be suspected in patients presenting with a severe respiratory illness within 10 days of travel to a country with avian influenza activity.[98] Contact and airborne precautions should be used for patients with suspected avian influenza (see **Tables 1** and **2**).[99] In addition, all health care workers should wear eye protection when entering the patient's room. Transmission-based precautions for avian influenza should be continued for 14 days after the onset of illness. Antiviral chemoprophylaxis for 7 to 10 days should also be considered for health care workers with unprotected exposures.[100]

OTHER VIRUSES
Adenovirus

Health care–associated outbreaks of respiratory tract infections caused by adenovirus have been reported from pediatric and adult health care settings.[101–104] Attack rates among patients have ranged from 15% to 56%.[101,102] Health care workers were often infected, and many continued to provide patient care while ill.[103] Similar to influenza, adenovirus is transmitted through large respiratory droplets. Transmission also occurs via self-inoculation after contact with contaminated fomites because adenovirus can survive on nonporous environmental surfaces for up to 49 days.[105] In one outbreak, adenovirus was recovered from 19% of environmental surfaces before terminal cleaning.[104] In addition to the standard precautions, the CDC recommends contact and droplet precautions to prevent health care–associated adenovirus infection (see **Tables 1** and **2**).[1,29]

Parainfluenza

Transmission of parainfluenza has been documented in pediatric wards,[5] neonatal nurseries,[8] and adult transplant units.[106] Transmission of parainfluenza is similar to that of RSV and primarily occurs by direct person-to-person contact. Parainfluenza can survive for up to 4 hours on porous surfaces and up to 10 hours on nonporous surfaces.[107] However, viral recovery from hand decreases rapidly, with only 5% detected after 10 minutes.[108] The CDC recommends contact precautions, in addition to standard precautions, for the prevention of health care–associated parainfluenza infection (see **Tables 1** and **2**).[1,29]

SUMMARY

Transmission of viral respiratory infections occurs in a variety of pediatric and adult health care settings, resulting in increased patient morbidity and health care costs. Transmission may occur via aerosol, large respiratory droplets, or self-inoculation after touching contaminated fomites. Different viruses have different modes of transmission, and prevention of transmission requires early recognition of symptomatic patients and prompt institution of appropriate transmission-based precautions in addition to adherence to basic infection control practices such as hand hygiene. In addition to administrative and environmental controls, influenza vaccination of health care workers is an effective means of prevention of health care–associated influenza infection.

REFERENCES

1. Tablan OC, Anderson LJ, Besser R, et al. Guidelines for preventing health-care-associated pneumonia, 2003: recommendations of CDC and the Healthcare Infection Control Practices Advisory Committee. MMWR Recomm Rep 2004; 53(RR-3):1–36.
2. Hall CB. Nosocomial viral respiratory infections: perennial weeds on pediatric wards. Am J Med 1981;70(3):670–6.
3. Shay DK, Holman RC, Newman RD, et al. Bronchiolitis-associated hospitalizations among US children, 1980–1996. JAMA 1999;282(15):1440–6.
4. Falsey AR, Hennessey PA, Formica MA, et al. Respiratory syncytial virus infection in elderly and high-risk adults. N Engl J Med 2005;352(17):1749–59.
5. Gardner PS, Court SD, Brocklebank JT, et al. Virus cross-infection in paediatric wards. Br Med J 1973;2(5866):571–5.
6. Hall CB, Douglas RG Jr, Geiman JM, et al. Nosocomial respiratory syncytial virus infections. N Engl J Med 1975;293(26):1343–6.
7. Hall CB, Kopelman AE, Douglas RG Jr, et al. Neonatal respiratory syncytial virus infection. N Engl J Med 1979;300(8):393–6.
8. Meissner HC, Murray SA, Kiernan MA, et al. A simultaneous outbreak of respiratory syncytial virus and parainfluenza virus type 3 in a newborn nursery. J Pediatr 1984;104(5):680–4.
9. Halasa NB, Williams JV, Wilson GJ, et al. Medical and economic impact of a respiratory syncytial virus outbreak in a neonatal intensive care unit. Pediatr Infect Dis J 2005;24(12):1040–4.

10. Guidry GG, Black-Payne CA, Payne DK, et al. Respiratory syncytial virus infection among intubated adults in a university medical intensive care unit. Chest 1991;100(5):1377–84.
11. Englund JA, Anderson LJ, Rhame FS. Nosocomial transmission of respiratory syncytial virus in immunocompromised adults. J Clin Microbiol 1991;29(1): 115–9.
12. Mathur U, Bentley DW, Hall CB. Concurrent respiratory syncytial virus and influenza A infections in the institutionalized elderly and chronically ill. Ann Intern Med 1980;93(1):49–52.
13. Hall CB, Geiman JM, Douglas RG Jr, et al. Control of nosocomial respiratory syncytial viral infections. Pediatrics 1978;62(5):728–32.
14. Hall CB. Nosocomial respiratory syncytial virus infections: the "Cold War" has not ended. Clin Infect Dis 2000;31(2):590–6.
15. Hall CB. Respiratory syncytial virus: its transmission in the hospital environment. Yale J Biol Med 1982;55(3/4):219–23.
16. Hall CB, Douglas RG Jr, Schnabel KC, et al. Infectivity of respiratory syncytial virus by various routes of inoculation. Infect Immun 1981;33(3):779–83.
17. Hall CB, Douglas RG Jr. Modes of transmission of respiratory syncytial virus. J Pediatr 1981;99(1):100–3.
18. Hall CB, Douglas RG Jr, Geiman JM. Possible transmission by fomites of respiratory syncytial virus. J Infect Dis 1980;141(1):98–102.
19. Hall CB, Douglas RG Jr, Geiman JM. Respiratory syncytial virus infections in infants: quantitation and duration of shedding. J Pediatr 1976;89(1):11–5.
20. Hall CB, Douglas RG Jr. Nosocomial respiratory syncytial viral infections. Should gowns and masks be used? Am J Dis Child 1981;135(6):512–5.
21. Murphy D, Todd JK, Chao RK, et al. The use of gowns and masks to control respiratory illness in pediatric hospital personnel. J Pediatr 1981;99(5): 746–50.
22. Leclair JM, Freeman J, Sullivan BF, et al. Prevention of nosocomial respiratory syncytial virus infections through compliance with glove and gown isolation precautions. N Engl J Med 1987;317(6):329–34.
23. Langley JM, LeBlanc JC, Wang EE, et al. Nosocomial respiratory syncytial virus infection in Canadian pediatric hospitals: a Pediatric Investigators Collaborative Network on Infections in Canada Study. Pediatrics 1997;100(6):943–6.
24. Gala CL, Hall CB, Schnabel KC, et al. The use of eye-nose goggles to control nosocomial respiratory syncytial virus infection. JAMA 1986;256(19):2706–8.
25. Agah R, Cherry JD, Garakian AJ, et al. Respiratory syncytial virus (RSV) infection rate in personnel caring for children with RSV infections. Routine isolation procedure vs routine procedure supplemented by use of masks and goggles. Am J Dis Child 1987;141(6):695–7.
26. Madge P, Paton JY, McColl JH, et al. Prospective controlled study of four infection-control procedures to prevent nosocomial infection with respiratory syncytial virus. Lancet 1992;340(8827):1079–83.
27. Macartney KK, Gorelick MH, Manning ML, et al. Nosocomial respiratory syncytial virus infections: the cost-effectiveness and cost-benefit of infection control. Pediatrics 2000;106(3):520–6.
28. Snydman DR, Greer C, Meissner HC, et al. Prevention of nosocomial transmission of respiratory syncytial virus in a newborn nursery. Infect Control Hosp Epidemiol 1988;9(3):105–8.
29. Siegel JD, Rhinehart E, Jackson M, et al. 2007 guideline for isolation precautions: preventing transmission of infectious agents in health care settings.

Available at: http://www.cdc.gov/hicpac/2007IP/2007isolationPrecautions.html. Accessed December 3, 2010.

30. Karanfil LV, Conlon M, Lykens K, et al. Reducing the rate of nosocomially transmitted respiratory syncytial virus. Am J Infect Control 1999;27(2):91–6.

31. Krasinski K, LaCouture R, Holzman RS, et al. Screening for respiratory syncytial virus and assignment to a cohort at admission to reduce nosocomial transmission. J Pediatr 1990;116(6):894–8.

32. Falsey AR, McCann RM, Hall WJ, et al. Evaluation of four methods for the diagnosis of respiratory syncytial virus infection in older adults. J Am Geriatr Soc 1996;44(1):71–3.

33. Kurz H, Herbich K, Janata O, et al. Experience with the use of palivizumab together with infection control measures to prevent respiratory syncytial virus outbreaks in neonatal intensive care units. J Hosp Infect 2008;70(3):246–52.

34. The IMpact-RSV Study Group. Palivizumab, a humanized respiratory syncytial virus monoclonal antibody, reduces hospitalization from respiratory syncytial virus infection in high-risk infants. Pediatrics 1998;102(3):531–7.

35. Feltes TF, Cabalka AK, Meissner HC, et al. Palivizumab prophylaxis reduces hospitalization due to respiratory syncytial virus in young children with hemodynamically significant congenital heart disease. J Pediatr 2003;143(4): 532–40.

36. Sullivan KM, Monto AS, Longini IM Jr. Estimates of the US health impact of influenza. Am J Public Health 1993;83(12):1712–6.

37. Talbot TR, Bradley SE, Cosgrove SE, et al. Influenza vaccination of healthcare workers and vaccine allocation for healthcare workers during vaccine shortages. Infect Control Hosp Epidemiol 2005;26(11):882–90.

38. Salgado CD, Farr BM, Hall KK, et al. Influenza in the acute hospital setting. Lancet Infect Dis 2002;2(3):145–55.

39. Elder AG, O'Donnell B, McCruden EA, et al. Incidence and recall of influenza in a cohort of Glasgow healthcare workers during the 1993-4 epidemic: results of serum testing and questionnaire. BMJ 1996;313(7067):1241–2.

40. Douglas RG Jr. Influenza in man. In: Kilbourne ED, editor. The influenza viruses and influenza. New York: Academic Press; 1975. p. 395–447.

41. Lester RT, McGeer A, Tomlinson G, et al. Use of, effectiveness of, and attitudes regarding influenza vaccine among house staff. Infect Control Hosp Epidemiol 2003;24(11):839–44.

42. Weingarten S, Riedinger M, Bolton LB, et al. Barriers to influenza vaccine acceptance. A survey of physicians and nurses. Am J Infect Control 1989; 17(4):202–7.

43. Poland GA, Tosh P, Jacobson RM. Requiring influenza vaccination for health care workers: seven truths we must accept. Vaccine 2005;23(17/18):2251–5.

44. Murphy BR, Chalhub EG, Nusinoff SR, et al. Temperature-sensitive mutants of influenza virus. III. Further characterization of the ts-1[E] influenza A recombinant (H3N2) virus in man. J Infect Dis 1973;128(4):479–87.

45. Hayden FG, Fritz R, Lobo MC, et al. Local and systemic cytokine responses during experimental human influenza A virus infection. Relation to symptom formation and host defense. J Clin Invest 1998;101(3):643–9.

46. Hall CB, Douglas RG Jr. Nosocomial influenza infection as a cause of intercurrent fevers in infants. Pediatrics 1975;55(5):673–7.

47. Englund JA, Champlin RE, Wyde PR, et al. Common emergence of amantadine- and rimantadine-resistant influenza A viruses in symptomatic immunocompromised adults. Clin Infect Dis 1998;26(6):1418–24.

48. Bean B, Moore BM, Sterner B, et al. Survival of influenza viruses on environmental surfaces. J Infect Dis 1982;146(1):47–51.
49. Boone SA, Gerba CP. The occurrence of influenza A virus on household and day care center fomites. J Infect 2005;51(2):103–9.
50. Morens DM, Rash VM. Lessons from a nursing home outbreak of influenza A. Infect Control Hosp Epidemiol 1995;16(5):275–80.
51. Andrewes CH, Glover RE. Spread of infection from the respiratory tract of the ferret. I. Transmission of influenza A virus. Br J Exp Pathol 1941;22(2):91–7.
52. Schulman JL, Kilbourne ED. Airborne transmission of influenza virus infection in mice. Nature 1962;195:1129–30.
53. Schulman JL. Experimental transmission of influenza virus infection in mice. IV. Relationship of transmissibility of different strains of virus and recovery of airborne virus in the environment of infector mice. J Exp Med 1967;125(3):479–88.
54. Alford RH, Kasel JA, Gerone PJ, et al. Human influenza resulting from aerosol inhalation. Proc Soc Exp Biol Med 1966;122(3):800–4.
55. Knight V. Viruses as agents of airborne contagion. Ann N Y Acad Sci 1980;353: 147–56.
56. Loudon RG, Roberts RM. Droplet expulsion from the respiratory tract. Am Rev Respir Dis 1967;95(3):435–42.
57. Papineni RS, Rosenthal FS. The size distribution of droplets in the exhaled breath of healthy human subjects. J Aerosol Med 1997;10(2):105–16.
58. Blachere FM, Lindsley WG, Pearce TA, et al. Measurement of airborne influenza virus in a hospital emergency department. Clin Infect Dis 2009;48(4):438–40.
59. McLean RL. The effect of ultraviolet radiation upon the transmission of epidemic influenza in long-term hospital patients. Am Rev Respir Dis 1961;83(2):36–8.
60. Moser MR, Bender TR, Margolis HS, et al. An outbreak of influenza aboard a commercial airliner. Am J Epidemiol 1979;110(1):1–6.
61. Blumenfeld HL, Kilbourne ED, Louria DB, et al. Studies on influenza in the pandemic of 1957–1958. I. An epidemiologic, clinical and serologic investigation of an intrahospital epidemic, with a note on vaccination efficacy. J Clin Invest 1959;38(1 Pt 2):199–212.
62. Bridges CB, Kuehnert MJ, Hall CB. Transmission of influenza: implications for control in health care settings. Clin Infect Dis 2003;37(8):1094–101.
63. Steininger C, Kundi M, Aberle SW, et al. Effectiveness of reverse transcription-PCR, virus isolation, and enzyme-linked immunosorbent assay for diagnosis of influenza A virus infection in different age groups. J Clin Microbiol 2002;40(6): 2051–6.
64. Fiore AE, Shay DK, Broder K, et al. Prevention and control of seasonal influenza with vaccines: recommendations of the Advisory Committee on Immunization Practices (ACIP), 2009. MMWR Recomm Rep 2009;58(RR–8):1–52.
65. Wilde JA, McMillan JA, Serwint J, et al. Effectiveness of influenza vaccine in health care professionals: a randomized trial. JAMA 1999;281(10):908–13.
66. Saxen H, Virtanen M. Randomized, placebo-controlled double blind study on the efficacy of influenza immunization on absenteeism of health care workers. Pediatr Infect Dis J 1999;18(9):779–83.
67. Feery BJ, Evered MG, Morrison EI. Different protection rates in various groups of volunteers given subunit influenza virus vaccine in 1976. J Infect Dis 1979; 139(2):237–41.
68. Salgado CD, Giannetta ET, Hayden FG, et al. Preventing nosocomial influenza by improving the vaccine acceptance rate of clinicians. Infect Control Hosp Epidemiol 2004;25(11):923–8.

69. Potter J, Stott DJ, Roberts MA, et al. Influenza vaccination of health care workers in long-term-care hospitals reduces the mortality of elderly patients. J Infect Dis 1997;175(1):1–6.

70. Carman WF, Elder AG, Wallace LA, et al. Effects of influenza vaccination of health-care workers on mortality of elderly people in long-term care: a randomised controlled trial. Lancet 2000;355(9198):93–7.

71. Hayward AC, Harling R, Wetten S, et al. Effectiveness of an influenza vaccine programme for care home staff to prevent death, morbidity, and health service use among residents: cluster randomised controlled trial. BMJ 2006;333(7581): 1241.

72. Lemaitre M, Meret T, Rothan-Tondeur M, et al. Effect of influenza vaccination of nursing home staff on mortality of residents: a cluster-randomized trial. J Am Geriatr Soc 2009;57(9):1580–6.

73. Schiller JS, Euler GL. Centers for disease control and prevention. Vaccination coverage estimates from the National Health Interview Survey: United States, 2008. Available at: http://www.cdc.gov/nchs/data/hestat/vaccine_coverage. htm. Accessed October 8, 2009.

74. The Joint Commission. Providing a safer environment for health care personnel and patients through influenza vaccination: strategies from research and practice; 2009. Available at: http://www.jointcommission.org/assets/1/18/Flu_ Monograph.pdf. Accessed December 6, 2010.

75. Immunization Action Coalition. Honor roll for patient safety. Mandatory influenza vaccination policies for healthcare workers. Available at: http://www.immunize. org/laws/influenzahcw.asp. Accessed November 19, 2009.

76. New York State Department of Health. Health care personnel influenza vaccination requirements - emergency regulation. Available at: http://www.health.state. ny.us/regulations/emergency/2009-08-13_health_care_personnel_influenza_ vaccination_requirements.htm. Accessed November 19, 2009.

77. Fiore AE, Shay DK, Broder K, et al. Prevention and control of influenza: recommendations of the Advisory Committee on Immunization Practices (ACIP), 2008. MMWR Recomm Rep 2008;57(RR–7):1–60.

78. Harper SA, Bradley JS, Englund JA, et al. Seasonal influenza in adults and children–diagnosis, treatment, chemoprophylaxis, and institutional outbreak management: clinical practice guidelines of the Infectious Diseases Society of America. Clin Infect Dis 2009;48(8):1003–32.

79. Centers for Disease Control and Prevention. Updated interim recommendations for the use of antiviral medications in the treatment and prevention of influenza for the 2009–2010 season. Available at: http://www.cdc.gov/ h1n1flu/recommendations.htm. Accessed October 6, 2009.

80. Centers for Disease Control and Prevention. Swine influenza A (H1N1) infection in two children–Southern California, March-April 2009. MMWR Morb Mortal Wkly Rep 2009;58(15):400–2.

81. Centers for Disease Control and Prevention. Novel influenza A (H1N1) virus infections among health-care personnel - United States, April–May 2009. MMWR Morb Mortal Wkly Rep 2009;58(23):641–5.

82. Centers for Disease Control and Prevention. Interim guidance for infection control for care of patients with confirmed or suspected novel influenza A (H1N1) virus infection in a healthcare setting. Available at: http://www.cdc. gov/h1n1flu/guidelines_infection_control.htm. Accessed July 27, 2009.

83. The Society for Healthcare Epidemiology of America. SHEA position statement: interim guidance on infection control precautions for novel swine-origin influenza

A H1N1 in healthcare facilities. Available at: http://www.shea-online.org/Assets/files/policy/061209_H1N1_Statement.pdf. Accessed July 27, 2009.

84. Centers for Disease Control and Prevention. Summary of Healthcare Infection Control Practices Advisory Committee (HICPAC) recommendations for care of patients with confirmed or suspected 2009 H1N1 influenza infection in healthcare settings, July 23, 2009. Available at: http://www.cdc.gov/ncidod/dhqp/hicpac_h1n1.html. Accessed September 17, 2009.

85. World Health Organization. Infection prevention and control in health care for confirmed or suspected cases of pandemic (H1N1) 2009 and influenza-like illnesses, interim guidance. Available at: http://www.who.int/csr/resources/publications/20090429_infection_control_en.pdf. Accessed August 8, 2009.

86. IOM (Institute of Medicine). Respiratory protection for healthcare workers in the workplace against novel H1N1 influenza A: a letter report. Washington, DC: The National Academies Press; 2009.

87. Loeb M, Dafoe N, Mahony J, et al. Surgical mask vs N95 respirator for preventing influenza among health care workers: a randomized trial. JAMA 2009; 302(17):1865–71.

88. Macintyre CR, Wang Q, Cauchemez S, et al. The first randomised, controlled clinical trial of surgical masks compared to fit-tested and non-fit tested N95 masks in the prevention of respiratory virus infection in hospital health care workers in Beijing, China [abstract 1247]. In: Final program of the 47th Annual Meeting of the Infectious Diseases Society of America. Philadelphia, October 31, 2009. p. 40.

89. Centers for Disease Control and Prevention. Prevention strategies for seasonal influenza in healthcare settings. Available at: http://www.cdc.gov/flu/professionals/infectioncontrol/healthcaresettings.htm. Accessed December 6, 2010.

90. World Health Organization. H5N1 avian influenza: timeline of major events, March 23, 2009. Available at: http://www.who.int/csr/disease/avian_influenza/Timeline_09_03_23.pdf. Accessed July 27, 2009.

91. World Health Organization. Cumulative number of confirmed human cases of avian influenza A/(H5N1) reported to WHO, September 24, 2009. Available at: http://www.who.int/csr/disease/avian_influenza/country/cases_table_2009_09_24/en/index.html. Accessed October 8, 2009.

92. Ungchusak K, Auewarakul P, Dowell SF, et al. Probable person-to-person transmission of avian influenza A (H5N1). N Engl J Med 2005;352(4):333–40.

93. Wang H, Feng Z, Shu Y, et al. Probable limited person-to-person transmission of highly pathogenic avian influenza A (H5N1) virus in China. Lancet 2008; 371(9622):1427–34.

94. Buxton Bridges C, Katz JM, Seto WH, et al. Risk of influenza A (H5N1) infection among health care workers exposed to patients with influenza A (H5N1), Hong Kong. J Infect Dis 2000;181(1):344–8.

95. Liem NT, Lim W. Lack of H5N1 avian influenza transmission to hospital employees, Hanoi, 2004. Emerg Infect Dis 2005;11(2):210–5.

96. Schultsz C, Dong VC, Chau NV, et al. Avian influenza H5N1 and healthcare workers. Emerg Infect Dis 2005;11(7):1158–9.

97. Shinya K, Ebina M, Yamada S, et al. Avian flu: influenza virus receptors in the human airway. Nature 2006;440(7083):435–6.

98. Centers for Disease Control and Prevention. Interim recommendations for infection vontrol in health-care facilities caring for patients with known or suspected avian influenza. Available at: http://www.cdc.gov/flu/avian/professional/infect-control.htm. Accessed July 27, 2009.

99. World Health Organization. Infection control recommendations for avian influenza in health-care facilities. Available at: http://www.who.int/csr/disease/avian_influenza/guidelines/EPR_AM1_E5.pdf. Accessed July 27, 2009.

100. Beigel JH, Farrar J, Han AM, et al. Avian influenza A (H5N1) infection in humans. N Engl J Med 2005;353(13):1374–85.

101. Brummitt CF, Cherrington JM, Katzenstein DA, et al. Nosocomial adenovirus infections: molecular epidemiology of an outbreak due to adenovirus 3a. J Infect Dis 1988;158(2):423–32.

102. James L, Vernon MO, Jones RC, et al. Outbreak of human adenovirus type 3 infection in a pediatric long-term care facility–Illinois, 2005. Clin Infect Dis 2007;45(4):416–20.

103. Gerber SI, Erdman DD, Pur SL, et al. Outbreak of adenovirus genome type 7d2 infection in a pediatric chronic-care facility and tertiary-care hospital. Clin Infect Dis 2001;32(5):694–700.

104. Lessa FC, Gould PL, Pascoe N, et al. Health care transmission of a newly emergent adenovirus serotype in health care personnel at a military hospital in Texas, 2007. J Infect Dis 2009;200(11):1759–65.

105. Gordon YJ, Gordon RY, Romanowski E, et al. Prolonged recovery of desiccated adenoviral serotypes 5, 8, and 19 from plastic and metal surfaces in vitro. Ophthalmology 1993;100(12):1835–9 [discussion: 39–40].

106. Zambon M, Bull T, Sadler CJ, et al. Molecular epidemiology of two consecutive outbreaks of parainfluenza 3 in a bone marrow transplant unit. J Clin Microbiol 1998;36(8):2289–93.

107. Brady MT, Evans J, Cuartas J. Survival and disinfection of parainfluenza viruses on environmental surfaces. Am J Infect Control 1990;18(1):18–23.

108. Ansari SA, Springthorpe VS, Sattar SA, et al. Potential role of hands in the spread of respiratory viral infections: studies with human parainfluenza virus 3 and rhinovirus 14. J Clin Microbiol 1991;29(10):2115–9.

Antimicrobial Stewardship

Pranita D. Tamma, MD[a,*], Sara E. Cosgrove, MD, MS[b]

KEYWORDS

- Antimicrobial stewardship • Antibiotic management
- Formulary restriction

ANTIMICROBIAL STEWARDSHIP

The overuse and misuse of antimicrobial agents has detrimental effects on the individual patient, the health care system, and society as a whole. Amongst other negative consequences, inappropriate antimicrobial use contributes to the increasing costs of health care, the emergence of multidrug resistant organisms (MDROs), and unnecessary adverse drug reactions. The implementation of a monitoring and intervention system is vital to optimize the effectiveness of currently available antimicrobial agents and preserve our ability to use them in the future. This system is especially necessary because the pace of antimicrobial development has markedly slowed in the last 20 years. The US Food and Drug Administration's approval of new antimicrobial agents decreased 56% from 1983 to 2002.[1] If the current rate of increase in resistance to antimicrobial agents continues, some experts believe we may eventually enter a postantibiotic era.[2]

WHAT IS ANTIMICROBIAL STEWARDSHIP?

Antimicrobial stewardship refers to a program or series of interventions to monitor and direct antimicrobial use at a health care institution, thus providing a standard, evidence-based approach to judicious antimicrobial use. The most effective antimicrobial stewardship programs simultaneously incorporate multiple strategies after collaborating with the various specialties within a given health care facility, although interventions on a smaller scale to improve antimicrobial use are also valuable in some settings. This review summarizes the goals of an antimicrobial stewardship program, the essential members needed to initiate and sustain such a program, the various antimicrobial stewardship strategies, barriers to the implementation and

Funding support: no funding was obtained for this review.
[a] Department of Pediatric Infectious Diseases, The Johns Hopkins Medical Institution, 200 North Wolfe Street Suite 3095, Baltimore, MD 21287, USA
[b] Division of Infectious Diseases, Antimicrobial Stewardship Program, The Johns Hopkins Medical Institution, Osler 425, 600 North Wolfe Street, Baltimore, MD 21287, USA
* Corresponding author.
E-mail address: ptamma1@jhmi.edu

Infect Dis Clin N Am 25 (2011) 245–260
doi:10.1016/j.idc.2010.11.011
0891-5520/11/$ – see front matter © 2011 Elsevier Inc. All rights reserved.

maintenance of the program, approaches to measure its effect, and the basic steps needed to initiate it.

THE GOALS OF ANTIMICROBIAL STEWARDSHIP

There are multiple goals of antimicrobial stewardship programs. From a public health standpoint, reduction of emergence of antimicrobial resistance and preservation of existing and future antimicrobial agents are a priority. Although there are several examples of stewardship approaches in the literature that have led to decreases in unnecessary antimicrobial use, there are fewer that have reported short-term reductions in antimicrobial resistance, and even fewer, if any, that have reported long-term reductions.[3] The lack of evidence is likely related to difficulties in measuring these outcomes, rather than because stewardship programs are ineffective in meeting this goal.

Nevertheless, it is useful to consider benefits other than reduction in resistance when justifying the existence of a program. Improvements in patient safety and outcomes in the area of antimicrobial prescribing are easier to demonstrate and may be more palatable for individual providers as reasons to endorse stewardship. Optimizing antimicrobial selection, dose, route of administration, and duration of therapy to maximize clinical cure while limiting unintended consequences, such as the emergence of resistance at the patient level, *Clostridium difficle* infection, and adverse drug toxicities are important clinically justifiable reasons for antimicrobial stewardship.

An additional goal of antimicrobial stewardship, and one of particular interest to administrators, is to reduce health care costs without compromising the quality of medical care. Antimicrobials account for up to 20% of hospital pharmacy budgets.[4] It is estimated that up to 50% of antimicrobial use is inappropriate, adding considerable costs to patient care.[5] According to the Office of Technology Assessment, antibiotics are the second most commonly prescribed class of drugs in the United States.[6] More than 40% of all hospitalized patients receive antibiotics in the United States annually. Antimicrobial stewardship programs have demonstrated significant annual savings in large academic hospitals as well as smaller community hospitals in the range of $200,000 to $900,000, without sacrificing the quality of clinical care.[7–13]

ESSENTIAL PARTICIPANTS IN AN ANTIMICROBIAL STEWARDSHIP PROGRAM

The next sections detail some of the important members of the team needed to initiate and sustain a stewardship program. The final composition of the program depends on available resources as well as its activities and goals.

Infectious-diseases Physician

Essential to a successful antimicrobial stewardship program is the presence of at least one physician trained in infectious diseases who dedicates a portion of his or her time to the design, implementation, and evaluation of the program. Having a stewardship team led by an infectious-diseases physician may increase acceptance and compliance of the program by other physicians. This strategy may also reduce the perception that a stewardship program is a pharmacy-driven cost-saving scheme.[14] Even if the infectious-diseases physician does not perform most of the daily activities of the program, it is essential to have someone trained in infectious diseases available to provide clinical guidance to support those administering the program. In addition, the infectious-diseases physician has the role of establishing general consensus regarding the content of institutional guidelines by all infectious-diseases practitioners within an institution as well as physician leadership in other departments. In institutions in which there is no physician trained in infectious diseases, a physician with a clinical interest in infectious diseases and antimicrobial use should be sought to lead the program. For example, at some institutions, hospitalists have successfully implemented stewardship activities.[15]

Clinical Pharmacist

One or more clinical pharmacists with specialized training in infectious diseases are recommended for establishing and maintaining a stewardship program. Infectious-diseases pharmacists can perform most of the day-to-day activities of a stewardship program, including antimicrobial education, pre- and postprescription review, and guideline development. However, an infectious-diseases pharmacist needs support from an infectious-diseases physician to assist with clinical decisions regarding the interpretation of laboratory, radiographic, history, and physical examination findings of individual patients. Gross and colleagues[16] implemented an antimicrobial stewardship program in which physicians were required to receive approval through a paging system operated by a clinical pharmacist trained in infectious diseases, with as-needed support from an infectious-diseases attending from 8 AM to 5 PM on week days. An infectious-diseases fellow-in-training responded to antimicrobial request pages at all other times. The study compared the appropriateness of antimicrobials as well as clinical outcomes resulting from recommendations made by the pharmacist or the fellows. The clinical pharmacists trained in infectious diseases outperformed the fellows in these outcomes, including appropriateness (87% vs 47%; $P<.001$), cure rate (64% vs 42%; $P = .007$), and reduction in treatment failures (15% vs 28%; $P = .03$).

Because many institutions do not currently have access to clinical pharmacists trained in infectious diseases, pharmacists without training in infectious diseases can also play an important part in antimicrobial stewardship.[17] Their role should be tailored based on the structure of the stewardship program. If there is support from an infectious-diseases pharmacist or physician, general pharmacists can flag certain cases for review or communicate recommendations to providers from the stewardship team. If guidelines for use of some antibiotics are in place, clinical pharmacists with advanced training in other specialties, such as oncology or critical care, can perform pre- or postprescription review for the patients for whom they have direct care based on the guidelines. If limited infectious-diseases resources are available, clinical pharmacists can perform cost-saving interventions such as recommending intravenous to oral agent conversions, monitoring for appropriate dosing, notifying physicians of multiple antibiotics being used for the same patient with overlapping spectrums of activity, and identifying the use of a prescribed antimicrobial agent to which the microorganism being targeted is resistant.

Microbiology Laboratory

The clinical microbiology laboratory plays a critical role in antimicrobial stewardship by providing patient-specific culture and susceptibility data to optimize individual therapy. A stewardship program and the microbiology laboratory should work collaboratively on the institution's antibiogram. Local antibiograms with microbe-specific susceptibility data updated at least annually can assist with developing treatment guidelines for certain infections within an institution.[4]

In addition, because the stewardship program directly observes how providers use and interpret microbiology data, it can provide important feedback to the laboratory regarding optimal mechanisms for communication of laboratory tests and testing modalities that should be considered to enhance patient care. For example, prioritization of tested antimicrobials and selective reporting of susceptibility profiles can aid in prudent antibiotic use by discouraging unnecessary broad-spectrum therapy (eg, masking susceptibility to meropenem for ampicillin-susceptible *Escherichia coli*) as well as inappropriate monotherapy (eg, masking susceptibility to rifampin for methicillin-resistant *Staphylococcus aureus* [MRSA]).[18] Hidden susceptibility results should be made available on request in situations in which potential drug toxicities, allergies, coinfections, or other considerations make first-line agents suboptimal.

Advanced molecular diagnostics have become increasingly popular; however, clinicians often need guidance in interpreting the results. In one institution, an antimicrobial stewardship program was notified with the results of peptide nucleic acid fluorescence in situ hybridization testing for the rapid identification of several organisms in blood cultures and then interacted with providers to interpret the results of these tests and recommend appropriate therapy. The program was able to reduce unnecessary vancomycin therapy for coagulase-negative *Staphylococci* spp isolated from blood cultures, decrease use of caspofungin for the treatment of *Candida albicans* fungemia, and decrease the time to appropriate therapy for *Enterococcus faecium* bacteremia.[19–21]

Information Technology

Access to experts in information technology (IT) is critical when developing and managing a stewardship program, both to assist with harnessing microbiology and antimicrobial use data from existing electronic sources for the purpose of detecting instances needing intervention by the program and to assist with measuring the effect of the program. Optimally, the budget of a stewardship program should include at least a portion of the salary for a data analyst, both to interface with the institutional IT group and to generate reports for the program.

Hospital Administration

An antimicrobial stewardship program is unlikely to be successfully implemented without at least passive endorsement by the hospital administration.[22] Commitment to implementation of antimicrobial stewardship programs must come from upper levels of hospital administration that are willing to invest resources in program development; otherwise funding for initiating and sustaining a stewardship program may be inadequate. If support from hospital leadership is lacking, some physicians may be less likely to comply with antimicrobial recommendations.

Pharmacy and Therapeutics Committee

The Pharmacy and Therapeutics (P & T) Committee determines which drugs, including antibiotics, should be placed on an institution's formulary. Antimicrobials are chosen based on costs, safety profiles, and pathogen resistance profiles.[23] An effective committee limits the number of agents that have a similar antimicrobial spectrum to simplify therapeutic options, reduce the effect of pharmaceutical detailing on antimicrobial selection by physicians, and reduce antimicrobial costs through contract negotiation. Members of the stewardship team should be involved in the P & T Committee to assist in antimicrobial formulary selection. If the program plans to establish standardized institutional guidelines for antimicrobial use, it is important to decide whether these should be approved or endorsed by the P & T Committee. In some institutions, endorsement by the P & T Committee can be an effective way of providing institutional endorsement of these guidelines.

Infection Control and Hospital Epidemiology Staff

The combination of effective antimicrobial stewardship with a comprehensive infection control program has been shown to limit the emergence and transmission of antimicrobial-resistant bacteria.[4] Although some resistant organisms have primarily been believed to be infection-control problems and others related more to antibiotic use and misuse, an absolute distinction can generally not be made. The development and spread of MDROs is likely a combination of both transmission and selection of resistant organisms. For example, the prevention of increasing MRSA rates in institutions seems to require stringent infection-control practices as well as restriction of antimicrobial usage.[24,25] Hospital epidemiologists have expertise in surveillance and study design, which may be useful in studying outcomes related to antimicrobial stewardship programs. Any antimicrobial stewardship program should work in close collaboration with the infection-control staff in the medical facility.

ANTIMICROBIAL STEWARDSHIP STRATEGIES

Several interventions have been evaluated to promote the judicious use of antimicrobials, including education, clinical guidelines, preprescription approval, postprescription review, computer-based decision support, and antibiotic cycling. Health care institutions with stewardship programs in place often use various combinations of these strategies, making strict classification, as well as evaluation, of stewardship programs not always feasible.

Development of Clinical Guidelines and Education Approaches

Development of institution-specific guidelines and algorithms for antimicrobial use is an important step in developing an antimicrobial stewardship program. Not only do they allow incorporation of relevant microbiologic trends and formulary agents but they also provide a backbone to support recommendations made by members of the stewardship program and an evidence-based educational resource for prescribers. Compliance with national guidelines may be suboptimal if they are perceived to be significantly different from local practices and local microbiological resistance patterns; input from institutional health care leaders to adapt national guidelines to local circumstances may increase acceptance.[22] In teaching hospitals, acceptance of guidelines by senior physicians is similarly important. The influence of senior physicians' antimicrobial prescribing practices may strongly influence compliance by house staff, and adherence to guidelines may be poor without acceptance from superiors.[26]

In a prospective study conducted at a surgical intensive care unit (ICU) in a community-based teaching hospital, clinical practice guidelines were developed by a multidisciplinary team for 6 diagnoses of infectious diseases: intraabdominal infections; complicated skin infections; lower respiratory tract infections; urinary tract infections; sepsis of undetermined cause; and intravenous catheter-related infections.[27] Mortality was significantly reduced (20% vs 5.6%; $P = .02$) and antibiotic costs were reduced from $676.54 per patient to $157.88 per patient ($P = .001$) in the postguideline period compared with the period before guideline implementation. The use of clinical practice guidelines for patients was shown to reduce costs, without a detrimental effect on patients' outcomes.

Another strategy that similarly addressed the inappropriate consumption of antimicrobials in the ICU setting used an algorithm incorporating the clinical pulmonary infection score (CPIS) as an operational criterion for decision making regarding antibiotic therapy.[28] Patients with a CPIS score of 6 or less (indicating low likelihood of pneumonia) were randomized to receive either a short course of therapy with ciprofloxacin for 3 days or standard care (broad-spectrum antibiotics for 10–21 days). Mortality and length of ICU stay did not differ despite a shorter duration ($P = .0001$) and lower cost ($P = .003$) of antimicrobial therapy in the experimental compared with the standard therapy arm. Antimicrobial resistance developed in 15% (5 of 37) of the patients in the experimental versus 35% (14 of 37) of the patients in the standard therapy group ($P = .017$).

In most institutions, guideline development must be accompanied by education initiatives. There is little argument that education is a cornerstone of any antimicrobial stewardship program. It can provide a foundation of knowledge that enhances and increases the acceptance of stewardship strategies, as well as reducing future inappropriate prescribing behavior. However, what constitutes an ideal educational program is debatable and can vary between passive approaches such as posters and newsletters to more active approaches such as one-on-one instruction and information sessions. Although passive educational strategies are easy to implement, if not combined with more active approaches, they are only marginally effective in changing antimicrobial prescribing practices and have not had a sustained effect.[29,30]

Preprescription Approval

Antimicrobial restriction, either through formulary limitation or by requirement of pre-authorization form from a physician or pharmacist is used to guide prescribers to make appropriate empirical antimicrobial choices. Besides simply denying or approving antimicrobial requests, the clinician or pharmacist can also assist with appropriate dosing, route of administration, duration, drug interactions, and interpretation of microbiological results. Results from before and after a policy change at a Veterans Administration Medical Center requiring prior approval from an infectious-diseases team for select antimicrobials showed a 24% decrease in the mean number of antibiotic doses per study patient ($P = .005$) and a 32% reduction in drug costs ($P = .004$).[31] The implementation of preprescription approval led to a significant and sustained decrease in antibiotic costs without adversely affecting length of therapy or mortality. The cost benefits with preprescription approval have similarly been reported in several other studies.[32–38] The cost savings do not take into account the effect the educational interactions have on future antimicrobial requests.

Evidence that preprescription approval reduces antimicrobial resistance is more elusive. A retrospective review of antimicrobial use assessing rates of select nosocomial infections before and after initiation of a prior approval program at a university hospital showed that in addition to reducing antimicrobial use and expenditures, prior approval was associated with significantly lower rates of *Stenotrophomonas* colonization or infection (0.35 vs 0.17; $P = .019$) and MRSA colonization or infection (0.66 vs 0.20; $P<.0001$).[38] Similarly, after implementation of a preprescription approval program at an urban teaching hospital, susceptibilities to all β-lactam and quinolone antibiotics increased, with increased susceptibilities to isolates in both the ICU and other inpatient wards, without compromising clinical outcomes.[37] However, other studies have either not reported decreases in resistance or have not evaluated this as an outcome.[3]

However, the challenge of antimicrobial restriction and its effect on antimicrobial resistance is exemplified in a study evaluating the effect of aggressive restriction of cephalosporins in response to an outbreak of cephalosporin-resistant *Klebsiella*.[39] This extreme restriction led to an 80% reduction in institution-wide cephalosporin use and a subsequent 44% reduction in the incidence of ceftazidime-resistant *Klebsiella*. However, imipenem use increased concomitantly 141%, with an accompanying

69% increase in the incidence of imipenem-resistant *Pseudomonas aeruginosa*. Stewardship programs should monitor proportions of antimicrobial agents prescribed to ensure that there is some diversity in the drugs recommended for specific indications to avoid development of resistance to antibiotic classes.

Preprescription approval methods can be labor intensive, particularly if the approval must be obtained from a pharmacist or a physician. In addition, the approver must be available to provide immediate, real-time service to prevent delays in initiation of appropriate therapy. In settings in which resources are more constrained, a modified restriction strategy can be implemented. In one institution, a 3-tier classification system was used. There were unrestricted agents, controlled agents, and restricted agents. Controlled agents could be dispensed for a limited period of time without approval but if prolonged durations of antimicrobials were desired (ie, of more than 24 to 72 hours), authorization by an infectious-diseases physician was needed. Restricted agents could not be dispensed without prior approval.[35] Another option is allowing certain antimicrobials to be used for documented indications (eg, vancomycin and ceftriaxone for bacterial meningitis, piperacillin-tazobactam for febrile neutropenia) via a form or order set. A secured Internet-based approach can also facilitate preprescription approval, as was shown at a pediatric teaching hospital where such a program resulted in improved communication and increased user satisfaction, and still retained the goals of efficient antibiotic prescription and cost savings.[40] Restriction strategies, when used alone, do not consider the appropriateness of prescribing nonrestricted antimicrobials, and a window of opportunity for teaching may be lost.

Postprescription Review

When faced with requests for broad-spectrum coverage in ill patients, an infectious-diseases specialist is likely to grant permission for use of broad-spectrum antibiotics out of concern for failing to cover MDROs, making preprescription approval less valuable in these settings. Postprescription review of antimicrobial therapy can be carried out in addition to preprescription approval; in these cases it is usually performed at 48 to 72 hours, after additional microbiology data are available and the patient's clinical course is further elucidated. It can also be conducted instead of preprescription approval; in these cases an earlier review within 24 hours can be considered to ensure appropriate empiric therapy and dosing and avoid a complicated on-demand system of preprescription approval.[41] Different methods have been used to provide postprescription review feedback, including one-on-one conversation in person or by phone, notes in the medical chart, or electronic notification. The optimal method has not been determined. Although existing data show that active, personalized interventions are more effective than more passive educational approaches, it has also been noted that for more complicated recommendations, written recommendations may allow for more accurate adherence to recommended drugs and doses.[3,42] Specific targets for postprescription review are outlined in **Box 1**.

In a large teaching hospital, house staff were randomized to receive either no intervention or one-on-one education by an infectious-diseases specialist on a patient-specific basis, discussing microbiological data, local resistance patterns, and clinical literature, prompted by orders for either levofloxacin or ceftazidime.[43] This strategy resulted in an almost 40% reduction in inappropriate use of levofloxacin or ceftazidime compared with controls (*P*<.001). Length of stay, ICU transfers, readmission rates, and in-hospital death rates were similar in both groups.

Gums and colleagues[44] conducted a prospective study in which consecutive patients who were receiving suboptimal therapy, after review by a clinical pharmacist,

---

Box 1
Targets for postprescription review

Streamlining (modification of initial empiric antibiotic regimen after more data are available)

Discontinuation of empiric therapy when cause of illness does not require antimicrobial therapy (eg, viral upper respiratory tract illness)

Dose optimization

Parenteral to oral antimicrobial conversion

Organism and antimicrobial mismatch

Drug-drug interactions

Therapeutic monitoring

---

were randomized to standard of care or to an intervention by a multidisciplinary antimicrobial treatment team. Physicians received timely, detailed reviews of relevant microbiologic and clinical data with recommendations of possible optimal antibiotic choices, dosages, and rationales. There was a 3-day difference when comparing median length of stay after randomization for control and intervention groups ($P = .0001$). Physician acceptance of suggestions was 89%. Substantial cost savings were noticed in the intervention group. Similarly, postprescription review was conducted using a before-and-after study design at a medium-sized community hospital.[8] This review resulted in a 22% decrease in the use of parenteral broad-spectrum antimicrobials. Concomitantly, there was a significant ($P = .002$) decrease in nosocomial infections caused by *Clostridium difficile* and a significant ($P = .02$) decrease in nosocomial infections caused by MDR Enterobacteriaceae.

In hospitals with more limited resources in which daily review of antimicrobial use is not feasible, a scaled-down postprescription review can still have a significant effect. This finding was depicted in a 120-bed community hospital that used an infectious-diseases physician and clinical pharmacist 3 days per week to review patients receiving multiple, prolonged, or costly courses of antimicrobial therapy.[9] Almost 70% of recommendations were implemented, resulting in a 19% reduction in antimicrobial expenditures, compared with the preintervention period.

Other considerations when implementing postprescription review include whether the stewardship program has authority to discontinue antibiotics regardless of the wishes of the treating provider. Many programs have opted not to implement this authority out of concern that it implies dictatorship rather than stewardship. However, it is reasonable to consider an approach for situations in which inappropriate use of antibiotics is causing significant individual patient harm. A variant of this approach is using automatic stop orders after a prespecified course of therapy has been given; reinitiation of therapy generally requires further approval. Automatic stop orders after 72 hours of empiric vancomycin therapy were used at a large academic center without harmful consequences, and if continuation of vancomycin was desired it required a discussion with the antimicrobial stewardship team.[45]

Computer-based Decision Support

Computers have become increasingly commonplace in medical institutions, and they can be used to facilitate the implementation of comprehensive antimicrobial stewardship programs. Antimicrobial stewardship incorporating computer programs may be as simple as linking the institution's antimicrobial guidelines to computerized physician order entry or may be more sophisticated. For example, computer-based decision support might provide individualized recommendations by assessing various patient-specific factors.

Glowacki and colleagues[46] created a computer program that alerted them to antimicrobial combinations that had an overlapping spectrum of activity. Those patients who were receiving any of these combinations were brought to the attention of an infectious-diseases pharmacist, who then made recommendations to the health care providers to consider altering therapy. Ninety-eight percent of the time, adjustments were made to the antimicrobial regimen based on the pharmacist's recommendations.

The most well-described computer decision-support system related to antimicrobial prescribing is from the Latter Day Saints (LDS) Hospital in Salt Lake City, UT, USA.[47–49] This program is linked to computer-based patient records and can make recommendations for antimicrobial regimens and assist with potential drug interactions as well as dosage and interval based on the patient's hepatic and renal function. It presents epidemiologic information, along with detailed recommendations and warnings regarding allergies in a specific patient. The program was studied prospectively for 1 year during which 545 patients in the ICU were cared for with the assistance of the antimicrobial computer program, and outcomes were compared with 2 years of data before use of the computer system.[48] The implementation of the program led to significant reductions in orders for medications to which the patients had reported allergies (35 vs 146 during the preintervention period; $P<.01$), excess medication dosages (87 vs 405, $P<.01$), and antibiotic-susceptibility mismatches (12 vs 206, $P<.01$). There were also significant reductions in total hospital costs and lengths of hospital stay. Incorporation of preoperative practice guidelines into the system increased the percentage of surgical patients receiving appropriately timed perioperative antimicrobials from 40% to 99.1%.[49]

Although advanced computer-assisted programs, such as that used at LDS Hospital are attractive options, merging medical records, electronic orders, and an antibiotic approval system can be a daunting task unless there are IT personnel dedicated to this duty. Once the system is established, close monitoring is still needed. In addition, it is important to assess whether providers at a particular institution are willing to receive and accept recommendations generated by a computer, preferably before extensive resources are dedicated to this task.

Antibiotic Cycling

Antibiotic cycling refers to the scheduled rotation of antibiotics with similar spectrums of activity, with a return to the original antibiotic after a defined period of time and reinitiation of the rotation.[50] The basic premise of this intervention is that during periods when an antibiotic is out of rotation, resistance to that agent declines because of reduced selective pressure on that antibiotic class. However, compliance with the recommended cycling protocol may be decreased based on concerns about adverse drug effects, beliefs that there is a more optimal antibiotic agent, and so forth. It is estimated that up to 50% of patients in cycling programs receive off-cycle antibiotics, with multiple antimicrobials being used simultaneously in different patients.[51]

Studies of true antimicrobial cycling are limited and differ in terms of antibiotic class selection, cycling duration, other therapies and practices introduced during cycling periods, and cycling by time period versus by patient. At the University of Virginia, a study was undertaken comparing the standard approach to antibiotic selection with a year of antibiotic cycling.[52] Antibiotics included in the rotating schedule during the second year include ciprofloxacin, piperacillin-tazobactam, carbapenems, and cefepime. Data from the second year showed significant reductions in MDROs and mortality. There were markedly different baseline characteristics between the groups (the antibiotic-cycling group had significantly fewer MDROs in their past medical history), and alcohol-based hand hygiene was introduced during the second year. It is unclear whether the outcomes seen were a result of the drug interventions, changes in patient population, low adherence rates to the protocol, or a result of improved hand hygiene.

A cycling experience from a surgical ICU (SICU) in The Netherlands of 4-month periods rotating between β-lactams and quinolones had a 96% adherence rate to the protocol.[53] Overall antibiotic use in the SICU increased 24%. There was a significant increase in MDROs; acquisition rates of resistant bacteria were highest during levofloxacin exposure (relative risk [RR] 3.2; 95% CI 1.4–7.1) and piperacillin-tazobactam exposure (RR 2.4; 95% CI 1.2–4.8). Even institutions that strictly adhere to antibiotic cycling, rotations may not see a benefit in rates of MDROs.

Mathematical models of antimicrobial resistance suggest that cycling antimicrobials are poor strategies for preventing the emergence of resistance. Such modeling suggests that the simultaneous mixed use of different antimicrobial classes in a heterogeneous fashion may slow the spread of resistance.[54,55] A recent systematic review of studies examining the efficacy of antibiotic cycling concluded that the current evidence is too weak to support the advocacy of this intervention as a means of reducing antibiotic resistance rates.[56]

BARRIERS TO IMPLEMENTATION AND MAINTENANCE OF STEWARDSHIP PROGRAMS

There are several barriers that may interfere with the initiation as well as continued maintenance of a stewardship program. Although most physicians recognize emergence of MDROs as an important problem, they are primarily concerned with their individual patients' clinical outcomes related to antibiotics and rate the risk of development of antimicrobial resistance as the factor least likely to influence their antimicrobial choices.[57] Because rates of antimicrobial resistance continue to increase and treating patients with resistant organisms is often a difficult endeavor, it is important that efforts exist to encourage prescribers to consider this public health challenge when they make decisions about antimicrobial use. However, resistance data alone are likely not sufficient as end points to gain interest and acceptance of an antimicrobial stewardship program amongst other physicians, and attention should be focused on the benefits of improved patient outcomes and safety.

Directing an intensive antimicrobial stewardship program may leave little time for an infectious-diseases specialist for clinical consultation and research. Thus it generally requires a dedicated infectious-diseases physician who should receive significant salary support for this task. Similarly, pharmacists trained in infectious diseases and other involved staff also need compensation. Only 18% of infectious-diseases physicians participating in antimicrobial stewardship programs acknowledge being reimbursed for their services.[58] This finding may represent a lost opportunity for hospitals, because cost savings from most published stewardship programs are significant and would likely offset the costs needed to employ personnel dedicated to the management of this system. Endorsement from hospital administration is vital to ensure adequate financial compensation.

Another barrier relates to infectious-diseases physicians sometimes accommodating antimicrobial requests to make their daily interactions with the requesting physicians more collegial. A key pharmaceutical marketing strategy entails identifying and involving local physician opinion leaders, in addition to infectious-diseases physicians, who adopt the proposed strategies and serve as respected sources of influence for other physicians.[59] A similar strategy should be used when initiating a stewardship program to overcome concerns of alienating colleagues.

Forty-five percent of infectious-diseases physicians believe that participation in antimicrobial stewardship programs leads to a loss of consultation requests.[58] Antimicrobial stewardship programs should augment and not interfere with the activities of an infectious-diseases consultation service. Stewardship programs should encourage physicians to request formal infectious-diseases consultations in medically complex cases and thus can potentially generate increased consultation requests. A prospective intervention performed to identify and modify inappropriate antimicrobial therapy at a large academic center showed that only about 5% of patients receiving broad-spectrum antimicrobial therapy had requested a formal infectious-diseases consultation.[41] This finding shows that a stewardship program has the potential to generate many infectious-diseases consultations. Other barriers related to stewardship programs include the need to educate incoming house staff and other new recruits on a routine basis and finding mechanisms to change long-standing antimicrobial prescribing practices. Both these barriers likely require significant education efforts.

MAKING A BUSINESS CASE FOR ANTIMICROBIAL STEWARDSHIP

There is currently no direct reimbursement to hospitals for establishing an antimicrobial stewardship program. Therefore, it is often necessary to make a business case to hospital administration for such a program to be created. The plans put forth from physicians, pharmacists, and others interested in initiating a stewardship program cannot be materialized without at least passive endorsement by hospital leadership. It may also be helpful to remind hospital administrators that the Joint Commission lists "reducing the risk of health care associated infections" as National Patient Safety Goal 7 and it is recommended that "antibiotic resistance and appropriate antibiotic use should be reviewed by the consulting pharmacist, IC [infection control] professional, director of nursing, and the medical director."[60,61] **Box 2** outlines steps to consider when approaching administration for support for a stewardship program based on a similar approach suggested for justifying infection control programs.[62]

MEASURING THE EFFECT OF THE PROGRAM

Most stewardship programs need to provide some evidence to institutional administration that they are improving care and/or reducing costs. It is important to establish at the time of initiation of the program what goals are expected. As changing behavior regarding antimicrobial use is challenging, the initial goals should be modest and directed at a reduction in use of one or a few antimicrobial agents rather than decreasing the use of all agents or decreasing antimicrobial resistance rates. If improving patient safety is an acceptable institutional goal, then data focusing on the acceptance rate of interventions could be considered in lieu of data on decreased antimicrobial use. It is also worth considering measuring improvements in antimicrobial use associated with a specific disease state, such as community-acquired pneumonia, rather than trying to assess antibiotic use for all indications. Significant cost reduction realized by changes in formulary antibiotics that are less expensive can often be at least partially attributed to efforts of the stewardship program. Approaches for quantifying antimicrobial use include defined daily doses and days of antibiotic therapy; the relative advantages of these approaches are detailed elsewhere.[63] Collection of antimicrobial use data in a standardized way allows institutions to

Box 2
Steps necessary to implement an antimicrobial stewardship program

Step 1: Frame the problem that needs to be addressed

Decide which problem needs to be targeted (eg, failure to discontinue surgical antibiotic perioperative orders, vancomycin therapy for a single coagulase-negative *Staphylococcus* spp [CoNS] blood culture, combination therapy for all Gram-negative infections)

Step 2: Consider potential solutions to the problem

What can be done to solve this problem (eg, programming automatic antibiotic stop orders to prevent unnecessary continuation of surgical perioperative orders, distributing guidelines stating that a single-positive blood culture for CoNS spp most likely does not warrant antibiotic therapy, implementing a postprescription review program for patients receiving more than one antimicrobial agent for more than 48 hours)?

Step 3: Decide what needs to occur to achieve the solution

How can this solution be achieved (eg, providing salary support to a computer-support person to implement automatic stop orders, obtaining funding for educational materials displaying guidelines for interpreting blood culture results, hiring a pharmacist trained in infectious diseases and an infectious-diseases physician to conduct postprescription reviews)?

Step 4: Meet key administrators

Schedule a meeting with key administrators (eg, chief medical officer, hospital epidemiologist, hospital safety control officer)

When meeting these individuals, determine if the issue is of institutional concern and if you have the support of leadership; determine critical leaders in various hospital departments who are affected by the proposal and may need to be involved in the decision making; ascertain what data they would like you to produce to determine cost-effectiveness

Step 5: Determine the annual cost

Determine the costs of hiring additional personnel (salary and benefits), which can be determined from institutional budgets

Include additional costs such as purchasing and installing additional computers, publishing antimicrobial management handbooks for house staff

Step 6: Determine the costs associated with the infection of interest in your institution

Determine the attributable cost of the problem with which you are concerned by using either hospital data or published literature (eg, costs of prolonged perioperative antibiotics, cost of treating a contaminated blood culture, excess costs of prescribing 2 antibiotics when one agent is likely sufficient)

Use this attributable cost data to determine your estimated cost savings (eg, multiply the cost of treating one contaminated blood culture by the annual number of contaminated blood cultures in your institution)

Step 7: Calculate the financial effect

Subtract the costs needed in advance from the estimated cost savings

Step 8: Include additional benefits

Provide additional data supported by literature citing the effect of an antimicrobial stewardship program on patient clinical outcomes and satisfaction, on the emergence of MDROs, and so forth.

Step 9: Prospectively collect outcome data

Intervention-specific outcome data should be collected after the intervention is implemented to demonstrate the continued benefit of the program

Outcomes can include costs, days on antibiotics, changes in prescription practices of a specific antibiotic, trends in MDROs or *Clostridium difficile* benchmark their progress internally and with peer institutions.[64] Regardless of what measures are chosen, all programs should plan to measure some process or outcome measure and report these results annually to the relevant stakeholders.

SUMMARY

Antimicrobial stewardship programs consist of ongoing efforts by health care institutions to optimize antimicrobial use, with the goals of improving patient outcomes, promoting cost-effective therapy, reducing untoward effects of unnecessary antimicrobials, and limiting the production of MDROs. Antimicrobial resistance is a serious threat that is exacerbated by the gradual withdrawal of the pharmaceutical industry from new antibiotic agent development. We are currently faced with a serious need to preserve the effectiveness of our existing antimicrobial arsenal. Although antimicrobial stewardship may be one mechanism for decreasing the emergence of MDROs, to have a real effect on the emergence of resistance, monitoring and restricting unnecessary and inappropriate use should be extended to longer-term care facilities, the outpatient setting, and the animal industry. Otherwise, stewardship programs may fail to affect hospital resistance rates if there is continuous importation of MDROs from these arenas.

REFERENCES

1. Spellberg B, Powers JH, Brass EP, et al. Trends in antimicrobial drug development: implications for the future. Clin Infect Dis 2004;38:1279–86.
2. Tenover FC, Hughes JM. The challenges of emerging infectious diseases. Development and spread of multiply-resistant bacterial pathogens. JAMA 1996;275(4): 300–4.
3. Davey P, Brown E, Fenelon L, et al. Interventions to improve antibiotic prescribing practices for hospital inpatients. The Cochrane Library 2005;4:1–117.
4. Dellit TH, Owens RC, McGowan JE, et al. Infectious Disease Society of American and the Society for Healthcare Epidemiology of America guidelines for developing an institutional program to enhance antimicrobial susceptibility. Clin Infect Dis 2007;44:159–77.
5. Reimann HA, D'Ambola J. The use and cost of antimicrobials in hospitals. Arch Environ Health 1966;13:631–6.
6. Office of Technology Assessment USC. Impacts of antibiotic-resistant bacteria. OTA-H-629. Washington, DC: Government Printing Office; 1995.
7. Schentag JJ, Ballow CH, Fritz AL, et al. Changes in antimicrobial agent usage resulting from interactions among clinical pharmacy, the infectious disease division, and the microbiology laboratory. Diagn Microbiol Infect Dis 1993;16:255–64.
8. Carling P, Fung T, Killion A, et al. Favorable impact of a multidisciplinary antibiotic management program conducted during 7 years. Infect Control Hosp Epidemiol 2003;24:699–706.
9. LaRocco A Jr. Concurrent antibiotic review programs–a role for infectious diseases specialists at small community hospitals. Clin Infect Dis 2003;37:742–3.
10. Ansari F, Gray K, Nathwani D, et al. Outcomes of an intervention to improve hospital antibiotic prescribing: interrupted time series with segmented regression analysis. J Antimicrob Chemother 2003;52:842–8.
11. Ruttimann S, Keck B, Hartmeier C, et al. Long-term antibiotic cost savings from a comprehensive intervention program in a medical department of a university-affiliated hospital. Clin Infect Dis 2004;38:348–56.

12. Lutters M, Harbarth S, Janssens JP, et al. Effect of a comprehensive, multidisciplinary, educational program on the use of antibiotics in a geriatric university hospital. J Am Geriatr Soc 2004;52:112–6.

13. Scheckler WE, Bennett JV. Antibiotic usage in seven community hospitals. JAMA 1970;213(2):264–7.

14. MacDougall C, Polk RE. Antimicrobial stewardship programs in health care systems. Clin Microbiol Rev 2005;18(4):638–56.

15. Kisuule F, Wright S, Barreto J, et al. Improving antibiotic utilization among hospitalists: a pilot academic detailing project with a public health approach. J Hosp Med 2007;10:93–101.

16. Gross R, Morgan AS, Kinky DE, et al. Impact of a hospital-based antimicrobial management program on clinical and economic outcomes. Clin Infect Dis 2001;33:289–95.

17. MacLaren R, Devlin JW, Martin SJ, et al. Critical care pharmacy services in United States hospitals. Ann Pharmacother 2006;40:612–8.

18. Steffee CH, Morrell RM, Wasilauskas BL. Clinical use of rifampicin during routine reporting of rifampicin susceptibilities: a lesson in selective reporting of antimicrobial susceptibility data. J Antimicrob Chemother 1997;40:595–8.

19. Forrest GN, Mehta S, Weekes E, et al. Impact of rapid in situ hybridization testing on coagulase-negative staphylococci positive blood cultures. J Antimicrob Chemother 2006;58:154–8.

20. Forrest GN, Mankes K, Jabra-Rizk A, et al. Peptide nucleic acid fluorescence in situ hybridization-based identification of *Candida albicans* and its impact on mortality and antifungal therapy costs. J Clin Microbiol 2006; 44(9):3381–3.

21. Forrest GN, Roghmann M, Toombs LS, et al. Peptide nucleic acid fluorescent in situ hybridization for hospital-acquired enterococcal bacteremia: delivering earlier effective antimicrobial therapy. Antimicrob Agents Chemother 2008; 52(10):3558–63.

22. Goldmann DA, Weinstein RA, Wenzel RP, et al. Strategies to prevent and control the emergence and spread of antimicrobial-resistant microorganisms in hospitals: a challenge to hospital leadership. JAMA 1996;275(3):234–40.

23. Paskovaty A, Pflomm JM, Myke N, et al. A multidisciplinary approach to antimicrobial stewardship: evolution into the 21st century. Int J Antimicrob Agents 2005;25:1–10.

24. Safdar N, Maki DG. The commonality of risk factors for nosocomial colonization and infection with antimicrobial-resistant *Staphylococcus aureus*, enterococcus, gram-negative bacilli, *Clostridium difficile*, and *Candida*. Ann Intern Med 2002; 136:834–44.

25. Monnet DL. Methicillin-resistant *Staphylococcus aureus* and its relationship to antimicrobial use: possible implications for control. Infect Control Hosp Epidemiol 1998;19:552–9.

26. Mol PG, Rutten WJ, Gans RO, et al. Adherence barriers to antimicrobial treatment guidelines in teaching hospitals, The Netherlands. Emerg Infect Dis 2004;10(3): 522–5.

27. Price J, Ekleberry A, Grover A, et al. Evaluation of clinical practice guidelines on outcome of infection in patients in the surgical intensive care unit. Crit Care Med 1999;27(10):2118–24.

28. Singh N, Rogers P, Atwood CW, et al. Short-course empiric antibiotic therapy for patients with pulmonary infiltrates in the intensive care unit. Am J Respir Crit Care Med 2000;162:505–11.

29. Bantar C, Sartori B, Vesco E, et al. A hospitalwide intervention program to optimize the quality of antibiotic use: impact on prescribing practice, antibiotic consumption, cost savings, and bacterial resistance. Clin Infect Dis 2003;37:180–6.
30. Belongia EA, Knobloch MJ, Kieke BA, et al. Impact of statewide program to promote appropriate antimicrobial drug use. Emerg Infect Dis 2005;11(6):912–20.
31. Coleman RW, Rodondi LC, Kaubisch S, et al. Cost-effectiveness of prospective and continuous parenteral antibiotic control: experience at the Palo Alto Veterans Affairs Medical Center from 1987 to 1989. Am J Med 1991;90:439–44.
32. Seligman SJ. Reduction in antibiotic costs by restricting use of an oral cephalosporin. Am J Med 1981;71:941–4.
33. Britton HL, Schwinghammer TL, Romano MJ. Cost containment through restriction of cephalosporins. Am J Hosp Pharm 1981;38(12):1897–900.
34. Hayman JN, Sbravati EC. Controlling cephalosporins and aminoglycoside costs through pharmacy and therapeutics committee restrictions. Am J Hosp Pharm 1985;42(6):1343–7.
35. Woodward RS, Medoff G, Smith MD, et al. Antibiotic cost savings from formulary restrictions and physician monitoring in a medical-school-affiliated hospital. Am J Med 1987;83:817–23.
36. Maswoswe JJ, Okpara AU. Enforcing a policy for restricting antimicrobial use. Am J Health Syst Pharm 1995;52(13):1433–5.
37. White AC, Atmar RL, Wilson J, et al. Effects of requiring prior authorization for selected antimicrobials: expenditures, susceptibilities, and clinical outcomes. Clin Infect Dis 1997;25:230–9.
38. Frank MO, Batteiger BE, Sorensen SJ, et al. Decrease in expenditures and selected nosocomial infections following implementation of an antimicrobial-prescribing improvement program. Clin Perform Qual Health Care 1997;5(4):180–8.
39. Rahal JJ, Urban C, Horn D, et al. Class restriction of cephalosporin use to control total cephalosporin resistance in nosocomial *Klebsiella*. JAMA 1998;280(14):1233–7.
40. Agwu AL, Lee CK, Jain SK, et al. A world wide web-based antimicrobial stewardship program improves efficiency, communication, and user satisfaction and reduces cost in a tertiary care pediatric medical center. Clin Infect Dis 2008;47:747–53.
41. Cosgrove SE, Patel A, Song X, et al. Impact of different methods of feedback to clinicians after post prescription antimicrobial review based on the Centers for Disease Control and Prevention's 12 steps to prevent antimicrobial resistance among hospitalized adults. Infect Control Hosp Epidemiol 2007;28:641–6.
42. Grimshaw JM, Shirran L, Thomas R, et al. Changing provider behavior: an overview of systematic reviews of interventions. Med Care 2001;39:112–45.
43. Solomon DH, Van Houten L, Glynn RJ. Academic detailing to improve use of broad-spectrum antibiotics at an academic medical center. Arch Intern Med 2001;161:1897–902.
44. Gums JG, Yancey RW, Hamilton CA, et al. A randomized, prospective study measuring outcomes after antibiotic therapy intervention by a multidisciplinary consult team. Pharmacotherapy 1999;19(12):1369–77.
45. Connor DM, Binkley S, Fishman NO, et al. Impact of automatic orders to discontinue vancomycin therapy on vancomycin use in an antimicrobial stewardship program. Infect Control Hosp Epidemiol 2007;28(12):1408–10.
46. Glowacki RC, Schwartz DN, Itokazu GS, et al. Antibiotic combinations with redundant antimicrobial spectra: clinical epidemiology and pilot intervention of computer-assisted surveillance. Clin Infect Dis 2003;37:59–64.

47. Evans RS, Pestotnik SL, Classen DC, et al. Evaluation of a computer-assisted antibiotic-dose monitor. Ann Pharmacother 1999;33:1026–31.
48. Evans RS, Pestotnik SL, Classen DC, et al. A computer-assisted management program for antibiotics and other antiinfectives agents. N Engl J Med 1998; 338:232–8.
49. Pestotnik SL, Classen DL, Evans RS, et al. Implementing antibiotic practice guidelines through computer-assisted decision support: clinical and financial outcomes. Ann Intern Med 1996;124:884–90.
50. Fishman N. Antimicrobial stewardship. Am J Infect Control 2006;34:S65–73.
51. Fridkin SK. Routine cycling of antimicrobial agents as an infection-control measure. Clin Infect Dis 2003;36:1438–44.
52. Raymond DP, Pelletier SJ, Crabtree TD, et al. Impact of a rotating empiric schedule on infectious mortality in an intensive care unit. Crit Care Med 2001; 29(6):1101–8.
53. Van Loon HJ, Vriens MR, Fluit AC, et al. Antibiotic rotation and development of Gram-negative antibiotic resistance. Am J Respir Crit Care Med 2005;171:480–7.
54. Bonhoeffer S, Lipsitch M, Levin BR. Evaluating treatment protocols to prevent antibiotic resistance. Proc Natl Acad Sci U S A 1997;94:12106–11.
55. Bergstrom CT, Lo M, Lipsitch M. Ecological theory suggests that antimicrobial cycling will not reduce antimicrobial resistance in hospitals. Proc Natl Acad Sci U S A 2004;7:13101–2.
56. Brown EM, Nathwani D. Antibiotic cycling or rotation: a systematic review of the evidence of efficacy. J Antimicrob Chemother 2005;55:6–9.
57. Metlay JP, Shea JA, Crossette LB, et al. Tensions in antibiotic prescribing: pitting social concerns against interests of individual patients. J Gen Intern Med 2002; 17:87–94.
58. Sunenshine RH, Kiedkte LA, Jernigan DB, et al. Role of infectious diseases consultants in management of antimicrobial use in hospitals. Clin Infect Dis 2004;38:934–8.
59. Soumerai SB, Avorn J. Principles of educational outreach ('academic detailing') to improve clinical decision making. JAMA 1990;263(4):549–56.
60. Pritchard V. Joint Commission standards for long-term care infection control: putting together the process elements. Am J Infect Control 1999;27:27–34.
61. The Joint Commission. Available at: http://www.jcrinc.com/2009-NPSGs-Goal-7/. Accessed February 10, 2010.
62. Perencevich EN, Stone PW, Wright SB, et al. Raising standards while watching the bottom line: making a business case for infection control. Infect Control Hosp Epidemiol 2007;28(10):1121–33.
63. Polk RE, Fox C, Mahoney A, et al. Measurement of adult antibacterial drug use in 130 US hospitals: comparison of defined daily dose and days of therapy. Clin Infect Dis 2007;44(5):664–70.
64. Pakyz AL, MacDougall C, Oinonen M, et al. Trends in antibacterial use in US health centers. Arch Intern Med 2008;168(20):2254–60.

Informatics and Epidemiology in Infection Control

Keith F. Woeltje, MD, PhD[a],*, Ebbing Lautenbach, MD, MPH, MSCE[b]

KEYWORDS

- HAIs • Electronic surveillance • Infection prevention
- Epidemiology

Surveillance for health care–associated infections (HAIs) and the epidemiologic evaluation of the resulting data are the cornerstones of any infection prevention activity. Of course, these activities alone are not enough; interventions must be implemented to actually reduce infection rates. But surveillance and analysis are essential for designing worthwhile interventions and determining whether infection prevention activities are achieving their goals.

MEDICAL INFORMATICS FOR HEALTH CARE EPIDEMIOLOGY
Background

Historically, surveillance and analysis activities were largely manual processes, consuming a large proportion of the time of an infection preventionist or a health care epidemiologist. Although still time-consuming, the introduction of computers into health care epidemiology has reduced the amount of time needed for surveillance and analysis activities in many hospitals and promises even more time-savings in the future. Likewise, statistical software has become easier to use, and statistical functions are built into many infection-control software packages. The ready availability of good surveillance data, along with the means to perform appropriate analysis, can easily help guide better interventions and allow more time to implement those interventions.

The personal computer revolution of the past 2 decades has made capable computers affordable. Even a basic spreadsheet program can greatly improve the efficiency of surveillance; more sophisticated software helps even more. Internet access and electronic mail round out the basic computer needs for infection prevention.

[a] Center for Clinical Excellence, BJC HealthCare and Washington University School of Medicine, 660 South Euclid Avenue, Campus Box 8051, St Louis, MO 63110, USA
[b] Department of Healthcare Epidemiology and Infection Control, Center for Clinical Epidemiology and Biostatistics, University of Pennsylvania School of Medicine, 825 Blockley Hall, 423 Guardian Drive, Philadelphia, PA 19104-6021, USA
* Corresponding author.
E-mail address: KWoeltje@DOM.wustl.edu

Infect Dis Clin N Am 25 (2011) 261–270
doi:10.1016/j.idc.2010.11.013
0891-5520/11/$ – see front matter © 2011 Elsevier Inc. All rights reserved.

Sources of Data

At the most basic level, surveillance data can be manually entered into a software package. The time spent on data entry will be recouped by the time saved in data retrieval and analysis. However, the biggest gains come from the systems that provide more automated entry. Periodic reports that have been specifically formatted for ease of import into the infection prevention software can be used. These reports may be sent monthly, weekly, or daily, depending on the needs of the user and the capabilities of the system generating the reports. At a more sophisticated level, direct data feeds into the software can be developed. Such feeds may include demographic information from the admission, discharge, and transfer system and culture data from the microbiology laboratory system. The operating room software may be able to send data on patient procedures, and many of these systems capture the information needed for the risk stratification of a surgical site infection (SSI), such as the length of the procedure and American Society of Anesthesiologists (ASA) score of the patient. As electronic medical records become more commonplace, even more patient data may be available. Although direct data feeds require a lot of time and assistance from the hospital's information technology department, the time-savings and completeness of the data make the efforts worthwhile.

Data Management

As data are gathered from hospital systems, decisions must be made on how it is stored. Although simple spreadsheets can be used for basic information, as data become more complex, the storage needs become more complex. Desktop general-purpose databases (eg, Microsoft Access) can be used for some information, and more sophisticated enterprise-level databases can be used as the desktop software is outgrown. Most health care epidemiologists need to consult with database-design specialists to develop these systems. Commercial infection prevention applications have their own storage mechanisms.

A variety of standards exist regarding terms to describe organisms, culture types, and procedures. When deciding on a system to store data for surveillance use, the user may be constrained by the terms used by the data sources. However, translation into other standard terms can be done and may be desirable. Commercial surveillance software may require the incoming data to be in a particular format. "Homegrown" systems may elect to use standardized terminology rather than vendor-specific terms used by the data sources because it makes migration to different vendors easier and also facilitates merging and benchmarking data from multiple facilities.

Mechanisms must be put into place to ensure ongoing data integrity. If an upstream data source changes terminology or adds new kinds of data, there must be a way to ensure that the database receiving the information handles it appropriately. Using an old example, if the system provides an alert to the infection preventionist when a patient has a positive culture for *Xanthomonas maltophilia*, what happens when the microbiology laboratory software gets updated and the new name *Stenotrophomonas maltophilia* is used instead? Will the alerts simply fail? Or more significantly, if microbiology reports fail to be sent altogether, will this failure be recognized? And is there a mechanism to recover the positive culture information that was not sent?

What data are needed?

Numerator data To assist in surveillance for HAIs, an electronic system should be able to assist in finding patients who have such infections (ie, patients in the numerator of the HAI rates). Many surveillance systems are organized around microbiology data, so positive cultures from a particular site (such as in blood) can be used to trigger further investigation. Other data that can be helpful in making surveillance fully automated include whether a given patient had a central venous catheter or other devices on a given day, antibiotic usage, information on negative culture results, and patient temperatures.

Denominator data To calculate infection rates, denominator data are necessary. For device-associated infections, device days for a given unit are necessary. The traditional method (and the method required by the Centers for Disease Control [CDC]'s National Healthcare Safety Network [NHSN][1]) is to have a nurse or other health care worker check at the same time each day for the number of patients who have a central venous catheter, urinary catheter, or other device. This number is then summed up for the month. Device days can be calculated automatically if the device usage is available electronically for each patient everyday. These data generally yield somewhat higher counts of device days because the day is usually counted if the device was present at any point during the day. Device use can often be extracted from nursing notes but it requires consistent charting by the caregivers.[2]

For SSIs, the appropriate procedures must be counted. For risk-adjustment, the ASA score, duration of procedure, and final wound classification must be also available for each patient. The hospital's operating room management software may capture all the required information. One potential pitfall is that the procedure codes are often entered before the case, so they may not reflect the actual final procedure. Likewise, wound classification (eg, clean, clean-contaminated) may be entered before the case, depending on the type of procedure. Care must be taken so that the designation is updated if there was an event during the procedure (eg, a breach of the sterile field that changed what is normally categorized as a clean procedure to a clean-contaminated procedure).

Examples of Electronic Surveillance

Wholly automated surveillance

A surveillance system that is fully automated is the "holy grail" in infection prevention informatics. Work is furthest along with central line–associated bloodstream infections (CLABSIs) because surveillance for these infections is the most amenable to straightforward rules. Early work by several investigators was promising for the detection of all nosocomial bloodstream infections[3–5]; however, these studies were not catheter specific. Trick and colleagues[6] demonstrated that a relatively simple electronic rule-based system for determining CLABSI performed at least as well as surveillance by infection preventionists, with a sensitivity of 81% and a specificity of 72% compared with investigator review. However, the hospitals in that study did not have access to central line usage electronically, so it had to be manually determined. At some hospitals in the BJC HealthCare system, central line data are electronically available; this system is beginning to implement fully electronic surveillance for CLABSI in patient-care areas that are not part of the intensive care unit (ICU), where there is no manual surveillance process in place at present.[7]

Fully automated surveillance systems are likely to raise several concerns. The accuracy of the surveillance is certainly an issue. Automated systems will inevitably have a lower sensitivity and specificity than manual surveillance if current surveillance by infection preventionists is used as a gold standard. However, as noted in the study by Trick and colleagues,[6] surveillance by infection preventionists is also not perfect. Current surveillance definitions have some subjective component to them, and case finding by individual infection preventionists can be variable. Several studies have found significant interrater variability in determining what an HAI is.[6,8–10] In one CDC study for the National Nosocomial Infection Surveillance System (the predecessor of NHSN), study personnel reported twice as many infections as the infection prevention-ists in hospitals did. However, even these specially trained personnel missed infec-tions that the hospitals had reported; 37% of such missed infections were determined by CDC staff as true HAIs.[11] The point here is not to belittle the consider-able efforts of infection preventionists; it is simply to indicate the difficulty of the surveillance for HAI. Automated surveillance may have advantages in being fully objective and perhaps more thorough in case finding.

In considering automated surveillance, the goals of surveillance should be consid-ered. The goal is not necessarily to identify each individual patient with or without an HAI. The goals may be to generate rates at the unit level to focus on improvement efforts and measure the effect of these efforts. Epidemiologists are comfortable with the notion that meeting a surveillance definition is not the same thing as a clinical diagnosis. A good surveillance definition is one that can be applied consistently and objectively. Automated surveillance fits in nicely with this concept. However, if auto-mated surveillance is to become more common, a broader acceptance of this notion in the health care community is necessary.

Augmented surveillance

Manual surveillance for HAI is unlikely to be replaced any time soon. In many states, mandatory reporting of HAI requires following NHSN definitions, which require manual evaluation of patients. However, electronic systems can significantly assist infection preventionists in their surveillance activities.

Many commercial and homegrown software systems for infection prevention can send alerts or generate lists of patients with positive cultures of interest. Although this advancement is certainly a big improvement from scanning paper microbiology reports, these simple systems still leave a lot of manual work for the infection preven-tionists in determining the patients who may truly have HAIs. By focusing on rules that have a high negative predictive value for a true infection, the Barnes-Jewish hospital has been able to implement a system that eliminated 68% of positive blood culture results of patients in ICU, with a negative predictive value of 99.2%. The infection pre-ventionists can then focus on a much smaller number of patients to determine whether they meet NHSN criteria for a CLABSI.[12]

Similar approaches could be used to identify other HAIs. Antibiotic usage with or without diagnostic codes may be suggestive of SSIs.[13–18] Using electronically avail-able laboratory data and ventilator settings may also allow for reliable detection of ventilator-associated pneumonia.[19] Augmented surveillance may be more acceptable to hospital administrators, physicians, infection preventionists, and other medical personnel involved because it offers the advantage of thorough case finding, while still allowing manual determination of factors that are hard to evaluate automatically that may exclude an infection from being considered an HAI (eg, the presence of an infec-tion elsewhere that would mean an infection is secondary, not a primary HAI).

Data for Investigations

In addition to automated or augmented routine surveillance, electronic data can assist with investigations of outbreak. Some homegrown and commercial systems have options to help detect clusters of infections. This assistance can vary from simple reports that indicate the aggregate number of infections or organism in a unit to a more sophisticated automated analysis.[20–22] To assist with the investigation of a potential cluster or outbreak, a software package should provide basic functions such as preparing a line list. Even if a commercial software package does basic statistical analysis, it should also be able to export data for analysis by more specialized statistical software.

BASIC EPIDEMIOLOGY FOR INFECTION CONTROL

A good working knowledge of the basic epidemiologic and statistical principles is critical for the health care epidemiologist and infection preventionist. The ability to gather, access, and organize data is critical to the practice of health care epidemiology. As noted earlier, many new approaches to these tasks are now available and continue to be refined. Once these data have been obtained, the next question is how to use them. The ability to accurately quantify new patterns of infectious diseases, design rigorous studies to characterize the factors associated with disease, and devise and evaluate interventions to address emerging issues are vital to effective health care epidemiology.

Epidemiology is commonly defined as the study of the distribution and determinants of disease frequency in human populations. This definition encompasses the 3 main components of the discipline of epidemiology: (1) disease frequency, involves identifying the existence of a disease and quantifying its occurrence; (2) distribution of disease, characterizes in whom, when, and where the disease is occurring; (3) determinants of disease, focuses on formulating and testing hypotheses with regard to the possible risk factors for disease.

After organized data has been gathered, the next step is typically to quantify the frequency with which certain outcomes occur. This is a critical first step and must occur before setting about to identify the possible causes of a disease (eg, a specific HAI). This step is important for both measuring the scope of the problem (ie, how many people are affected by the HAI) and subsequently allowing comparison between different groups (ie, those with and without a particular risk factor of interest). The most commonly used measures of disease frequency in epidemiology are prevalence and incidence.

Prevalence

Prevalence is defined as the proportion of people with disease at a given point in time (eg, the proportion of hospitalized patients with a specific HAI) and is also sometimes referred to as point prevalence.

$$\text{Prevalence} = \frac{\text{Number of diseased individuals}}{\text{Total population}}$$

A related measure, although infrequently used, is the period prevalence, which is defined as the number of persons with disease in a given period divided by the number of persons observed during the period. Prevalence is a proportion and as such has no units. This measure of disease frequency depends on both the incidence (ie, the number of new cases which develop) and the duration of disease (ie, how long a diseases lasts once it has developed). The greater the incidence and the duration of disease, the higher is the prevalence. Prevalence is useful for measuring the burden of disease in a population (ie, the overall proportion of persons affected by the disease), which may in turn inform decisions regarding issues such as the allocation of resources and funding of research initiatives.

All populations are dynamic, perhaps few more so than the hospitalized patient population. Individuals are constantly entering and leaving the population. Depending on the population, the prevalence may vary depending on when it is measured. If a dynamic population is at steady state (ie, cases leaving = cases entering), the prevalence is constant over time.

Incidence

Incidence is defined as the number of new cases of diseases occurring in a specified period. Incidence may be described in several ways. Cumulative incidence is defined as the number of new cases of disease in a particular time period divided by the total number of disease-free individuals at risk of the disease at the beginning of the time period (eg, the proportion of patients who develop a nosocomial infection during hospitalization). In infectious diseases epidemiology, cumulative incidence traditionally has been termed as the attack rate.

$$\text{Cumulative Incidence} = \frac{\text{Number of new cases of disease between t0 and t1}}{\text{Total disease-free individuals at risk of disease at t0}}$$

The cumulative incidence, similar to prevalence, is a proportion and thus has no unit. To calculate the cumulative incidence, a complete follow-up on all observed individuals must be performed such that their final disposition regarding the presence or absence of the disease may be determined. Although this measure describes the total proportion of new cases occurring in a time period, it does not describe when in the time period the cases occurred.

For the cumulative incidence of HAIs, the time period implied is the course of hospitalization until a first event or discharge without a first event. However, patients do not all stay in hospital and remain at risk for exactly the same period. Furthermore, most HAIs are time related, and comparing the cumulative incidence of nosocomial infection among patient groups with differing lengths of stay may be misleading. By contrast, if events that come from a point source are investigated and are not time related (eg, tuberculosis acquired from a contaminated bronchoscope), then the cumulative incidence is an excellent measure of incidence. SSIs are also usually thought of as having a point source (ie, the operation).

Historically, HAI rates have often been reported as a cumulative incidence (ie, the number of infections per 100 discharges). This definition had no unique quantitative meaning because it did not separate first infections from multiple infections in the same patient and allowed undefined multiple counting of individuals. The implications of 5 infections per 100 discharges would be entirely different, depending on whether it represented 5 sequential infections in a single moribund patient or 5 first infections in 5 different but healthy patients such as women with normal deliveries.

The incidence rate (or incidence density) is defined as the number of new cases of disease in a specified quantity of person-time of observation among individuals at risk (eg, the number of central line–associated bloodstream infections per 1000 catheter-days).

$$\text{Incidence} = \frac{\text{Number of new cases of disease during given time period}}{\text{Total person-time of observation among individuals at risk}}$$

The primary value of this measure can be seen when comparing HAI rates in groups that differ in their time at risk (eg, short- vs long-stay patients). When the time at risk in one group is much greater than the time at risk in another, the incidence rate, or risk per day, is the most convenient way to correct for time and thus separate the effect of time (duration of exposure) from the effect of daily risk. For convenience in hospital epidemiology, incidence rates for HAIs are usually expressed as the number of first events in a certain number of days at risk (eg, infections per 1000 hospital days) because this value usually produces a small single- or double-digit number.

Incidence rate is usually restricted to first events (eg, the first episode of HAI). It is standard to consider only first events because second events are not statistically independent from first events in the same individuals (ie, patients with a first event are more likely to suffer a second event). For example, all hospitalized patients who have not yet developed a nosocomial infection would comprise the at-risk population. After a patient develops an infection, that patient would then be withdrawn and would not be a part of the population still at risk for a first event. Each hospitalized patient who never develops an infection would contribute all hospital days (ie, the sum of days the patient is in the hospital) to the pool of days at risk for a first event. However, a patient who develops an infection would contribute only those days before the onset of the infection.

Unlike cumulative incidence, the incidence rate does not assume complete follow-up of subjects and thus accounts for different entry and dropout rates. However, even when follow-up is complete (and thus cumulative incidence could be calculated), reporting the incidence rate may still be preferable. Cumulative incidence reports only the overall number of new cases occurring during the time period (regardless of whether they occur early or late in the time period). By comparison, the incidence rate, by incorporating the time at risk, accounts for potential difference in time to occurrence of the event.

Because the incidence rate counts time at risk in the denominator, the implicit assumption is that all the at-risk time periods are equal (eg, the likelihood developing a HAI infection in the first 3 days after hospital admission is the same as the likelihood of developing an infection during days 4 through 6 of hospitalization). If all time periods are not equal, the incidence rate may be misleading, depending on when, in the course of their time at risk, the patients are observed for the outcome.

Once the frequency of disease has been clearly characterized, subsequent steps may include focusing on the second and third components of the definition of epidemiology. As noted earlier, this definition includes describing the distribution of disease (ie, characterizing in whom, where, and when it is occurring), and the determinants of disease (ie, focusing on formulating and testing hypotheses with regard to the possible risk factors for disease). These next steps might include calculating measures of effect (eg, relative risk, odds ratios) to compare diseases in patient populations with different risk-factor profiles. Subsequent analytical studies to further define the epidemiology of a given disease could include study designs, such as case-control studies, cohort studies, or randomized controlled trials.

A detailed discussion of various study designs and statistical tests is beyond the scope of this article. Depending on the question being asked and the study design chosen, various statistical tests are required to compare patient groups. Before embarking on such a project, close collaboration or consultation with an epidemiologist and potentially a biostatistician is of great value. The choice of study design and statistical approaches require careful consideration to ensure proper conduct of the study and valid interpretation of the results. Time spent initially in designing such studies pays off immeasurably.

The importance of epidemiologic methods in the study of HAIs has been recognized for some time.[9,23–25] Indeed, the past 10 years has seen a renewed focus on efforts to explore previously unstudied aspects of epidemiologic methods in the study of HAIs and antimicrobial resistance.[26–31] Although this article is meant to provide a broad overview, the reader is also directed to numerous published textbooks that are solely dedicated to general epidemiology, infectious diseases epidemiology, and statistical analysis.[32–38]

SUMMARY

Technology offers the promise of increased efficiency in surveillance, but the trade-offs inherent in adopting new methods must be understood. The understanding of these trade-offs requires a firm grounding in basic principles of epidemiology. Just as health care epidemiologists must balance surveillance efforts with interventions, they must also balance new technology with traditional techniques. The challenge is determining how to strike the proper balance and the success is achieving an efficient and effective infection prevention program. Such a program leads to the best patient outcomes, which is the real reward.

REFERENCES

1. CDC. NHSN key terms. Available at: http://www.cdc.gov/nhsn/PDFs/pscManual/16pscKeyTerms_current.pdf. Accessed November 27, 2009.
2. Wright MO, Fisher A, John M, et al. The electronic medical record as a tool for infection surveillance: successful automation of device-days. Am J Infect Control 2009;37:364–70.
3. Leth RA, Moller JK. Surveillance of hospital-acquired infections based on electronic hospital registries. J Hosp Infect 2006;62:71–9.
4. Wang SJ, Kuperman GJ, Ohno-Machado L, et al. Using electronic data to predict the probability of true bacteremia from positive blood cultures. Proc AMIA Symp 2000;893–7.
5. Graham PL III, San Gabriel P, Lutwick S, et al. Validation of a multicenter computer-based surveillance system for hospital-acquired bloodstream infections in neonatal intensive care departments. Am J Infect Control 2004;32:232–4.
6. Trick WE, Zagorski BM, Tokars JI, et al. Computer algorithms to detect bloodstream infections. Emerg Infect Dis 2004;10:1612–20.
7. Woeltje KF, Goris AJ, Butler AM, et al. Automated surveillance for catheter-associated bloodstream infections outside of the intensive care unit. Presented at the 17th Annual Scientific Meeting of the Society for Healthcare Epidemiology of America. Baltimore (MD), April 2007.
8. Wenzel RP, Osterman CA, Hunting KJ. Hospital-acquired infections. II. Infection rates by site, service and common procedures in a university hospital. Am J Epidemiol 1976;104:645–51.
9. Haley RW, Schaberg DR, McClish DK, et al. The accuracy of retrospective chart review in measuring nosocomial infection rates: results of validation studies in pilot hospitals. Am J Epidemiol 1980;111:516–33.
10. Burke JP. Infection control—a problem for patient safety. N Engl J Med 2003;348:651–6.
11. Emori TG, Edwards JR, Culver DH, et al. Accuracy of reporting nosocomial infections in intensive-care-unit patients to the National Nosocomial Infections Surveillance System: a pilot study. Infect Control Hosp Epidemiol 1998;19:308–16.
12. Woeltje KF, Butler AM, Goris AJ, et al. Automated surveillance for central line–associated bloodstream infection in intensive care units. Infect Control Hosp Epidemiol 2008;29:842–6.
13. Platt R, Yokoe DS, Sands KE. CDC Eastern Massachusetts Prevention Epicenter investigators. Automated methods for surveillance of surgical site infections. Emerg Infect Dis 2001;7:212–6.

14. Sands K, Vineyard G, Platt R. Surgical site infections occurring after hospital discharge. J Infect Dis 1996;173:963–70.
15. Sands K, Vineyard G, Livingston J. Efficient identification of postdischarge surgical site infections using automated medical records. J Infect Dis 1999; 179:434–41.
16. Sands KE, Yokoe DS, Hooper DC, et al. Detection of postoperative surgical-site infections: comparison of health plan-based surveillance with hospital-based programs. Infect Control Hosp Epidemiol 2003;24:741–3.
17. Yokoe DS, Noskin GA, Cunnigham SM, et al. Enhanced identification of postoperative infections among inpatients. Emerg Infect Dis 2004;10:1924–30.
18. Bolon MK, Hooper D, Stevenson KB, et al. Centers for Disease Control and Prevention Epicenters Program. Improved surveillance for surgical site infections after orthopedic implantation procedures: extending applications for automated data. Clin Infect Dis 2009;48:1223–9.
19. Klompas M, Kleinman K, Platt R. Development of an algorithm for surveillance of ventilator-associated pneumonia with electronic data and comparison of algorithm results with clinician diagnoses. Infect Control Hosp Epidemiol 2008;29:31–7.
20. Wright MO, Perencevich EN, Novak C, et al. Preliminary assessment of an automated surveillance system for infection control. Infect Control Hosp Epidemiol 2004;25:325–32.
21. Moser SA, Jones WT, Brossette SE. Application of data mining to intensive care unit microbiologic data. Emerg Infect Dis 1999;5:454–7.
22. Huang SS, Yokoe DS, Stelling J, et al. Automated cluster detection in hospitals. Presented at the Annual Meeting of the Infectious Diseases Society of America. Washington, DC, October 25–28, 2008.
23. Haley RW, Quade D, Freeman HE, et al. The SENIC Project. Study on the Efficacy of Nosocomial Infection Control (SENIC Project). Summary of study design. Am J Epidemiol 1980;111:472–85.
24. Freeman J, McGowan JE Jr. Methodologic issues in hospital epidemiology. I. Rates, case-finding, and interpretation. Rev Infect Dis 1981;3:658–67.
25. Freeman J, McGowan JE Jr. Methodologic issues in hospital epidemiology. II. Time and accuracy in estimation. Rev Infect Dis 1981;3:668–77.
26. D'Agata EM. Methodologic issues of case-control studies: a review of established and newly recognized limitations. Infect Control Hosp Epidemiol 2005;26:338–41.
27. Paterson DL. Looking for risk factors for the acquisition of antibiotic resistance: a 21st century approach. Clin Infect Dis 2002;34:1564–7.
28. Schwaber MJ, De-Medina T, Carmeli Y. Epidemiological interpretation of antibiotic resistance studies—what are we missing? Nat Rev Microbiol 2004;2:979–83.
29. Harbarth S, Samore M. Antimicrobial resistance determinants and future control. Emerg Infect Dis 2005;11:794–801.
30. Hyle EP, Bilker WB, Gasink LB, et al. Impact of different methods for describing the extent of prior antibiotic exposure on the association between antibiotic use and antibiotic-resistant infection. Infect Control Hosp Epidemiol 2007;28:647–54.
31. Gasink LB, Zaoutis TE, Bilker WB, et al. The categorization of prior antibiotic use: impact on the identification of risk factors for drug resistance in case control studies. Am J Infect Control 2007;35:638–42.
32. Agresti A. Categorical data analysis, vol 2. New York: Wiley Interscience; 2002.
33. Hennekens CH, Buring JE, Mayrent SL. Epidemiology in medicine. 1st edition. Philadelphia: Lippincott Williams & Wilkins; 1987.
34. Hosmer DW, Lemeshow SL. Applied logistic regression. 2nd edition. New York: Wiley Interscience; 2000.

35. Kleinbaum DG, Kupper LL, Morgenstern H. Epidemiologic research: principles and quantitative methods. New York: Van Nostrand Reinhold; 1982.
36. Nelson KE, Williams CM, Graham NMH. Infectious disease epidemiology: theory and practice. 1st edition. New York: Aspen Publishers; 2000.
37. Rothman KJ, Greenland S. Modern epidemiology. Philadelphia: Lippincott Williams & Wilkins; 1998.
38. Thomas JC, Weber DJ. Epidemiologic methods for the study of infectious diseases. 1st edition. Oxford (UK): Oxford University Press; 2001.

Infection Prevention in Alternative Health Care Settings

Elaine Flanagan, RN, BSN, MSA, CIC[a], Teena Chopra, MD[b],
Lona Mody, MD, MSc[c,d],*

KEYWORDS

- Infection prevention • Programs • Skilled nursing facilities
- Ambulatory care setting

Health care delivery in the United States has evolved significantly over the latter part of the twentieth century. Health care delivery has moved from acute care facilities to skilled nursing facilities (SNFs), rehabilitation units, assisted living, home, and outpatient settings. Measures to reduce health care costs have led to a reduced number of hospitalizations and shorter lengths of stay (with an increase in the severity of illness among hospitalized patients including more frequent intensive care unit admissions), along with increased outpatient, home care, and SNF stays for older adults.[1–3]

This review focuses on infection control issues in SNFs and ambulatory clinics.

INFECTION PREVENTION PROGRAMS IN SNFs

SNFs are emerging as a major health care delivery site. Approximately 1.43 million older adults reside in Centers for Medicare and Medicaid Services certified SNFs (2006 data). About 3% to 15% of such patients acquire an infection in these facilities. In a year, there are approximately 2.1 million discharges from SNFs, with the primary reason for discharge being death or transfers to hospitals. These numbers are expected to grow as the population ages.[2]

SNFs provide 2 distinct types of care for older patients: (a) long-term care for older adults with irreversible functional and cognitive deficits and (b) subacute care for patients who require a short admission to complete their medical treatment plan and regain their functional strength before returning to their independent living.

[a] Department of Infection Prevention and Hospital Epidemiology, Detroit Medical Center, Detroit, MI, USA
[b] Division of Infectious Diseases and Infection Control ,Wayne State University, Detroit, MI, USA
[c] Division of Geriatric Medicine, University of Michigan Medical School, Ann Arbor, MI, USA
[d] Geriatrics Research, Education and Clinical Center, Veterans Affairs Ann Arbor Healthcare System, Ann Arbor, MI, USA
* Corresponding author. 11-G GRECC, Veterans Affairs Ann Arbor Healthcare System, 2215 Fuller Drive, Ann Arbor, MI 48105.
E-mail address: lonamody@umich.edu

Infect Dis Clin N Am 25 (2011) 271–283
doi:10.1016/j.idc.2010.11.008
0891-5520/11/$ – see front matter. Published by Elsevier Inc.

id.theclinics.com

Because SNFs accept increasingly complex patients from acute care settings, infection prevention becomes crucial. Infection prevention research in the SNF setting has made enormous strides in the last 2 decades. There is an increasing recognition that infection prevention strategies have to be more individualized than in hospital settings, and residents' social well-being remains paramount.

However, SNFs have unique characteristics that create special challenges in implementing an effective infection prevention program. First, SNF residents are particularly susceptible to infections because of multimorbidity, greater severity of illness, functional impairment, cognitive impairment, incontinence, and the frequent use of short-term and long-term indwelling devices such as urinary catheters and feeding tubes. Second, SNF residents may also serve as host reservoirs for antimicrobial resistant pathogens such as methicillin-resistant *Staphylococcus aureus* (MRSA) and vancomycin-resistant enterococci (VRE). With reduction in the length of hospital stay, the severity of illness among residents of the subacute care nursing unit has increased with resultant inherent rapid transfers to a hospital. Older adults serve as vectors, transmitting pathogens from one setting to another. Third, utility of diagnostic specimens is often limited because of the difficulty in obtaining specimens from older adults (such as a clean catch urine sample or a sputum sample) and the lag time between specimen acquisition and clinical evaluation. Conversely, some tests might be more frequently performed and might lead to inappropriate antibiotic usage. All these factors combined create an environment where vulnerable residents are highly prone to infections and acquisition of resistant pathogens. The diagnostic dilemmas often lead to suboptimal management of infections in older adults and make infection prevention programs even more crucial.

INFECTION PREVENTION PROGRAM IN SNFs: FUNCTIONS, COMPONENTS, AND OVERSIGHT

Main functions of an infection prevention program include (a) obtaining and managing critical data, including surveillance information for endemic infections and outbreaks; (b) developing and updating policies and procedures; (c) developing individualized interventions to prevent infections and antimicrobial resistance; and (d) educating and training health care workers (HCWs), patients, visitors, and nonmedical caregivers.[1]

An effective infection prevention program includes a method of surveillance for infections and antimicrobial resistant pathogens, an outbreak control plan for epidemics, isolation and standard precautions, hand hygiene, staff education, an employee health program, a resident health program, policy formation and periodic review with audits, and a policy to communicate reportable diseases to public health authorities. An infection preventionist (IP) is crucial in developing and executing an infection prevention program.

Information Transfer During Care Transitions

Transitional care is defined as "a set of actions designed to ensure the coordination and continuity of health care as patients transfer between different locations or different levels of care in the same location."[4] For older adults, these locations include acute care hospitals, nursing homes, SNFs, rehabilitation units, assisted living facilities, inpatient hospice care, home care, and outpatient primary and specialty clinics. During these care transitions, older adults are particularly prone to fragmented care that can lead to errors and omissions in health care delivery. These transitions also provide an opportunity for pathogens to be transferred from one setting to another.

It then becomes important for the SNFs to request clinical information from the transferring facility regarding current culture reports of the resident's body sites that may be infected or colonized with pathogenic organisms, especially multidrug-resistant organisms. This action enables the physician providers and HCWs to determine the nursing care interventions necessary to meet the resident's needs and to prevent spread of pathogens in the facility.

Hand Hygiene

Hand hygiene remains the most effective and least expensive measure to prevent transmission of pathogenic organisms in a health care setting. Despite calls from numerous local, national, and international organizations and infection prevention societies, compliance with hand hygiene remains dismal averaging only 30% to 50%.[5–8] Reasons frequently reported for poor compliance with hand hygiene measures by HCWs include skin irritation from frequent washing, too little time because of high workload, and simply forgetting.

The World Health Organization (WHO) launched its first Global Patient Safety Challenge, 'Clean Care is Safer Care,' in October 2005.[9] The objective of this initiative is to reduce health care–associated infections around the globe. The program's initial focus is the promotion of hand hygiene practices in diverse health care systems. WHO has also developed an innovative core theme, 'My five moments of hand hygiene,' which details appropriate situations for compliance with hand hygiene measures during health care delivery. This approach provides guidelines and specific recommendations to enhance hand hygiene compliance and is targeted at a broad audience of HCWs, hospital administrators, and health authorities.

The use of waterless alcohol-based hand rubs as an adjunct to washing hands with soap and water has become a routine practice by HCWs in many acute care facilities.[10] Introduction of alcohol-based hand rubs has been shown to significantly improve hand hygiene compliance among HCWs in acute care hospitals and to decrease overall nosocomial infection rates and transmission of MRSA infections. Alcohol-based hand rubs have also been shown to enhance compliance with hand hygiene in SNFs and should be used to complement educational initiatives.[6] Although the cost of introducing alcohol-based hand rubs could be a concern of SNFs, recent data in acute care have shown that the total costs of a hand hygiene promotion campaign, including alcohol-based hand rubs, corresponded to less than 1% of costs that could be attributed to nosocomial infections.[7]

Although introducing alcohol-based hand rub in health care settings is a prudent cost-effective measure, several issues need to be considered. Alcohol-based hand rubs should not be used if hands are visibly soiled, in which case hand hygiene with antimicrobial soap and water is recommended. Alcohol-based hand rubs can cause dryness of skin; however, recent data on rubs containing emollients have shown that hand rubs cause significantly less skin irritation and dryness than soap and water.[11] Facilities should be aware that alcohols are flammable. Facilities have reported difficulties in implementing the current hand hygiene guidelines pertaining to the use of alcohol-based hand rubs because of the fire safety concerns. Existing national fire codes permit the use of alcohol-based hand rub dispensers in patient rooms but not in egress or exit corridors. Because the state and local fire codes may differ from national codes, facilities should work with their local fire marshals to ensure that installation of alcohol-based hand rub containers is consistent with local fire codes.

Multidrug-Resistant Organisms

Infection and colonization with antimicrobial resistant pathogens are important concerns in SNFs and they develop primarily because of the widespread use of empiric antibiotics, functional impairment, the use of indwelling devices, mediocre adherence to hand hygiene programs among HCWs, and cross-transmission during group activities. An SNF can reduce infections and colonization with resistant pathogens by emphasizing hand hygiene, developing an antimicrobial use program, encouraging evidence-based clinical evaluation and management of infections, and ensuring that the facility has a well-established individualized infection prevention program. Guidelines and expert reviews to control MRSA and VRE infections provide a good base for developing facility-specific policies.[1,12–14]

There has been some debate on the role and effect of active surveillance cultures (cultures used to detect asymptomatic colonization of a patient with an organism) on isolation policies in acute care hospitals. The Society for Healthcare Epidemiology of America (SHEA) guidelines for preventing nosocomial transmission of multidrug-resistant organisms advocate the use of active surveillance cultures,[15] whereas the recent draft of Healthcare Infection Control and Prevention Advisory Committee (HICPAC) guidelines call for individual facilities to assess their own needs and conduct surveillance cultures as they deem necessary.[16] These guidelines refer to studies from acute care hospitals serving a sicker shorter-staying population than those served by SNFs. The role of active surveillance cultures in SNFs has not been clearly defined. Facilities should evaluate these guidelines and individualize their plan to obtain active surveillance cultures based on the population they serve, the baseline rates of MRSA and VRE, and any recent outbreaks.

Isolation Precautions

The Centers for Disease Control and Prevention's (CDC's) HICPAC has proposed a 2-tiered structure for isolation precautions. In the first tier, HICPAC proposes the use of standard precautions that have been designed for the care of all patients in hospitals, regardless of their diagnosis, infections, or otherwise. Standard precautions constitute the primary strategy for preventing the transmission of organisms between patients and HCWs. In the second tier are transmission-based precautions that have been designed for the care of patients suspected or known to be infected with epidemiologically important pathogens that have been acquired by physical contact or airborne or droplet transmission.[17]

Standard precautions apply to blood; all body fluids; secretions and excretions, regardless of whether they contain visible blood; nonintact skin; and/or mucous membrane material. Designed to reduce the risk of transmission of pathogens, both from apparent and ambiguous sources of infection, these precautions include hand hygiene compliance; using gloves, masks, gowns; and eye protection, as well as avoiding injuries from sharps. Two new elements of standard precautions added in the new HICPAC isolation precautions guidelines and also applicable to SNFs include respiratory hygiene/cough etiquette and safe injection practices. The elements of respiratory hygiene/cough etiquette include education of health care facility staff, patients, and visitors; display of appropriate language and education on posters and signs; source control measures such as covering the mouth/nose with a tissue and prompt disposal of used tissues; hand hygiene compliance after contact with respiratory secretions; and spatial separation of symptomatic patients by more than 3 ft in common areas, if possible. Safe injection practices include the use of single-use, sterile, disposable needles and syringes for each injection and the prevention of contamination of any injection equipment and medication.[17]

Transmission-based precautions are intended for use in patients who may be infected with highly transmissible or epidemiologically significant pathogens. These include airborne precautions (eg, for tuberculosis), droplet precautions (eg, for influenza), and contact precautions (eg, for *Clostridium difficile* infections). Although these guidelines were designed for acute care settings, several of them, especially the universal precautions, apply to SNFs as well. These recommendations have to be adapted to the needs of the individual facility. A single-patient room is preferred for residents who require contact precautions. Often, SNFs have high occupancy rates and a paucity of single-resident rooms. In such situations, residents should be cohorted or retained with the same roommate. A spatial separation of 3 ft or more between beds is advised to reduce the opportunities for inadvertent sharing of items between a colonized or infected patient and an uncolonized patient.[17]

Private rooms are generally indicated for residents with uncontrolled excretions (diarrhea), secretions, excessive coughing, heavy wound drainage, or widespread skin disease; if these conditions are active, single-resident rooms are preferable. However, if no private rooms are available, the resident can be admitted in a semiprivate room, preferably with a resident who is at low risk of developing an infection (such as one who is well nourished, is ambulatory, can perform daily activities independently, and has no indwelling catheters/lines or open wounds).

Residents, colonized or infected with a specific pathogen, should participate in facility activities and eat in the dining hall. Because there are both recognized and unrecognized pathogen carriers participating in these group activities, all residents should have their wounds or invasive sites cleansed and covered and their hands washed before leaving their rooms.

Surveillance for Infections and Antimicrobial Usage

Infection surveillance in SNFs involves collection of data on facility-acquired infections. Surveillance is defined as "ongoing, systematic collection, analysis, and interpretation of health data essential to the planning, implementation, and evaluation of public health practice, closely integrated with timely dissemination of these data to those who need to know."[18] Surveillance can be limited based on a particular objective, a particular ward, or an unusual organism or it may be facility wide.

For surveillance to be conducted correctly, use of standardized SNF-appropriate definitions of infections is crucial.[19,20] Besides using valid surveillance definitions, a facility must have clear goals and aims for setting up a surveillance program. These goals, as with other elements of an infection control program, have to be reviewed periodically to reflect changes in the facility's population, pathogens of interest, and changing antimicrobial resistance patterns. Plans to analyze the data and the use of these data to design and implement proved preventive measures must be clearly delineated in advance. The analysis and reporting of infection rates in SNFs are typically conducted monthly, quarterly, and annually to detect trends. Infection rates (preferably reported as infections per 1000 resident-days) can be calculated by using resident-days or average resident census for the surveillance period as the denominator.

These data can then be used to establish endemic baseline infection rates and to recognize variations from the baseline that could represent an outbreak. This information should eventually lead to specific targeted infection control initiatives. Additionally, a facility's surveillance system should include monitoring for appropriate antibiotic use. For example, a person with positive culture results but without clinical symptoms rarely requires treatment with antibiotics.

Outbreak Management

An illness in a community or region is considered an outbreak when the frequency of the illness clearly exceeds the normal rate of expectancy. The existence of an outbreak is thus always defined relative to the number of cases that are expected to occur in a specific population in a specific period.

The main objectives of an outbreak investigation are control and elimination of the source, prevention of new cases, prevention of future outbreaks, research to gain additional knowledge about the infectious agent and its mode of transmission, program evaluation, and strategies for improvement.

It is vital that the IP, in conjunction with physician support, has the skills to recognize an outbreak, conduct appropriate data collection methods, analyze and interpret the data using simple epidemiologic measures, conduct an initial outbreak investigation efficiently, and institute emergent, effective, and appropriate outbreak control measures. Although local health departments are available for counseling, it may also be beneficial for the IP to have access to a hospital epidemiologist for consultation.

Rehabilitation Services

SNFs increasingly are responsible for postacute care rehabilitation, including physical therapy (PT), occupational therapy (OT), and wound care with or without hydrotherapy. The therapists providing these therapies, like other clinical staff such as nurses and nurses' aides, frequently come into contact with residents and thus have many opportunities to transmit pathogens. In an SNF, PT and OT services can be provided either at the bedside or in a central therapy unit. For bedside therapy, therapists may move between rooms and units and do not routinely wear gloves and gowns. For care at a central therapy unit, residents are transported to an open unit where hand washing sinks may not be readily available. Although therapists have not been implicated in any major outbreaks, hydrotherapy for wounds has been shown to facilitate outbreaks of resistant pathogens.[21]

A detailed infection control program for rehabilitation services should be prepared and should focus on facility design to promote hand hygiene compliance, including convenient and easy access to sinks and the use of alcohol-based hand rubs. Patients who are infectious should not be treated at the central therapy facility. Facilities providing hydrotherapy should consider providing the service in a dedicated room with a separate resident entrance.

Resident and Employee Health Program

The resident health program should focus on immunizations, tuberculin testing, and infection control policies to prevent specific infections. The program should include skin care, oral hygiene, prevention of aspiration, and catheter care to prevent urinary tract infections. Adults older than 65 years should receive pneumococcal vaccination at least once, influenza vaccination every year, and a tetanus booster every 10 years.

The employee health program mainly concerns employees with potentially communicable diseases, policies for sick leave, immunizations, and Occupational Health and Safety Administration (OSHA) regulations to protect the employees from blood-borne pathogens. It is a requirement that SNFs bar employees with known communicable diseases or infected skin lesions from being in direct contact with the residents and that employees with infected skin lesions or infectious diarrhea be prevented from having direct contact with residents' food. Moreover, when hiring new employees, an initial medical history must be obtained along with a physical examination and screening for tuberculosis.

Infection control policies and measures in SNFs must be in place to address post-exposure prophylaxis for infections such as AIDS and hepatitis B. Varicella vaccine should be given to employees not immune to the virus. Employees are expected to be up-to-date with their tetanus boosters and to receive influenza vaccinations every year. The influenza vaccine effective in preventing influenza and reducing absenteeism in HCWs and it also has been associated with a decrease in mortality caused by influenza in residents.[22] Annual influenza vaccination campaigns play a central role in deterring and preventing nosocomial transmission of the influenza virus and should be promoted by the IP and SNF leadership.

Role of IP

An IP, usually a staff nurse, is assigned the responsibility of directing infection control activities in an SNF. The IP is responsible for implementing, monitoring, and evaluating the infection control program. Often, an IP also functions as an assistant director of nursing or is involved in staff recruitment and education. For an infection control program to succeed, the IP should be empowered with sufficient time and resources to carry out infection control activities. The IP should also be familiar with the federal, state, and local regulations regarding infection control. Collaborating with an infectious diseases epidemiologist should be encouraged. Such collaborations could also provide assistance with outbreak investigations, emergency preparedness in the event of bioterrorism and vaccine shortages, and the use of microbiological and molecular methods for infection prevention. Resources available to the IP are discussed in **Box 1**.

Box 1
Resources for IPs

1. Both SHEA and the Association for Professionals in Infection Control and Epidemiology (APIC) have long-term care committees that publish and approve SNF infection guidelines and publish periodic position papers related to pertinent infection control issues. Their Web sites have several educational resources for staff education and in-service training. In addition, APIC also publishes a quarterly long-term care newsletter.

2. Local APIC articles provide a network for infection control practitioners to socialize, discuss infection control challenges and practical solutions to overcome them, and provide access to educational resources and services. Infection control practitioners should become members of APIC at both the local and national levels to remain up-to-date with practice guidelines, position statements, information technology resources, and changes in policies and regulations.

3. Glen Mayhall C, editor. Hospital epidemiology and infection control. 3rd edition. Philadelphia: Lippincott Williams & Wilkins; 2004.

4. Selected Internet Web sites:

   CDC: http://www.cdc.gov

   SHEA: http://www.shea-online.org/

   APIC: http://www.apic.org

   OSHA: http://www.osha.gov

   Joint Commission on Accreditation of Healthcare Organizations (JCAHO) Infection Control Initiatives: http://www.jcaho.org/accredited+organizations/patient+safety/infection+control/ic+index.htm.

Environmental rounds

The IP should conduct walk rounds on a regular basis to make observations regarding (1) equipment decontamination and cleaning procedures in bathroom/tub areas; (2) adherence to infection control guidelines by physical therapists, in medication/treatment rooms, and in kitchen and laundry areas; (3) availability of soap and paper towels, handling of sharps and infectious waste, and storage of health care supplies, medications, and food.

Staff education

The IP plays a vital role in meeting these requirements and in educating SNF personnel on various infection control measures, particularly in view of rapid staff turnover that occurs at many SNFs. Informal education during infection control and quality improvement meetings as well as during infection control walk rounds should be complemented with in-service education on hand hygiene, appropriate and early diagnosis of infections, indications for antibiotic usage and antimicrobial resistance, and isolation precautions and policies.

Ongoing staff education is important because of the new research data and guidelines published every year, advancements in technology, and regulatory demands. Joint Commission on Accreditation of Healthcare Organizations expects new employee orientation to include the facility's infection prevention program, and the employee's individual responsibility is to prevent infections. In addition, OSHA requires training for handling blood-borne pathogens and patients with tuberculosis for any employee who is expected to come into contact with potentially infectious agents.

Oversight Committee

The Federal Nursing Home Reform Act from the Omnibus Budget Reconciliation Act (OBRA) of 1987 mandated the formation of a formal infection control committee to evaluate infection rates, implement infection control programs, and review policies and procedures. Although still required by some states, this mandate has been dropped by OBRA at the federal level A small subcommittee or a working group that is composed of the medical director, administrator or nursing supervisor, and infection control practitioner should evaluate the SNF infection rates on a regular basis and present the data at quality control meetings, review policies and any relevant research, and make decisions regarding infection control changes. This subcommittee can review and analyze the surveillance data, assure that these data are presented to the nursing and physician staff, and approve targeted recommendations to reduce the incidence of infections. Records pertaining to these activities and infection data should be kept and filed for future reference.

Principles guiding infection control practices also provide a model for enhancing quality of care and patient safety for other noninfectious adverse outcomes such as falls, delirium, inappropriate medication usage, and adverse drug events.

AMBULATORY CARE CENTERS

Ambulatory care settings have the same infection prevention and control requirements as inpatient hospital settings, but the method of application to comply with the standards varies depending on the type of care provided by that clinic to their population. The settings range from clinics that provide medical specialty expertise to clinics that perform invasive procedures, such as hemodialysis, endoscopy, and surgical centers. There are many challenges in ambulatory care to reduce infection risk and improve patient safety. Infection control oversight and accountability is often lacking, especially if the clinics are not part of a hospital or system.

Communicable Diseases and Isolation Management

Patients may be exposed to infectious diseases in the ambulatory waiting rooms. HCWs need to use standard precautions in the care of all patients, but patients exhibiting communicable disease symptoms should be managed per the CDC isolation precautions.[17] Because most ambulatory centers do not have adequate private rooms, a triage policy should be followed. The goal is to promptly identify and handle patients with symptoms compatible with communicable disease in order to protect other patients and ambulatory care staff from exposure or infection. Symptoms of a communicable disease may include tuberculosis symptoms such as cough, bloody sputum, night sweats, weight loss, anorexia, and fever. Symptoms of other communicable diseases might include rash of unknown origin or persistent cough. Patients with respiratory symptoms should wear a mask and should be promptly directed to a separate waiting area or examination room apart from other patients. If the ambulatory site has negative pressure rooms for acid-fast bacillus (AFB) and airborne isolation, patients with suspected tuberculosis and other communicable diseases transmitted by airborne route should be triaged to these rooms as soon as possible.[23] When entering the room of a patient with suspected or confirmed tuberculosis, all ambulatory staff should wear a fit-tested particulate respirator. Cough-inducing procedures such as aerosol administration of medication, bronchoscopy, and sputum inductions in patients with a respiratory illness pose a high risk of aerosolization of organisms and infection of staff and other patients. Rooms where these aerosol-producing procedures are performed must be modified to meet airborne isolation standards to protect ambulatory care staff and other patients. Ambulatory surgery centers must provide particulate respirators to staff caring for patients maintained in AFB and airborne isolation. Dental clinics should defer treatment in a patient with known or suspected *Mycobacterium tuberculosis* infection or other potentially communicable airborne diseases unless it is determined that the procedure is an emergency.

Respiratory hygiene/cough etiquette is an infection control component of the CDC standard precautions in care of patients. The protocol is optimized by giving tissues to patients and instructing them to cover their mouth and nose when coughing or sneezing and to dispose used tissues in the trash. Hand washing must be reinforced with accessible hand washing facilities or waterless hand hygiene agents. Patients with persistent cough should be given a surgical mask while in a waiting room or other common areas and instructed to ask for a new mask if their old mask becomes soiled or moistened. Respiratory etiquette signage is a Joint Commission requirement for ambulatory centers within hospital institutions but is encouraged to be used in all ambulatory centers especially during flu season.

Environmental Hygiene: Cleaning, Disinfection, and Sterilization

Cleaning and disinfection of frequently touched surfaces reduce the risk of transmission of multidrug-resistant organism and *C difficile*. Ambulatory settings need to standardize cleaning procedures and types of chemicals used and establish a monitoring system to assure that the patient care equipment and environment are cleaned and disinfected and the equipment stored appropriately so that patient safety is optimized.[22,24–26] Staff should be educated on the use of the chemicals, and annual competencies are recommended for specific disinfection and sterilization procedures. All cleaning, disinfection, and sterilization processes should comply with the CDC guidelines.[24]

High-level disinfection and sterilization of patient care equipment is an important area of infection control in many ambulatory settings and is discussed by W. Rutala, in the following section as well as in detail elsewhere in this issue.

Ambulatory surgical centers

The same aseptic techniques and environmental standards apply to all surgical settings. The National Patient Safety Goals (NPSGs) for ambulatory and office-based surgery provide the elements of performance to achieve safe patient care.[27] One of the elements of NPSGs requires improvement in hand hygiene compliance. Another element requires evidence-based practices for preventing surgical site infections (SSIs). The IP can provide guidance to implement the practices. Major components include hair removal only with clippers and no shaving at the surgical site, administration of antimicrobial agents for prophylaxis for a particular procedure or disease according to guidelines, and providing education regarding prevention of SSIs to patients and families as well as staff and licensed independent practitioners involved in surgical procedures. Process and outcome measures need to be documented and reviewed as determined by the ambulatory site's risk assessment. These measures might include incidence of SSIs, compliance with antibiotic prophylaxis, time-out practices by the operating room team, or compliance with hair removal methods. The IP can collaborate with the surgery team in identifying the high-risk or most frequent surgical procedures performed, so that the surveillance program can be targeted to address key components of operative care. Currently, there are no external benchmarks available for SSIs or other process measures for surgeries performed in ambulatory centers. It is recommended that internal benchmarks be used (ie, ambulatory centers track SSIs and compliance rates at their institution and look for changes over time). Overall, surgical infection rates and procedure specific rates (for procedures primarily performed in hospitals), as published by the CDC, may be used.[28]

IPs and other HCWs who clean and process patient care equipment should be familiar with the basic principles for sterilization and disinfection outlined by Earle H. Spaulding. The principles classify patient care items and equipment into 3 categories based on the degree of risk of infection involved in the use of the items: critical, semicritical, and noncritical.[26] This classification provides guidance for determining the level of disinfection required and items requiring sterilization. Flash sterilization must be performed at a minimum and should not be used as a reason for shortage of instruments per Association for the Advancement of Medical Instrumentation guidelines.[25] The Joint Commission Infection Control Standards are now focusing on flash sterilization procedures in the operating room to assure procedural compliance.[22] A major challenge to ambulatory surgical centers and the IP is to remain current with changes in sterilization technology and disinfectant products. New surgical equipment is frequently becoming available and the manufacturer's processing guidelines need to be followed to prevent damage to the instruments as well as for adequate disinfection or sterilization.

Safe Injection Practices

The CDC has implemented recommendations related to safe injection practices as part of their standard precautions to provide safety to both the HCW and the patient. Injuries caused by needles and other sharps have been associated with the transmission of hepatitis B virus, hepatitis C virus, and human immunodeficiency virus. The federal Needlestick Safety and Prevention Act signed into law in November 2000 authorized OSHA's revision of its Bloodborne Pathogens Standard to require the use of safety-engineered sharp devices.[29] Ambulatory services need to provide policies and infection control to in-service staff, regarding aseptic techniques and correct management of sharps in patient care.

Syringes, needles, insulin pens, and all sharps must be single use. Changing a needle or cannula and using the same syringe may still support transmission of pathogens. Fluid infusion and administration should be single use. Single-dose vials should be used whenever possible and clearly dedicated to a single patient. If multiple-dose vials are used, they must be stored appropriately according to manufacturer recommendations and kept in the immediate patient treatment areas. Using bags or bottles of intravenous solution as a common source for multiple patients is an unsafe practice and has been associated with outbreaks.[30]

Inappropriate use of products among multiple patients has resulted in many large and harmful outbreaks. Examples include a hepatitis B outbreak in New York City in 2001 because of multidose use for injections and contaminated syringes left on the table where medications were prepared, a hepatitis C outbreak in a Nevada endoscopy clinic in 2007 due to reuse of same syringe for propofol administration, and hepatitis B and C transmission caused by the reuse of glucometers and insulin pens.[31–33]

Bioterrorism and Disaster Planning

A risk assessment of the clinic location and the community it serves provides guidance for emergency preparedness and emergency plans. Factors to consider in emergency planning are the socioeconomic level and vaccine status of the population, natural disasters the area may be prone to, and access routes to the clinic. Clinics associated with health systems should be included in the emergency plans of the health system. Independent clinics need to collaborate with a local hospital, public health department, and government agencies. The plans should provide a process by which the facility can use mitigation strategies to become prepared to respond to and recover from all types of disasters. IPs should actively participate in the planning process.[34]

SUMMARY

Outpatient services are continually increasing and changing with the expansion of new technologies. Increased use of invasive devices and procedures provides new and challenging risks for infection. Risks associated with contaminated equipment can be decreased by knowledge and maintenance of aseptic techniques and disinfection practices. The challenge to infection control and ambulatory staff is to remain updated and familiar with these emerging technologies to increase the likelihood of preventing health care–associated infections and providing safe patient care. More patients with a high acuity of illness are now being encountered in ambulatory instead of inpatient settings, and these patients often spend prolonged periods in waiting rooms, in close proximity to others. The risk of communicable disease transmission and presence of multidrug-resistant organisms necessitate standard and transmission-based precautions for all patient care settings, including ambulatory settings. The HCWs, patients, and family members of patients need to be educated to support patient safety and minimize risk for infection. The IP has unique challenges in providing the ambulatory clinic both infection prevention and regulatory strategies.

REFERENCES

1. Smith PW, Bennett G, Bradley SF, et al. Infection prevention and control in long-term care facilities. Infect Control Hosp Epidemiol 2008;29:785–814.
2. Friedman C, Barnette M, Buck AS, et al. Requirement for infrastructure and essential activities of infection control and epidemiology in out-of-hospital settings: a consensus panel report. Infect Control Hosp Epidemiol 1999;20: 695–705.
3. Jarvis WR. Infection control and changing health-care delivery systems. Emerg Infect Dis 2001;7:170–3.

4. Coleman EA. Falling through cracks: challenges and opportunities for improving transitional care for persons with continuous complex care needs. J Am Geriatr Soc 2003;51:549–55.

5. Aiello A, Malinis M, Knapp J, et al. Hand hygiene practices in nursing homes: does knowledge influence practice? Am J Infect Control 2009;37:164–7.

6. Mody L, McNeil SA, Sun R, et al. Introduction of a waterless alcohol-based hand rub in a long-term care facility. Infect Control Hosp Epidemiol 2003;24:165–71.

7. Pittet D, Sax H, Hugonnet S, et al. Cost implications of successful hand hygiene promotion. Infect Control Hosp Epidemiol 2004;25:264–6.

8. Centers for Disease Control and Prevention. Guideline for hand hygiene in health-care settings: recommendations of the Healthcare Infection Control Practices Advisory Committee and the HICPAC/SHEA/APIC/IDSA hand hygiene task force. MMWR 2002;51:S3–40.

9. Pittet D, Allegranzi B, Boyce J. The World Health Organization guidelines on hand hygiene in health care and their consensus recommendations. Infect Control Hosp Epidemiol 2009;30:611–22.

10. Mody L, Saint S, Kaufman S, et al. Adoption of alcohol-based handrub by United States hospitals: a national survey. Infect Control Hosp Epidemiol 2008;29:1177–80.

11. Pedersen LK, Held E, Johansen JD, et al. Less skin irritation from alcohol-based disinfectant than from detergent used for hand disinfection. Br J Dermatol 2005;153:1142–6.

12. Bradley SF. Issues in management of resistant bacteria in long-term care facilities. Infect Control Hosp Epidemiol 1999;20:362–6.

13. Hujer AM, Bether CR, Hujer KM, et al. Antibiotic resistance in the institutionalized elderly. Clin Lab Med 2004;24:343–61.

14. Goldrick BA. MRSA, VRE, and VRSA: how do we control them in nursing homes? Am J Nurs 2004;104:50–1.

15. Muto CA, Jernigan JA, Ostrowsky BE, et al. SHEA guideline for preventing nosocomial transmission of multidrug-resistant strains of *Staphylococcus aureus* and *Enterococcus*. Infect Control Hosp Epidemiol 2003;24:362–86.

16. Siegel JD, Rhinehart E, Jackson M, et al. Management of multi-drug resistant organisms in healthcare settings. 2006. Available at: http://www.cdc.gov/ncidod/dhqp/pdf/ar/MDROGuideline2006.pdf. Accessed February, 2010.

17. Siegel JD, Rhinehart E, Jackson M, et al. Guideline for isolation precautions: preventing transmission of infectious agents in healthcare settings. 2007. Available at: http://www.cdc.gov/ncidod.dhqp/pdf/isolation2007.pdf. Accessed February, 2010.

18. Horan TC, Gaynes RP. Surveillance of nosocomial infections. In: Mayhall CG, editor. Hospital epidemiology and infection control. 3rd edition. Philadelphia: Lippincott Williams & Wilkins; 2004. p. 1661–702.

19. McGeer A, Campbell B, Emori TG, et al. Definitions of infection for surveillance in long-term care facilities. Am J Infect Control 1991;19:1–7.

20. Stevenson KB, Moore J, Colwell H, et al. Standardized infection surveillance in long-term care: interfacility comparisons from a regional cohort of facilities. Infect Control Hosp Epidemiol 2005;26:231–8.

21. Embril JM, McLeod JA, AL-Barrak AM, et al. An outbreak of methicillin-resistant *Staphylococcus aureus* on a burn unit: potential role of contaminated hydrotherapy equipment. Burns 2001;27:681–8.

22. Steam sterilization–update on the Joint Commission's position. Available at: www.jointcommission.org/Library/WhatsNew/steam_sterilization.htm. Accessed November 3, 2010.

23. Centers for Disease Control and Prevention. Guideline for preventing the transmission of *Mycobacterium tuberculosis* in healthcare settings. Atlanta (GA): Centers for Disease Control and Prevention; 2005.
24. Rutala W, Weber D, Healthcare Infection Control Practices Advisory Committee (HICPAC). Guideline for disinfection and sterilization in healthcare facilities. Atlanta (GA): Centers for Disease Control and Prevention; 2008.
25. Connor R, Spry C. Comprehensive guide to steam sterilization and sterility assurance in health care facilities. Arlington (VA): Association for the Advancement of Medical Instrumentation; July 2006.
26. Spaulding EH. Chemical disinfection of medical and surgical materials. In: Lawrence C, Block SS, editors. Disinfection sterilization and preservation. Philadelphia: Lea & Febiger; 1968. p. 517–31.
27. Ambulatory Health Care Accreditation Program. Chapter: National Patient Safety Goals. The Joint Commission on Accreditation of Healthcare Organizations. 2010. Available at: www.jointcommission.org/standards. Accessed November 3, 2010.
28. Edwards JR, Peterson KD, Mu Y, et al. National Healthcare Safety Network (NHSN) report: data summary for 2006 through 2008, issued December 2009. Am J Infect Control 2009;37:783–805.
29. Needlestick Safety and Prevention Act (Public Law 106-430), November 6, 2000.
30. Centers for Disease Control and Prevention (CDC). Transmission of hepatitis B and C viruses in outpatient settings-New York, Oklahoma, and Nebraska, 2000–2002. MMWR Morb Mortal Wkly Rep 2003;52(38):901–6.
31. Hepatitis B outbreak in New York City, 2001. Infect Control Hosp Epidemiol 2005; 26:745–60.
32. Centers for Disease Control and Prevention (CDC). Acute hepatitis C virus infections attributed to unsafe injection practices at an endoscopy clinic-Nevada, 2007. MMWR Morb Mortal Wkly Rep 2008;57:513–7.
33. US Food and Drug Administration alert: insulin pens and insulin cartridges must not be shared [news release]. Silver Spring (MD): FDA; March 19, 2009.
34. Chapter 117: emergency management and Chapter 118: infectious disease disasters: bioterrorism, emerging infections, and pandemics. In: APIC text of infection control and epidemiology. 3rd edition. Scientific and practice elements, vol. 2. Washington, DC: Association for Professionals in Infection Control and Epidemiology, Inc; 2009.

Index

Note: Page numbers of article titles are in **boldface** type.

A

Accelerated hydrogen peroxide, for sterilization and high-level disinfection, 53
Active surveillance, in MDRO control, 187–189
Active surveillance cultures, in MRSA control, 164–170
Adenovirus, 237–238
AERs. See *Automated endoscope reprocessors (AERs)*.
Alcohol-based hand rubs, 24–26
Alternative health care settings, infection prevention in, **271–283**. See also specific settings
    and *Infection prevention and control program(s)*.
Ambulatory care centers, infection prevention programs in, 278–281
    bioterrorism and disaster planning, 281
    communicable diseases and isolation management, 279
    environmental hygiene, 279–280
    safe injection practices, 280–281
Antibiotic(s). See also *Antimicrobial.*
Antibiotic-impregnated central venous catheters, in CLA-BSI prevention, 82–85
Anti-infective catheters, in CAUTI prevention, 111–112
Anti-infective "locks," in CLA-BSI prevention, 86
Antimicrobial prophylaxis, perioperative, in surgical site infection prevention, 142–143
Antimicrobial stewardship, **245–260**
    described, 245–246
    goals of, 246
    in MDRO control, 189–191
    in MRSA control, 171–172
    making business case for, 255
    strategies in, 249–254
        antibiotic cycling, 253–254
        clinical guidelines development and education approaches, 249–250
        computer-based decision support, 252–253
        postprescription review, 251–252
        preprescription approval, 250–251
Antimicrobial stewardship program
    essential participants in, 246–249
        clinical pharmacist, 247
        hospital administration, 247–248
        infection control and hospital epidemiology staff, 249
        infectious-disease physician, 246–247
        information technology, 247–248
        microbiology laboratory, 247–248
        Pharmacy and Therapeutics Committee, 248
    implementation and maintenance of, barriers to, 254–255
    measuring effect of, 255–257

Infect Dis Clin N Am 25 (2011) 285–293
doi:10.1016/S0891-5520(10)00110-8
0891-5520/11/$ – see front matter © 2011 Elsevier Inc. All rights reserved.

id.theclinics.com

Moving?

Make sure your subscription moves with you!

To notify us of your new address, find your **Clinics Account Number** (located on your mailing label above your name), and contact customer service at:

Email: journalscustomerservice-usa@elsevier.com

800-654-2452 (subscribers in the U.S. & Canada)
314-447-8871 (subscribers outside of the U.S. & Canada)

Fax number: 314-447-8029

Elsevier Health Sciences Division
Subscription Customer Service
3251 Riverport Lane
Maryland Heights, MO 63043

*To ensure uninterrupted delivery of your subscription,
please notify us at least 4 weeks in advance of move.

Printed and bound by CPI Group (UK) Ltd, Croydon, CR0 4YY

03/10/2024

01040448-0008